1983

ACTUALIZING THERAPY

ACTUALIZING THERAPY
Foundations for a Scientific Ethic

EVERETT L. SHOSTROM
Director, Institute of Actualizing Therapy
Diplomate in Clinical Psychology
American Board of Professional Psychology

with Lila Knapp and Robert R. Knapp

LIBRARY
College of St. Francis
JOLIET, ILL.

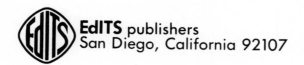
EdITS publishers
San Diego, California 92107

The quotations on pages 32 and 309 are from *The Farther Reaches of Human Nature* by Abraham Maslow, published by Viking Press, copyright 1971.

The quotations on pages 65 and 306 are from *Toward a Psychology of Being* by Abraham Maslow, published by Harper & Row, copyright 1968.

The quotations on pages 88 to 92 are from *To a Dancing God* by Sam Keen. Copyright © 1970 by Sam Keen. Reprinted by permission of Harper & Row, Publishers, Inc.

The quotation on page 94 is from an editorial by Robert Graves, published in *Life* magazine. Copyright 1972.

The quotation on page 95 is from *A Fire On the Moon* by Norman Mailer, copyright 1969. Reprinted by permission of the author and the author's agents, Scott Meredith Literary Agency, Inc., 845 Third Avenue, New York, New York 10022.

The quotation on pages 107 to 109 is from Buhler and Goldenberg's contribution to *The Course of Human Life,* edited by Buhler and Massarik, published by Springer Publishing Co., copyright 1968.

The quotation on page 124 is from "How U.S. Men Can Live Longer" by W. Crampton, published in *This Week,* copyright 1955.

The quotations on pages 125, 126, and 129 are from *Modern Man in Search of a Soul* by C. Jung, published by Harcourt Brace Jovanovich, copyright 1933.

The quotation on page 131 is from *A Few Buttons Missing* by J. Fisher, published by J. B. Lippincott, copyright 1951.

The quotation on page 133 is from "The Golden Mean of Roberto Assagioli" by Sam Keen, published in *Psychology Today,* copyright 1974 by Ziff-Davis Publishing Company. Reprinted by permission.

The quotation on page 165 is from "Rational Psychotherapy" by Albert Ellis, published in the *Journal of General Psychology,* copyright 1958.

The quotation on pages 284 to 286 is from *The Manipulator and the Church* by Dunham, Herbertson, and Shostrom, published by Abingdon Press, copyright 1968.

The quotation on page 308 is from "Is Creativity Akin to Madness" by F. Barron, published in *Psychology Today,* copyright 1972.

First printing, January 1976

ISBN: 912736-14-3

Library of Congress catalog card number: 75-17255

To Nealika, Eden L'ia, Lisa, Marta,
and Clark, who have demonstrated the
meaning of actualizing to us.

CONTENTS

LIST OF ILLUSTRATIONS

PREFACE

Actualizing Therapy is a process utilizing the principle of *Creative Synthesis*. Using the latest research and theories, one synthesizes new positions that have personal meaning, and one must be willing to revise present practices in light of new data. It is this position that we refer to as creative synthesis.

In this volume we attempt to establish that creative synthesis is essential not only to the sophisticated psychologist as a therapeutic tool but also to the lay person as an ideal philosophy governing his day-to-day life. In order to meet the challenge of daily existence, therapist and layman alike must gather *all* the data available and put this information to use through a constantly evolving personal synthesizing system.

Actualizing Therapy is a creative adventure. If the therapist or layman is open to new ideas and to continuing evolvement as a "creative synthesizer," he can experience the joy of creativity, but the source of growth is primarily from within the core of the self rather than from without, as an imitation of others.

The term "Actualizing Therapy" may be thought of as having three meanings. In one sense it identifies a particular viewpoint in therapy, but it also describes a method for enhancing or "actualizing" existing schools of therapy, which can use the processes presented in this book to further facilitate their own methods. Furthermore, Actualizing Therapy suggests a method for actualizing one's philosophy for daily living.

This book breaks fresh ground in the field of self-actualization, using Maslow essentially as a departure point from which to pursue a more therapeutic "process" approach, utilizing the term "actuali*zing*" in place of the static term "actualiza*tion*."

Most of Maslow's research focused on the public life of his lofty subjects. His self-actualizers included such people as Abraham Lincoln, Eleanor Roosevelt, and Thomas Jefferson. Maslow adduced greatness from the public, rather than the private, lives of his actualizers. Had he been more cognizant of the personal lives and humanness of his subjects, in addition to their obvious public achievements, he would have noted, for example, that Lincoln, a great president, had a chronically depressed personality and was essentially antifeminist. Eleanor Roosevelt, admittedly a distinguished humanitarian, is said to have privately refused to discuss sex with her children and apparently never came to grips with her own intimate problems with her famous husband. Jefferson, although a great intellect and humanitarian, was said to have had an unnatural affection for power, extraordinary sexual needs, and an extreme hunger for self-esteem. Neither

Lincoln, Jefferson, nor Eleanor Roosevelt could be said to be wholly actualizing in these aspects of their personal lives.

The point that Maslow missed about these great people is that while they were truly actualizing, they were so only because of their awareness of, and ability to work through, the limitations imposed by their handicaps. In their handicaps were the seeds of their own greatness. Actualizing Therapy, by focusing on weaknesses as well as strengths, creates the same potential for the person dedicated to his own growth.

Helen Keller, for example, because of her lack of sight and hearing, developed a greater awareness through her sense of touch. Anne Morrow Lindbergh's "hours of lead," or her hours of sorrow, produced her ability to experience her "hours of gold"—her peak experiences. Eleanor Roosevelt's limitations made her acutely empathic to the limitations and needs of all peoples in her work with the United Nations. Thomas Jefferson's own humanness is reflected in his authorship of the Declaration of Independence. Lincoln's trials and tribulations produced in him the ability to feel the plight of the black man in his day.

Actualizing one's strengths is possible only when one has the capacity for experiencing weaknesses as well. The person who knows that his capacity to express anger is the same capacity that motivated another person to commit murder can say, "There, but for the grace of God, go I." Actualizing people have the ability to balance their greatness with an awareness of their potential for failure. In addition to achieving potentials, self-actualizing involves accepting personal limitations and humanness and facing losses.

Self-actualizing is a process of moving toward full humanness, not perfection. The actualizing person is fundamentally nonmanipulating in interaction with others, rhythmically swinging between poles of expression—a flowing person whose core remains relatively stable but who retains a continuing capacity to maintain contact with others and to grow toward ultimate potential. Therapeutically, self-actualizing comes about by facing one's limitations and losses and by accepting one's lack of growth in specific areas, such as we believe Jefferson, Lincoln, and Eleanor Roosevelt did.

In these pages we attempt a unique merging of sophisticated psychological theory with what might be termed the psychology of the layman. The first two sections of the book deal with the foundations of Actualizing Therapy. This more academically oriented portion will still appeal to knowledgeable nonprofessionals bent on expanding their grasp of available source material. The book's third section emphasizes creative hunches, ideas that have a less formal validity than those previously described. We intend to hypothesize freely on the different applications of the basic theory to sex, love, marriage, values, and creativity, as well as to other areas.

This book has a deliberately constructed duality designed to aid professionals, as well as erudite laymen who wish to utilize actualizing principles in their daily living. The essential synthesis of the two approaches will be readily apparent to those who believe that professional and personal growth can be enhanced by the presentation of hypotheses not yet supported by systematic research.

Actualizing Therapy, as the authors conceive it, places a unique emphasis on research and data at the professional level, yet at the same time we hope it will have appeal and value to the perceptive nonprofessional.

(As a final note, we would like to point out that while the conventional terms "man" and "he" have been used generically in some parts of this book, they are intended to refer to both females and males and should not be construed as reflecting a biased attitude toward women in any contexts.)

ACKNOWLEDGMENTS

The authors would like to express gratitude to:

Jane Leonard, for her tireless dedication and assistance in editing the ideas expressed in this volume;

Dave Estrada, for his thorough work in the final copy editing of the manuscript;

the clients of the Institute of Actualizing Therapy and the staff members, especially William Pickering, Neil Matheson, Alan Levy, Roy Magden, and Mary Wells, who contributed their wisdom and their services;

also to Judy Marquart, Bruce Parsons and Wiley Johnson gratitude is expressed for the continuing development of the program in Actualizing Therapy;

the staff of EdITS, expecially Bea Neher, for typing the original manuscript;

Lawrence Brammer, for many ideas expressed through long association, and Alexander Lowen, Robert Hilton and Renato Monaco for the ideas on Bioenergetics;

Abraham Maslow and Frederick Perls, whose work has served as the foundation for Actualizing Therapy; and

each of the dedicated researchers who have contributed to the ever-growing body of knowledge supporting the Actualizing Assessment Battery.

CREATIVE SYNTHESIS: AN INTRODUCTION FOR PROFESSIONALS
By Everett L. Shostrom

I believe that for too long each therapeutic school has advertised itself as the only effective one. I also believe, however, that a new movement is taking place. This movement I have chosen to call *Creative Synthesis*. Historically, it is found in the emphases of Perls (1969) and Assagioli (in Keen, 1974) and more recently in the writings of Gendlin (1969), Schutz (1971), and myself. The writings of these creative synthesizers represent a new emphasis on bringing together specific aspects of various systems into new and creative wholes, rather than taking off on tangents, which has been the emphasis in the past two decades.

Fritz Perls is an excellent example of an early creative synthesizer. Perls' wide collection of influences was a continuous building process, as Shepard's recent volume, *Fritz* (1975), suggests. My own personal experience with him also attests to this fact. Every subsequent meeting after a two-year training program with him was a series of "new revelations" that he was incorporating into his system! His wide collection of influences included, as Shepard writes, Freud, Jung, Adler, and Reich; Schilder, Goldstein, and Lewin; Moreno, the founder of psychodrama; actors, directors, and dancers; writers and philosophers; Zen and Tao; existentialists and phenomenologists. This collection was itself a gestalt, a reorganization of selected elements in his experience and thought.

It can be seen from this that Perls was continuously open to new experiences. Perls told me, "I am not the *founder* of Gestalt Therapy, I am the *re-finder* of gestalt principles as applied to therapy. Just before his death he said, "There is much yet I have to do. I am still not satisfied."

Others, including Roberto Assagioli and Will Schutz, have stressed a creative synthesis approach. Schutz's Open Encounter model has, in fact, developed in a manner parallel to that of Actualizing Therapy. He has integrated the approaches of Freud, Reich, Lewin, and group dynamics as well as having developed a measurement approach to his group dynamics models.

Another spokesman for this new generation of therapeutic innovators who are seeking to unite current methods into new and meaningful wholes is Eugene Gendlin. Gendlin (1969) says, "Synthesizing is not the same as eclecticism." It is a creative process, whereas eclecticism is often only an imitative procedure with little or no creative integration involved. (A discussion of Gendlin's approach to creative synthesis will be found in Chapter 7 of this volume.)

Eclecticism sometimes takes the direction drifting toward mediocrity—characterized by the approach of many who simply take a casual smorgasboard, or "benevolently" eclectic, approach to personal learning, where ideas are swallowed whole and unsynthesized. Creative synthesis, on the other hand, may be described as the pursuit of excellence, of the kind advocated by Hans Strupp (1975). It is a continuous synthesizing in which one attempts to critically examine and integrate specific points of view into new wholes. Creative synthesis is a process of chewing on ideas and then digesting and applying only those that will facilitate therapeutic growth at the moment.

I believe that the more recent shift to eclecticism in therapy is a forerunner of creative synthesis. The fact that eclecticism is an established theoretical orientation is attested to by a study by Garfield and Kurtz (1975). This study surveyed 733 Ph.D. clinical psychologists with membership in Division 12 of the American Psychological Association. In this group, 211 had an academic and clinical-research orientation and 522 were primarily clinical practitioners or supervisors. Of this group of 733 clinical psychologists, 64 percent (470) identified their orientation as eclectic. One may conclude that eclecticism is therefore the primary theoretical orientation of a group of recognized clinical psychologists and not simply a casual orientation adopted by an undisciplined practitioner. Creative synthesis goes a step beyond eclecticism, but I believe that it can be embraced by most of the above "disciplined eclectics." The research by Garfield and Kurtz strongly suggests that the trend is away from fragmentation and toward a creative synthesis or integration in therapy.

The twin principles of *synergy* (summated systems create a new whole that exceeds the power of individual systems) and *potentiation* (the power of an individual system can be augmented by the power of a unified system) lead to the idea that therapy is most empowered when there is a continual creative synthesizing of all established and newly developing systems of therapy.

I wish to stress that creative synthesis is not simply an arrogant attempt to put down predecessors. I believe that great ideas are never single and solitary births but, rather, the result of many years of integration by many minds. Isaac Newton has put it another way: "If I have seen further, it is because I have stood on the shoulders of giants."

As each new gestalt emerges, it becomes more than the sum of its parts. Every new gestalt is a step beyond. And so, Actualizing Therapy is not simply an imitation of its predecessors. I believe it expands, extends or amplifies, and modifies the theories from which it builds—just as I hope students will expand and amplify the theories of this volume.

Thus, Actualizing Therapy is not so much a *school* as a *viewpoint* that, paradoxically, encourages an individual therapist *not* to rigidly follow a particular school of thought but rather to develop his own theory of creative synthesis. Every therapist is invited to be the architect of a unique synthesis of his own.

The following are the "building blocks" of Actualizing Therapy, built on the principle of the creative synthesis of various current systems of thought. The list is illustrative of how creative synthesis does not buy any system "wholesale," but rather is based on critically examining many systems and then building from specific aspects of various systems a new synthesis, organized into a new creative-whole.

1. Actualizing Therapy builds on the foundations of Sigmund Freud, who laid the foundation for all forms of therapy. I believe, however, in the positive elements of "transference" as a means whereby true caring may be learned by the client without the danger of sexual exploitation. "Negative transference" in Actualizing Therapy is represented by the *necessity* that the Actualizing Therapist receive anger as a basic polar dimension of expression without necessarily interpreting the anger as a client projection "onto an authority figure."

   Freud's "defense mechanisms" are roughly equivalent to my manipulative processes. The latter, however, produce the concept of "gains" that assist the client in the rational understanding of his "secret system." To make the unconscious conscious is parallel to the dictum of Actualizing Therapy that "awareness creates change."

   Freud stressed the first six years as developmentally significant. Actualizing Therapists believe *all* "turning points" or stages of life are important considerations for what is going on in therapy.

   Actualizing Therapy focuses on learning to live in the present, in contrast to the Freudian emphasis on the past. Thus the period of therapy is shortened considerably. Freud's therapy process continued over some six to eight years, while Actualizing Therapy usually lasts six months to two years.

2. Actualizing Therapy builds on the polarities that were so succinctly stressed by Jung as "thinking-feeling" and "intuition-sensation." These are both essentially intrapersonal. My polarities are both *inter*personal (anger-love) and *intra*personal (strength-weakness).

3. Actualizing Therapy also has its roots in the psychology of Alfred Adler in that the search for *power* is recognized as a primary motivation caused by the helplessness all people feel as children. The impotence of

children in a manipulatively controlled adult world causes people to seek to manipulate others and to manipulate and control themselves. Adler also focused on the importance of future goals, in contrast to the emphasis on the present in Actualizing Therapy.

4. From Erich Fromm's emphasis on the "marketplace orientation," I derive, in part, the concept of manipulation. Fromm says, "Man is not a thing," but manipulation is man's attempt to make himself and others into things.

5. From Karen Horney comes the emphasis on the "idealized image": We all idealize others and then become hostile and discard them because of our disappointment in their inevitable inability to live up to our expectations. Actualizing Therapy is an attempt to analyze high and low expectations.

6. Actualizing Therapy builds on, but goes beyond, the *theory* of Abraham Maslow in that it is a *therapy system.* Maslow remained a personality theorist; he never purported to be a therapist. In fact, he refused to go into therapy exclusively. He told me that he sought *not* to obtain an ABPP diploma, because he felt that would narrow his interests. Thus Maslow remained a general humanistic theorist. He sought to describe a specific, narrow group of well-functioning persons (with an average age of fifty-five) whom he characterized as magnificent and virtuous. He called such people self-actualiz*ed* persons. When actualizing becomes a *therapy* system, the emphasis is not only on the strengths but also on the weaknesses of the person seeking to use his potentials for fuller productivity and expression. In Actualizing Therapy, it is necessary to explore fully the depths of a man's weaknesses before one can appreciate the peaks of his strengths.

Maslow focused on the upper 1 percent of the population in his attempt to understand greatness. In Actualizing Therapy our attempt to help the average person seeking help has been to focus on the upper 50 percent, thus presenting hope for the great majority of the population that want to discover their untapped potentials within.

The normal person is subject to the sin of pride: he seeks only to accelerate his worth and to deny his deficiencies. He also seeks to be consistently strong and considers it a weakness to change his mind. Actualizing Therapy, on the other hand, maintains that the ability to change one's assumptions—to be inconsistent—is a higher form of being. It is only through the principle of polarities of expression that people discover the importance of inconsistency and of the rhythmic movement between one's strengths and weaknesses. As Thoreau said, "A foolish consistency is the hobgoblin of little minds."

To grow from the ashes of worthlessness, like the phoenix, requires accepting that man is in a continuous cycle of survival that does not end until death. As the lives of Maslow's "healthy champions" have more recently shown, no man remains king of the mountain. Actualizing requires that each person, no matter how strong, accept that he is equally weak, that he is often foolish, and that he makes many mistakes.

7. Carl Rogers' Client-Centered Therapy has stressed that the counselor be unconditionally permissive and accepting of the client. Actualizing Therapy extends this view in requiring that both therapist and client become profoundly aware of each other's weaknesses. This view demands a deeper acceptance of self than is implied in Rogers' "unconditional positive regard" for the client. Actualizing Therapy makes the therapist fully available as a person, in dialogue. He is not merely a mirror of empathy for the client.

8. Although appreciating and respecting the work of Martin Buber, who stresses the "I-Thou" dialogue, Actualizing Therapy also stresses what I call the "fool-fool" dialogue. The therapist is but a client a little further down the road, and sometimes the client even passes the therapist by.

Actualizing persons are not lovable angels—they are angel demons! All truly actualizing persons have unconditional negative regard as well as unconditional positive regard. They know that they are not simply lovable but that they are often unlovable scoundrels. And they must love their own unlovableness!

9. Actualizing Therapy also builds on the work of R. D. Laing, who sees psychoses as creative. I see all forms of "deviant behavior" as crudely creative attempts to actualize. The therapist must be able to recognize and appreciate the creativity in all "coping" behavior.

10. In accord with Harold Greenwald, Actualizing Therapists realize that people must all have a profound sense of humor regarding themselves, for the actualizing person knows that, while at any one moment he or she may be experiencing love or strength, at any future moment he or she may reverse polarities and become a scoundrel or a bitch.

At the same time, however, one must recognize that life is serious. To always focus on the humor of life is to see only one side of the coin. As Kierkegaard has stressed, "to become what one truly is" is the most profound developmental task of all, and actualizing persons take this job seriously.

Actualizing Therapists also agree with Greenwald that therapy must focus on decisions. Too often, therapists have focused only on feelings and not on problem solving. At the same time, however, I believe that current Behavior Therapy often stresses the importance of decision-making without the incubation necessary for *creative* decisions. I agree with Rilke that one must *live* the questions of life. Actualizing Therapy is an experiential therapy that does seek to live them, not simply to provide a quick answer for them.

11. Frederick Perls and Eric Berne are both geniuses of our time, but each stressed that autonomy and self-support should be the ultimate goals of therapy. I disagree. I believe that the journey of therapy, and of life itself, is from dependence to independence to *interdependence*. No person is an island, and thus a primary goal of living is to live together with one's fellows. Interdependence is a difficult and ongoing task of living.

12. I believe, with Albert Ellis, that many problems of living have to do with the inappropriate assumptions people make about life as they grow up. Therapy is a process of checking assumptions. The job of the therapist is not merely to note assumptions, but to challenge them. But attitudes are simply assumptions bolstered by strong feelings. Actualizing Therapy extends beyond Ellis' rational therapy to a process that focuses on the feelings behind the assumptions as well.

13. In agreement with Alexander Lowen, however, I believe that the focus on feelings is not enough. I believe that people often repress their feelings into their body-muscle structure and that bodily exercises such as Lowen prescribes have an important place in therapy. Actualizing Therapy utilizes much of Lowen's work on character personality types that result from chronic muscular tensions in living. But it goes further than Lowen in that it emphasizes the *inter*personal, as well as the *intra*personal. I believe that group therapy, with the interpersonal insights obtained from group work, is essential to the actualizing process.

14. I believe, with Rollo May, that love is one of the most important dimensions of human relationships. But my colleagues and I have *measured* the dimensions of love that he and others have stressed as a primary humanistic concern. The inventory that measures the various

aspects of love is the Caring Relationship Inventory, and recent research has demonstrated its clinical usefulness.

As a psychoanalyst, May typically refuses to permit the recording or filming of what analysts do in therapy. This book not only provides a film transcript of the process of an actualizing group, but also presents an analysis of the interventions made by the therapist in this film. I feel I have pioneered in presenting the most comprehensive series of films of various forms of therapy available. [These films are presented in the film list at the end of this book.]

15. I agree with Viktor Frankl that, in addition to love, work is an important dimension for achieving meaning in life. But I believe that the personality of the actualizing man becomes interchangeable with his work. Maslow, for instance, did not simply work on actualization—it is synonymous with his being. The personality of each man is more than an accumulation of his life tasks—it identifies the unique being of each person beyond any other.

16. In problems of marriage, I value the work of Robert Winch, whose theory of mate selection was that of complementarity: opposites attract. I also value Don Jackson's theory of symmetry: like selects like. I believe that complementarity and symmetry unite in the theory of the rhythmic relationship, wherein both partners rhythmically alternate in complementary *and* symmetrical ways to form an actualizing relationship.

17. I agree with George R. Bach that *creative aggression* is an important task for living. But the actualizing person also balances anger and aggression with the dimension of love. I believe that people must go beyond mere aggression to understand that love and anger are creatively intermingled in actualizing relationships.

18. I believe, with Paul Tillich, that the *courage to be* is a reasonable way of describing actualizing behavior. But the courage to be is a *dare*, and I extend this view to describe the *freedom to be*, which is a *right* belonging to each person, as a unique and irreplaceable human being.

19. Actualizing Therapy *utilizes* the Behavior Therapy principles of *modeling* (the therapist provides a model for the client's behavior in what he himself does as a member of the group), *reinforcement* (the therapist encourages behaviors that are thought to be self-actualizing), *problem solving* (the problem-solving process is part of the emphasis on the intellectual aspects of actualizing behavior), and *assigning priorities to*

values (the therapist encourages the client to set up a system of priorities for his own behavior in the later stages of therapy).

Actualizing Therapy *amplifies* Behavior Therapy by emphasizing the dimensions of *increasing awareness,* by stressing the importance of *developmental psychology* in the understanding of the person, and by stressing the importance of *personality theory* in the understanding of human nature.

20. In the area of religion, I go beyond traditional theologians and posit that discovering one's own *core being* is to discover the "Kingdom of God within." Unlike Freud, who was antireligious, or Adler, who emphasized social interest as a future goal, I go beyond to a here-and-now philosophy of secular valuing that is congruent with much religious philosophy.

21. I believe that the acceptance of the concepts expressed in my book *Man, the Manipulator* (1967) has shown the importance of manipulation as a relevant variable in understanding human behavior within ourselves and others. Furthermore, we need not stereotype ourselves and others as manipulators, but we must admit that we are manipulative or manipulating as we seek to grow.

22. I believe that the medical model of understanding human behavior has a limited value in that it takes the *responsibility* for a man's behavior away from him and puts it into the hands of the doctor, who simply treats the patient. Actualizing Therapy supplants the medical model to propose a system that holds that the understanding of man in terms of a positive system of actualizing is a more useful method for understanding man's creativity, which is the sine qua non of actualizing.

23. Unlike most systems of therapy, which are based solely on clinical insights, Actualizing Therapy is based on thirteen years of solid research, involving more than 200 studies in the measurement of actualizing, and on studies on group encounter employing the instruments developed by my coauthors and me. I believe this goes beyond current practice, which has ignored the importance of research as a necessary base for clinical practice.

24. Actualizing Therapy suggests a new horizon for the many contemporary therapists who have chosen not to use standardized tests, or who use only tests like the MMPI, which measures pathology. Thirteen years of research with the Personal Orientation Inventory and other instruments (making up the Actualizing Assessment Battery) has not only given convincing evidence of the value of standardized inventories, both intra-

personal and interpersonal, but has also presented persuasive evidence for the value of the concept of self-actualizing as a reasonable goal for all forms of therapy.

25. In accord with Roberto Assagioli, I believe a creative synthesis must be geared to the existential moment. *Who* the therapist is, *who* the client is, *what* is going on at the moment, and *where* in the total process of therapy they *each* are, all contribute to the existential decision on a thinking, feeling, or bodily approach.

I believe that no system of therapy worth its salt can ignore the great contributions that these giants have given us. The creative synthesizer must, however, develop a system that truly integrates rather than one that simply uses these contributions indiscriminately. A therapist needs to employ a variety of tools appropriate to the situation of the moment. I believe this is the primary challenge of Actualizing Therapy.

CHAPTER 1. ACTUALIZING THERAPY: AN EMERGING METHODOLOGY

Because modern man has identified with security, he has sought to rigidify and control his being. But living is a process of continuous change. Therapy, therefore, must be a process of helping man to continuously adapt and change. Research into the effects of Actualizing Therapy shows that man's core being *can* be revitalized.

Actualizing Therapy emphasizes progressive awareness through a *growth process*. The term "actualization" was originally used by Goldstein to describe the growing process of the organism, and the idea has been elaborated upon by Abraham Maslow, Rollo May, Carl Rogers, Frederick Perls, and others. The concept of actualizing is used here to stress the *process* of being what one is and of becoming more of what one can be, as opposed to being in a static state.

In this book we not only present a therapy of change, but we present a philosophy of life that embraces process and change as a central emphasis.

Actualizing Therapy is based on the belief that each person is a unique human being seeking fulfillment. It is a multidimensional approach used to assist the individual toward self-actualizing, which may be defined as *an ongoing process of growth toward utilizing one's potential.* "Potential" is one's ultimate capacity for creative expression, interpersonal effectiveness, and fulfillment in living. "Multidimensional" refers to the various means available for growth including individual therapy techniques and group therapy methods.

No one theory is yet sufficiently comprehensive or systematic to adequately guide the therapist through the multitudinous problems met in everyday practice. The Actualizing Therapist places chief emphasis on the moment-to-moment growth process. The here and now is the chief focus of the process, but this does not exclude the individual's past and future as they *relate* to the present.

From Maslow (1954) comes the emphasis on self-actualizing as a reasonable goal for psychotherapy. From Martin Buber (1951) and Gordon W. Allport (1937; 1961) comes the emphasis on the achievement of one's own "particularity" and the growth of unique, unprecedented, and never-recurring potentialities. Self-actualizing, not self-concept actualization, is the goal. The person who tries to become self-concept actualizing is simply trying to become some phony ideal, rather than be himself. In self-actualizing, each person is being and becoming what he or she *is*—discovering a unique identity and then risking being it.

Because the individual must practice actualizing in an interpersonal setting, the actualizing group, the encounter group, or group therapy becomes a primary means by which growth toward actualization takes place. The client learns the fundamental principle that "the group is the individual turned inside out." By observing the various maladaptive manipulative patterns and character styles of members of these "growth" groups, clients learn to see the manipulative patterns in themselves and the potentials that can grow from these manipulative processes.

EDUCATING THE POTENTIAL

A fundamental thesis of Actualizing Therapy is that the problem of change is not one of change from mental illness to mental health, but rather of change from deficiency to fulfillment and from deadness to aliveness. Actualizing Therapy is a fundamental process of educating the potential within and has little to do with the medical model of illness. To actually believe that out of one's self-defeating manipulations will come increased actualizing is to develop hope. As Erik Erikson (1964) says, "We recognize . . . an inner affinity between the . . . deepest mental disturbances and a radical loss of a basic kind of hope" (p. 112). For years it has been clear that such hope has been missing in contemporary psychiatry and psychology.

Actualizing Therapy, therefore, is a positively oriented system of therapy with innovative features particularly designed to motivate clients to move toward actualizing. Elements of this approach may be utilized by all therapists, regardless of their particular persuasion.

ROOTS OF ACTUALIZING THERAPY

Two roots underlie Actualizing Therapy: philosophy and research. The philosophical root is essential because of the emphasis on actualizing as growth. The model of the kind of person who evolves in this growth process incorporates a series of value judgments about the human condition. The research root is also essential to the actualizing point of view. The therapist is a true scientist; he is curious, critical, truthful, logical, objective, and precise in this role, as opposed to his more subjective emotional functioning as a human participant in the client's actualizing process. This means that Actualizing Therapy is in league with the behavioral as well as the humanistic school of psychotherapy. Observable results, which can be validated by recognized research procedures, are part of the actualizing model. The Actualizing Therapist must strive to reconcile his frequently contradictory roles by employing them in a kind of synergistic alternating of awareness— a check and balance system.

ASSUMPTIONS

Therapists are involved in deeply human growth processes and must constantly face questions of what values and goals to promote, how free the individual is or should be, and how much influence the Actualizing Therapist should have on the client's values.

Actualizing Therapy is based on the following assumptions:

1. *Individual Uniqueness.* Each person is a unique human being seeking self-fulfillment, although each has "human nature" shared in common with others. A better term is Buber's "particularity" principle, a unique "thou" seeking to be realized. We prefer to see each person as a unique tapestry or mosaic.

2. *Here-and-Now Emphasis.* Although the actualizing principle has a futuristic quality in the "becoming" sense, it takes place in the moment-to-moment growth process. Hence, the present is the most important of the time modalities, and the "here and now" becomes the focus of the process.

3. *Freedom.* Although much of a person's behavior is determined by personal history and by forces beyond his control, the actualizing process assumes that one's future is largely undetermined and that a person has a wide range of actions from which to choose.

4. *Responsibility.* The assumption of freedom places corresponding responsibility on the individual for his own actualizing. He cannot depend on others or blame others for his growth or lack of it. Even though growth takes place in a social context, the individual alone is responsible for his own life.

5. *Learning.* Although some primitive behaviors are reflexive and largely genetically determined and others are the result of chemical or neurological changes, a fundamental assumption of Actualizing Therapy is that social behavior is learned and that changes in behavior follow the learning process.

6. *Social Interaction.* Actualizing is achieved not merely by thinking, meditating, or reading about the goals of growth, but by social interaction with a therapist, teacher, minister, group, friend, or family. Social interaction becomes the vehicle for such conditions of actualizing as honesty with feelings, awareness of self, freedom of expression, and trust in oneself and others.

THE CONCEPT OF POLARITIES

The concept of polarities is central to Actualizing Therapy. A polarity is defined as a continuum with discrete variations, from a central zero-point of constriction of feeling, to fullness of feeling at the outward extremes.

The difference between a one-directional continuum and a polarity, or two-directional continuum, needs to be made clear. Most people think of life as having *discrete* qualities, such as trust, anger, and tenderness, each having strong or weak dimensions on a singular continuum. Polarity theory, on the other hand, assumes continua having zero-points between two distinct, but related, life qualities. Two of the most important of these continua are termed the *anger-love polarity* and the *strength-weakness polarity.* Other such polarities are conservatism-liberalism, activity-passivity, and dependence-independence. Within man's nature there is evidence to suggest the universality of such a two-party system of polarities.

The importance of full feeling on polarities is illustrated by the celebrated remark made by Dorothy Parker when criticizing what she felt was a weak performance by Katharine Hepburn. "Miss Hepburn," she wrote, "ran the gamut of emotions from A to B." An actualizing person expresses polarity feelings from A to Z. Such polarities have a *rhythmic* mean, as opposed to an *arithmetic* mean.

For most people, this is a new idea. The middle—the golden mean—is generally agreed upon as the place to be. The "middle of the road" metaphor is commonly used. Yet the poet Robert Frost complained that "the middle of the road is where the white line is—and that's the worst place to drive."

The middle may be all right for a society, striking balances between competing feelings strongly held between various groups, but for an individual it becomes a place of *indifference*—for *cancelling out* of feelings.

The middle becomes a natural hiding place for the *uninvolved* and the *disinterested*. If one feels, then one cares, and actualizing means involvement and caring. The actualizing person must be willing to express the natural extremes of feeling that come with involvement and interest in living.

Actualizing involves a willingness to risk expression of these internal feelings. To *be* is to be on the outside what one feels within. As Aristotle has said, this is to fluctuate in the farthest extreme of our feelings "between an assertion of strength that is truculent and a confession of helplessness that is cowardly." But actualizing still requires movement between both extremes and not simply a static "golden mean" of nothingness and indifference.

Such feelings are polarized on the anger-love continuum as well. To love someone is to be closely involved with them and "stroking" them the right way. But closeness also involves "rubbing each other the wrong way" from time to time. Thus, paradoxically, to love is also to be angry from time to time. Otherwise, people become locked in manipulative relationships in which they can only show their "loving" feelings.

The actualizing person is "centered"—not arithmetically, but rhythmically. A person who is being his core is able to move rhythmically outward from his center in accord with whatever feelings emerge in living; he does not constrict himself to the zero-point of indifference or fear, where no feelings are expressed.

Actualizing Therapy utilizes the polarities of anger-love and strength-weakness only as examples in defining the primary points of latitude and longitude in the world of feelings; but there are many other polarities and dimensions necessary for the journey of life, which involves finding one's way in contact with other human beings.

Homeostasis and Transtasis

Building on the concept of polarities, we hypothesize that man's nature is both homeostatic and transtatic and that growth of personality requires movement in the present along one's polarities in the manner described by Hegel. Hegel suggests that change comes about in a movement from thesis (polar dimension) to antithesis (opposite polar dimension) to synthesis (integration). From this integration the individual grows to a *higher* level of expression of his polarities, and this requires the concept of *transtasis*. This movement to higher and higher levels of integration of one's polarities is essential in the process of therapy. *Homeostasis,* or inner balance, is a necessary concept to restore balance to polarity theory. Instead of being passive *or* active, the client becomes synergistically balanced, that is, *both* strong and weak, *both* assertive and caring. Self-actualizing requires full expression of basic personality polarities in the present (Shostrom, 1967). Allport's (1960; 1961) concept of transtasis enlarges on homeostasis. This concept implies change and creation of tension, movement, and progress as well as homeostatic restoration of balance. The idea of transtasis is consistent with the idea of self-actualizing as a *process,* rather than as a fixed state. These processes, expressed coactively, are shown in Figure 1.

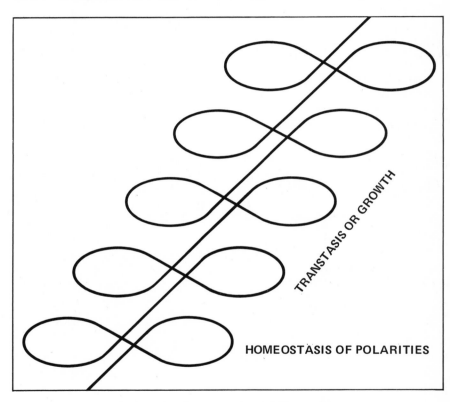

Figure 1. Homeostasis and Transtasis

Research Roots

The general points made in the foregoing discussion are supported to some extent by specific research. Research by Leary (1957), with Barron, Coffey, and MacKinnon, on more than 5,000 cases showed that all generic interpersonal factors could be expressed as combinations of the four nodal points of strength, weakness, anger, and love. Research based on the inventories composing the *Actualizing Assessment Battery* (AAB), especially the *Personal Orientation Inventory* (POI) (Shostrom, 1964) and the *Personal Orientation Dimensions* (POD)—both developed to measure self-actualizing—has shown that actualizing behavior is characteristic of those persons having completed psychotherapy and that such persons are more synergistically balanced on these four polar dimensions. (See Chapter 2 for a comprehensive discussion of the inventories that make up the Actualizing Assessment Battery.)

Figure 2 may be seen as representing the total sphere of a person's psychological being. We envision the polarities as major axes, following from the early research of Leary (1957) and extended in our own research.

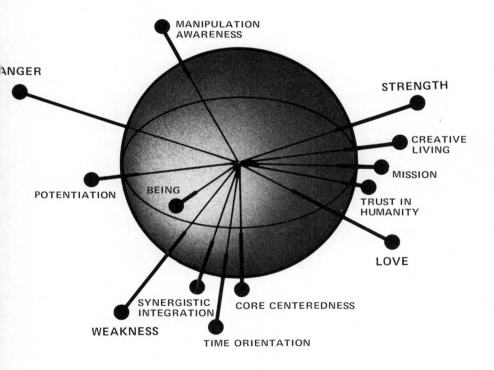

Figure 2. Three-Dimensional Representation of a Person's Total Psychological Being (dimensions shown are based on factor analytic research with the POD)

We consider the dimensions emerging from research with the Actualizing Assessment Battery to be psychometric approximations of vectors. *Vectors,* after Thurstone (1947), may be defined as quantities that have magnitude and direction, and they are commonly represented by a directed line whose length represents magnitude and whose orientation in space represents direction. Although we will speak throughout this volume of the polarities of anger-love and strength-weakness, the reader should be aware that we use them as primary reference points, positioned as poles, to make comprehensible a much more complex system. Just as street signs are used to give orientation and, thus, to aid in finding a particular address in space, so the basic polarities of anger-love and strength-weakness can be used as basic points of "latitude and longitude" of the personality.

LEVELS OF THERAPIST GROWTH

It is becoming increasingly clear that many contemporary psychotherapists do not rigidly adhere to a particular system or school of thought. As each clinician matures, he seems to go through a process of professional growth toward a unique style with definable parameters (the integral factors of systematic counseling and psychotherapy that are adopted by a particular therapist). The adopted combination of parameters would be descriptive of his unique style or approach to counseling and psychotherapy. The technique of "parametric analysis" corroborates the idea that the growing practitioner is committed to a unique combination of therapeutic parameters and applies them flexibly to the emerging therapeutic situation. A particular therapist's parameters can be identified and profiled hierarchically at each of four levels of development:

1. *General Level.* The therapist is heavily influenced by the parameters that are superimposed on the general psychological background by a teacher or supervisor.

2. *Personalized Level.* The therapist adapts the original training and further study to his own personality, evolving a more personalized parametric approach.

3. *Stylized Level.* Through training and experience, the therapist commits himself to selected stylized parameters that combine with his personality into a unique gestalt or style.

4. *Expressive Level.* The therapist goes beyond his personal style to create unique parameters that he is confident are worth sharing professionally and are worth subjecting to the critical evaluation of his colleagues.

Few practitioners achieve Level 4—most reach their peak of expression as performers rather than as creative writers.

It should be stressed that Actualizing Therapists grow through this hierarchy only by a long process of education and personal growth. There are no short cuts to this process. It seems that many young therapists, out of a need for security and a need to feel they "know" what to do, become attached to a narrow school of thought early in their professional development. As William Shutz has said, "I was a nondirective therapist until I learned what else to do!"

Actualizing Therapists: Creative Synthesizers

A study by Shostrom and Riley (1968) confirms the general hypothesis that experienced, seasoned therapists tend to become creative synthesizers. Following the dictum of Albert Einstein, who is reported to have said, "Never ask anyone what he does, follow him around and see what he does," a rating form was used to rate therapists on the degree to which their approach manifested each of ten parameters:

1. *Caring*—the therapist's attitude of loving regard for the individual, whether expressed by unconditional warmth or by aggressive critical caring (see, for example, Fromm, 1962).

2. *Ego strengthening*—helping clients to develop their thinking, feeling, and perceiving abilities so that they can cope with life more effectively (see, for example, Kris, Hartmann, & Rapaport, 1963).

3. *Encountering*—providing the experience of active encounter between client and therapist, each of whom is being and expressing real feelings (see, for example, May, 1958).

4. *Feeling*—helping the client to experience, in a psychologically safe relationship, feelings that heretofore have been found too threatening to experience freely (see, for example, Rogers, 1951).

5. *Interpersonal analyzing*—the analysis of the client's perceptions or manipulations of the therapeutic relationship and, therefore, of other interpersonal relationships in life (see, for example, Perls, Goodman, & Hefferline, 1951; Sullivan, 1953).

6. *Pattern analysis*—the analysis of unworkable patterns of functioning, and assistance in the development of adaptive patterns of functioning for the individual (see, for example, Frankl, 1963; Shostrom, 1967).

7. *Reinforcing*—the therapist's rewarding of behavior that is growth-enhancing as well as socially adaptive and punishing of behavior that is negative or self-defeating (see, for example, Ellis, 1962; Eysenck & Rachman, 1965; Wolpe, 1958).

8. *Self-disclosing*—the therapist's exposure of his own self-adaptive and self-defensive patterns of living, which encourages the client to do the same (see, for example, Jourard, 1964; Maslow, 1954).

9. *Value reorienting*—the reevaluation of the clients' loosely formulated value orientations (assumptions about self and others, for instance), which enables the clients to commit themselves to examined and operational values (see, for example, Brammer & Shostrom, 1968; Buhler, 1962).

10. *Reexperiencing*—the therapist's assistance in the client's reexperiencing of past influential learnings and in desensitizing the pathological effects of these learnings on present functioning (see, for example, Fenichel, 1945).

Analysis of the ratings based on these parameters showed that each of the therapists in the study, as judged by forty raters, utilized all of the parameters to some degree in their work. The therapists rated were Carl Rogers, Fritz Perls, and Albert Ellis, as they performed in the film *Three Approaches to Psychotherapy*. Even Rogers, who many feel is the most parochial, included several of the parameters in his work. According to the study, Rogers scored highest on the parameters of caring and feeling; Perls scored highest on encountering, feeling, and interpersonal analyzing; and Ellis scored highest on value reorienting and pattern analysis.

The importance of this research lies in the fact that Rogers, Perls, and Ellis, all of whom claim to be "founders" of specific schools, were each found to use several parameters in their work, indicating that they are not uniquely specific in their orientations. In fact, this research suggests that even these men are creative synthesizers, in that an impartial group of judges found them using overlapping parameters.

Therapists cannot explain the events of the interview by means of a single theoretical view of personality; no theory has yet been found that explains the process completely. Furthermore, clients respond differently to various approaches. Sometimes one approach works well in the initial phases, when the need for support overshadows all other therapeutic efforts, while at other times the client may respond well to a highly interpretive approach.

It is important that the therapist's theory match his style of counseling. That is, therapists must use a point of view and a therapeutic style with which they feel comfortable and effective. The trend appears to be toward individual variations and toward the position of creative synthesis.

Creative synthesis means that a therapist may use a combination of techniques, or different single techniques, for different clients. In the first instance, the psychologist might choose to use several different approaches with one client; in the second case, the therapist would use one model (such as Gestalt Therapy, Existential Therapy, or Behavior Modification) throughout the duration of one client's therapeutic experience but use a different technique consistently with another client. Actualizing Therapy offers the opportunity for the professional to use either one model or many models in combination.

Thus, the Actualizing Therapist is not concerned with restraining methodology but is, instead, a creative synthesizer—constantly expanding approaches to the technique of therapy. Innovative methods, as they are developed, must be integrated with traditional methodology. The therapist's personal growth requires a continual evolving and emerging, both personally and professionally.

A New Comprehensive System

Based on the principle of creative synthesis, Actualizing Therapy has grown to the point that it can be recognized as a unique system with its own unique identity. There are important features of Actualizing Therapy that are not contained in any other schools or systems. Actualizing Therapy represents a selective integration embracing the techniques and theories of many therapeutic systems.

Three separate therapeutic systems are illustrated in the film *Three Approaches to Psychotherapy,* and the following transcription from a recent condensation of the film (titled *Actualizing Therapy: An Integration of Rogers, Perls, and Ellis*) will illustrate how Actualizing Therapy has integrated elements of these three specific systems.

AN INTEGRATION OF ROGERS, PERLS, AND ELLIS

Interviewer: This is Gloria. She is troubled and in search of a psychotherapist. There is something very special about her situation. In a moment, Gloria will have a rare opportunity to interact with three of the most influential psychotherapists of our time: Dr. Carl Rogers, originator of "Client-Centered Therapy"; Dr. Frederick Perls, famed "Gestalt" Therapist; and Dr. Albert Ellis, creator of "Rational-Emotive Therapy."

There are many forms of psychotherapy. If you explore the subject, you may be surprised when you discover so many different theoretical assumptions—the divergent goals and the wide range of treatment techniques. While no single approach has been found to be effective for all persons, it is generally agreed that the effectiveness of psychotherapy is dependent upon the nature of the relationship between the patient and the therapist. Today we are going to focus on that ordinarily private relationship as we watch excerpts from a film series which many regard as a classic in the field of psychotherapy. We are fortunate to have Dr. Everett Shostrom, the creator of the series, as our special guest.

Recently we took our camera crew to the Institute of Actualizing Therapy where we asked Dr. Shostrom to provide the background to his classic experiment, which features Gloria and the three distinguished psychotherapists.

Dr. Shostrom, what significance does the series have for you?

Shostrom: When the American Psychological Association met in 1964, I knew that Rogers, Ellis, and Perls were going to be there and the thought came to me, wouldn't it be interesting to have these highly divergent points of view brought together with one patient, in one afternoon? And this was the birth of the series.

Interviewer: So we will have an opportunity to see the divergence of each view?

Shostrom: Yes. Great men, each with their own point of view and yet terribly different, as they interact with Gloria. So I think all three films will show these divergencies as we go along.

Interviewer: Good, now, let's go ahead and see the first segment. In this first excerpt the therapy session is already in progress. We meet Gloria, the client, as she interacts with the founder of Client-Centered Therapy, Dr. Carl Rogers.

[Cut to Gloria and Rogers.]

Gloria: Well, the main thing I want to talk to you about is, I'm just newly divorced, and I had gone in therapy before and I felt comfortable when I left, and all of a sudden now the biggest change is adjusting to my single life. And one of the things that bothered me the most is especially men, and having men to the house and how it affects the children. The biggest thing I want—the thing that keeps coming to my mind I want to tell you about is that I have a daughter, nine, who at one time I felt had a lot of emotional problems. I wish I could stop shaking. And I'm real conscious of things affecting her. I don't want her to get upset, I don't want to shock her. I want so badly for her to accept me. And we're real open with each other especially about sex. And the other day she saw a girl that was single but pregnant and she asked me all about "can girls get pregnant if they are single?" And the conversation was fine and I wasn't ill at ease at all with her until she asked me if I had ever made love to a man since I left her Daddy and I lied to her. And ever since that, it keeps coming up to my mind because I feel so guilty lying to her because I never lie and I want her to trust me. And I almost want an answer from you. I want you to tell me if the effect on her would be wrong if I told her the truth, or what.

Rogers: And it's this concern about her and the fact that you really aren't truthful, that this open relationship that has existed between you—now you feel it's kind of vanished?

Gloria: Yes, I feel like I have to be on guard about that because I remember when I was a little girl, when I first found out my mother and father made love, that was dirty and terrible, and I didn't like her any more, for awhile. And I don't want to lie to Pammy either and I don't know . . .

Rogers: I sure wish I could give you the answer as to what you should tell her.

Gloria: I was afraid you were going to say that.

Rogers: Because what you really want is an answer.

Gloria: I want to especially know if it would affect her if I was completely honest and open with her or if it would affect her because I lied. I feel like it is bound to make a strain because I lied to her.

Rogers: You feel she'll suspect that, or she'll know something is not quite right?

Gloria: I feel that in time she will distrust me, yes. And also I thought well, gee, what about when she gets a little older and she finds herself in touchy situations. She probably wouldn't want to admit it to me because she thinks I'm so good and so sweet. And yet I'm afraid she could think I'm really a devil. And I want so bad for her to accept me. And I don't know how much a nine-year-old can take.

Rogers: And really both alternatives concern you. That she may think you're too good or better than you really are.

Gloria: Yes.

Rogers: Or she may think you are worse than you are.

Gloria: Not worse than I am. I don't know if she can accept me the way I am. I think I paint a picture that I'm all sweet and motherly. I'm a little ashamed of my shady side, too.

Rogers: I see. It really cuts a little deeper. If she really knew you, would she, could she accept you.

Gloria: This is what I don't know. I don't want her to turn away from me. I don't even know how I feel about it because there are times when I feel so guilty like when I have a man over, I even try to make a special setup so that if I were ever alone with him, the children would never catch me in that sort of thing. Because I'm real leery about it. And yet I also know that I have these desires.

Rogers: And so it is quite clear that it isn't only her problem or the relationship with her, it's in you as well.

Gloria: In my guilt. I feel guilty so often.

Rogers: What can I accept myself as doing? And you realize that instead of some sort of subterfuges so as to make sure that you're not caught or something, you realize that you are acting from guilt, is that it?

Gloria: Yes, and I don't like the . . . I would like to feel comfortable with whatever I do. If I choose not to tell Pammy the truth, to feel comfortable that she can't handle it, and I don't. I want to be honest, and yet I feel there are some areas that *I* don't even accept.

Rogers: And if you can't accept them in yourself, how could you possibly be comfortable in telling them to her.

Gloria: Right.

Rogers: And yet, as you say, you do have these desires and you do have your feelings, but you don't feel good about them.

Gloria: Right. I have a feeling that you are just going to sit there and let me stew in it and I want more. I want you to help me get rid of my guilt feelings. If I can get rid of my guilt feeling about lying or going to bed with a single man, any of that, just so I can feel more comfortable.

Rogers: And I guess I'd like to say, "No, I don't want to let you just stew in your feelings," but on the other hand, I also feel that this is the kind of very private thing that I couldn't possibly answer for you. But I sure as anything will try to help you work toward your own answer. I don't know whether that makes any sense to you, but I mean it.

Gloria: Well, I appreciate you saying that. You sound like you mean it.

[Cut to Interviewer and Shostrom.]

Interviewer: Well, it seems as though the relationship was a real one.

Shostrom: Yes. I think that this is the real strength of Rogers' approach. That he really exuded warmth and Gloria received it and at the same time his warmth was communicated by his mirror of her, his reflection of her feelings and his refusal to answer her question. Yet he was also doing something which he has written about more recently, which is that he is encountering her with his feelings, his feelings of helplessness and not being able to give her advice or to tell her what to do. I think the other thing which, of course, interests me is that when she mentions her guilt, Perls or Ellis would have given some concrete formulation as to how to cope with that, whereas Rogers, again, places this in the same category of relationship, and simply says he wishes he could help her with this but it is up to Gloria to handle her own guilt.

Interviewer: He is certainly not going to give her the answers, but rather, she must . . .

Shostrom: Discover them for herself. Yes. But again this is a contrasting viewpoint, and as we see the others work, we'll see how differently they would handle specifics, like guilt, for example.

Interviewer: Before we see the next segment, which features Dr. Fritz Perls, how about a definition of the term "gestalt"? What does it mean?

Shostrom: "Gestalt" is a German word for whole, but the whole always has to be broken down into two parts, the figure and the ground. [Figure 3] shows a typical "gestalt" figure with two faces which are background, and yet, with a vase emerging between the figures of the faces. So what "Gestalt" psychologists are saying, is that one must always break the whole into two parts, the figure, which stands out, which is really brought out by the viewer, and then the background.

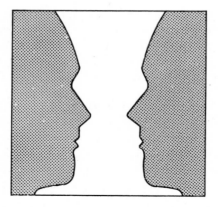

Figure 3. The Gestalt Figure and Ground Principle

You can make the figure or the background reverse themselves. You can focus either on the vase in the center or you can focus on the faces behind the vase. But figure and ground always are the two dimensions of the whole, which makes up the "gestalt."

Interviewer: Well, in reference to the dichotomy of mind and body, which really are inseparable, Perls tries to unify both elements.

Shostrom: Yes, I think this is true with Perls and a number of other therapists now, including myself. I think we really have to get rid of that mind and body dichotomy and realize that your body involves thinking, and feeling also . . . and that we don't just simply operate from the head or from below the head, but rather that we operate as a unified whole. And, again, we have this "gestalt" coming through with an integration of mind and body.

Interviewer: Then there is the possibility that man is really more than all of his parts, and I imagine that is what makes man so unique—that something more.

Shostrom: Yes. The word you are trying to give me is the sum—the total of man's being is greater than the sum of the parts. Just like an automobile is more than just a bunch of nuts and bolts and screws put together, when it comes together it becomes an automobile, which is *more* than these pieces separately.

Interviewer: Let's watch Dr. Fritz Perls in action, as he demonstrates Gestalt Therapy.

[Cut to Gloria and Perls.]

Perls: What would it do for you to be dumb and stupid? Look at it like this: what would it do to me, if you would play dumb and stupid?

Gloria: It makes you all the smarter and all the higher above me, and then I really have to look up to you because you are so smart.

Perls: Oh, you are bottling me up, right and left.

Gloria: No. I think you can do that all by yourself.

Perls: Oh, I think the other way around. If you play dumb and stupid, you force me to be more explicit.

Gloria: That has been said to me before, but I don't buy it. I don't like . . .

Perls: What are you doing with your feet now?

Gloria [laughing]: Wiggling!

Perls: You joke now.

Gloria: No. I'm afraid you are going to notice everything I do. Gee!

Perls: Don't you want me . . .

Gloria: I want you to help me become more relaxed. Yes. I don't want to be so defensive with you. I don't like to feel so defensive. You're acting like—you're treating me as if I am stronger than I am, and I want you to protect me more and be nicer to me.

Perls: Are you aware of your smile? You don't believe a word you are saying.

Gloria: I do too, and I know you are going to pick on me for it.

Perls: Sure, you're bluffing, you're a phony.

Gloria: Do you believe . . . are you meaning that seriously?

Perls: Yes. You say you are creative, you laugh and you giggle and you squirm. It is phony. You put on a performance for me.

Gloria: Oh, I resent that, very much.

Perls: Can you express this?

Gloria: Yes sir! I am most certainly not being a phony. I will admit this: It's hard for me to show my embarrassment and I hate to be embarrassed, but boy, I resent you calling me a phony. Just because I smile when I'm embarrassed or put in a corner, doesn't mean I'm being a phony.

Perls: Wonderful. Thank you. You didn't squirm for the last minute.

Gloria: Well, I'm mad at you.

Perls: That's right. You didn't have to cover up your anger with your smile. In that moment, in that minute, you were not a phony.

Gloria: Well, at that minute I was mad though, I wasn't embarrassed.

Perls: In other words, when you are mad, you are not a phony.

Gloria: I still resent that. I'm not a phony when I'm nervous.

Perls: Again.

Gloria: I want to get mad at you. I . . . I . . . You know what I'd like to do?

Perls: "I . . . I . . . I . . ."

Gloria: I want you on my level so I can pick on you just as much as you are picking on me.

Perls: O.K. Pick on me.

Gloria: Well, I have to wait until you say something that I can pick on. But . . .

Perls: What does this mean? Can you develop this movement?

Gloria: It's . . . I can't find words. I want to . . .

Perls: Develop it as if you were dancing.

Gloria: I want to start all over again with you.

Perls: O.K. Let's start all over again.

Gloria: I know a corner I'd like to put you in. I'd like to ask you a question because I have the feeling you don't like me, right off the bat, and I want to know if you do.

Perls: Can you now play Fritz Perls not liking Gloria? What would he say?

Gloria: He'd say that she is a phony, for one.

Perls: Say, "You are a phony."

Gloria: "You are a phony and you're a flip little girl, and you're a show-off."

Perls: What would Gloria answer to that?

Gloria: I know what I'd answer. I'd say, "I think you are, too!"

Perls: Now say, tell this to me. Tell me what a phony I am.

Gloria: Well, I . . .

Perls: Say, "Fritz, you are a phony."

Gloria: "Phony" is not quite the right word, but it's more like a show-off.

Perls: A show-off.

Gloria: Like you know all the answers.

Perls: Yeah.

Gloria: And I want you to be more human and that doesn't seem very human to me.

Perls: To know the answers is not really human?

Gloria: Yes. And right away to find out how I'm kicking my feet and why I am doing like this. Why are you doing that?

Perls: Oh, dear. I've got eyes. I can see you are kicking your feet. I don't need a scientific computer to see that you are kicking your feet. What's big about that? You don't need to be wise to see that you are kicking your feet.

Gloria: I know, but it seems like you're trying to find some reason for it.

Perls: I don't. It is your imagination.

Gloria: O.K. I know what I'd like from you. Can I tell you what I'd like from you?

Perls: Yes.

Gloria: I'd like you to be aware that I'm kicking my feet and to be aware that I'm giggling when I'm really nervous, and accept it instead of putting me on the defensive having to explain it. I don't want to have to explain why I'm doing these things.

Perls: Did I ask you to explain?

Gloria: You said, "Why am I," or "What am I doing?"

Perls: No.

Gloria: Well, "What am I doing?" you said.

Perls: That is right. Kicking your feet. I did not ask you to explain it. It's your imagination. That is not this Fritz, it is the Fritz of your imagination. There is a big difference.

Gloria: [Sighs]

Perls: Now do this again.

Gloria: [Sighs]

Perls: Again.

Gloria: [Sighs]

Perls: How do you feel now?

Gloria: I don't know.

Perls: Playing stupid.

Gloria: I'm not playing stupid. I don't know the right answer.

Perls: You said, "I don't know." This is playing stupid.

[Cut to Interviewer and Shostrom.]

Interviewer: Dr. Perls deliberately confronted and challenged Gloria. Why?

Shostrom: I think I would like to answer that indirectly if I can. I was impressed by the difference in pace, between Rogers and Perls, but it seems to me in some ways, Perls was more *with* Gloria than Rogers. Rogers has set the deliberateness of his slowly reflecting feeling, whereas Perls was *with* Gloria and all she was doing. For example, when she showed an obvious difference between her body and her verbal expression, he called attention to this, which frustrated her because she didn't know that this was happening; that her smile was ungenuine and phony and she really didn't want the help, in a sense, that he was suggesting to her.

Interviewer: When he suggested that Gloria was manipulating?

Shostrom: Yes. Of course. That word interests me because I have written about it. She was playing dumb and stupid. That is, she really wasn't dumb and stupid. She is a bright girl and yet, she played a little girl, hiding in the corner and he really attempted to point it out, and here and now, to make her aware of that. Of course, there is always a gain or an advantage if you play dumb and stupid. Then the expert, the authority, will do it for you. And she was attempting to get him to do this and he was not going to let her get away with it.

Interviewer: It seems as though he was trying to get Gloria to assume more responsibility for her own behavior.

Shostrom: Yes. In an entirely different way than Rogers, and yet, in a very profound way. That is, the average patient really does play dumb and stupid most of the time. He wants the problem solved for him. He thinks of psychotherapy as a helping process and in reality what one does is to project onto the therapist the expertness—the knowledge—and Perls simply frustrated her attempts to do this.

Interviewer: And he did it deliberately?

Shostrom: Deliberately. And so frustration is a deliberate part of Gestalt Therapy as opposed to the ease and the warmth that characterizes the Rogers approach.

Interviewer: Let's watch the third and final segment, which features the founder of "Rational-Emotive Therapy," Dr. Albert Ellis.

[Cut to Gloria and Ellis.]

Ellis: I believe that people only get emotions, such as negative emotions of shyness, embarrassment, shame, because they tell themselves something in simple exclamatory sentences. Now, let's try to find out what you're telling yourself. You're meeting this individual. Now what do you think you are saying to yourself, before you get flip?

Gloria: I know what it is, that I'm not . . . I don't stand up to his expectations. I'm not quite enough for him. He's superior to me. Although I want this type of man, I'm afraid I won't have enough to attract him.

Ellis: Well, that's the first part of the sentence. That might be a true one because maybe he could be superior to you in some ways, and maybe he wouldn't be attracted to you. But that would never upset you, if you were only saying that, "I think he may be superior to me." Now, you're adding a second sentence to that which is, "If this is so, that would be awful."

Gloria: Well, not quite so extreme as that because I've thought about that too. It's usually, "I've missed my chance again." Because when I want to show the very best of myself because I think I have self-confidence and I have enough to offer, then, I get afraid, then I show all the bad qualities—I'm flip. Then I'm so much on the defensive that I can't show my good qualities and it's like, "I missed my chance again. There was a good opportunity to be close to this man, and I loused it up again."

Ellis: All right. But let's suppose you *are* saying that, and I think you really are. You must be saying something else, too. Because if you were just saying, "Hell, I missed my chance again," you'd say, "All right, next time I'll take advantage of what I learned this time and do it a little better." Now you still must be saying, if you feel shame, embarrassment, shyness, that there's something pretty bad about your error in missing your chance again.

Gloria: I don't know if this follows in context with what you are saying, but the thing I do feel is that I get suspicious then. Am I the type of woman that will only appeal to the ones that are . . . to not my type of guy now anyway? Is there something wrong with me? Am I never going to find the kind of man I enjoy? I always seem to get the other ones.

Ellis: All right. Now you are getting closer to what I'm talking about because you are really saying, "If I am this type of woman that none of these good eligible males are going to appeal to, then that would be awful. I'd never get what I want and that would really be something frightful." Isn't that . . .

Gloria: Of course, I don't like thinking of myself that way. I want to put myself on a higher standard. I don't like to think that I may be just an average Jane Doe.

Ellis: Well, let's just suppose for the sake of argument at the moment, that that were so.

Gloria: All right.

Ellis: That you were an average Jane Doe. Now would that be so terrible? It would be inconvenient. It would be unpleasant. You wouldn't want it, but would you get an emotion like shyness, embarrassment, shame out of just believing that maybe I'm going to end up like Jane Doe?

Gloria: I don't know.

Ellis: Well, I don't think you could because you would still have to be saying on some level, as I think you've just said, "It would be very bad. It would be terrible. I would be a nogoodnik if I were just Jane Doe."

Gloria: Well, of course, I would never get what I want. If I were just a Jane Doe and if I were to have to accept it, I'd never get what I want and I don't want to live the rest of my life with just icky men.

Ellis: Well, it's not necessarily so, you would never . . . you really mean your chances would be reduced, because we know some icky girls who get some splendid men, don't we?

Gloria: Oh, that's so.

Ellis: So you are generalizing there. You are saying, "It probably would be that I'd have a more difficult time," but then you are jumping to, "Therefore, I'd never get it at all." You see the catastrophizing there, that you have jumped to?

Gloria: Yes, but it feels that way to me at the time. It seems like forever.

Ellis: That's right. But isn't that a vote of nonconfidence in you, an essential vote of nonconfidence?

Gloria: Yes.

Ellis: And the nonconfidence is because you are saying, "I don't want to miss out on things. I would like to get the kind of a man I want and be," in your words, "a superior kind of girl who gets a superior kind of man. But if I don't, then I'm practically on the other side of the chain completely, a nogoodnik, somebody who'll never get anything that I want." Which is quite an extreme away, isn't it?

Gloria: Yes.

Ellis: And that is what I call catastrophizing: taking a true statement—and there is a good deal of truth in what you are saying, if you didn't get the kind of man you wanted, it would be inconvenient, annoying, frustrating, which it really would be—and then saying, "I would never possibly get what I want" and even beyond that you are really saying, "And then I couldn't be a happy human being." Aren't you really saying that on some level?

Gloria: Yes.

Ellis: But let's just look at that. Let's just assume the worst. As Bertrand Russell once said years ago, assume the worst—that you never got at all, for whatever the reasons may be, the kind of man you want. Look at all the other things you could do in life to be happy.

[Cut to Interviewer and Shostrom.]

Interviewer: Well, according to Dr. Ellis, Gloria had a problem because she had irrational thoughts about herself.

Shostrom: Yes. I think sometimes there is a tendency for students to under-value Ellis. Freud used to say, "The voice of the intellect is a soft one, but it demands to be heard." I think all therapy is exciting and experi-ential in the way that Rogers and Perls bring things out. But I think from time to time in therapy, it is important to *coach,* getting at some of the *assumptions,* some of the values that are implicit in what's happening. So in Gloria, as I see it, her *assumption* was that she was shy and that she shouldn't be shy. She *should* be flippant. And that this would make her more attractive to a man. This underlying assump-tion that she didn't want to be an ordinary Jane Doe is a very important assumption. I think 90 percent of our problems are due to the un-realistic expectations we have about ourselves. Lack of a feeling of self-worth comes when we don't live up to those expectations. So it seems to me what Ellis is saying is a very important thing. Let's look at those expectations, let's look at those assumptions about yourself and re-evaluate those assumptions. This is the nuts and bolts part of psychotherapy.

Interviewer: How is it possible to integrate these divergent points of view?

Shostrom: Well, what you are asking now is what I have dedicated my life to doing, in a sense. Since we made this film it seems to me we have had to look at therapy as an enterprise, something like medicine. Many years ago, medicine used to have many specialties. You would have a bone specialist and you would have a person working on your eyes and other specialists working on different parts, but we never put it together until the general practitioner came along. And my theory is that, in therapy, we have to go beyond simply schools of thought, that most therapists today are what I call "creative synthesizers," that we have to not only look at the *methods* to learn from these men and others, but that we also have to have a goal for therapy, which I call "self-actualizing," from Maslow's writings. I think we not only have to learn methods of helping, but we have to have a clear picture of what we are attempting to do. As Maslow has said, psychotherapy has to be *for* something and not just to get rid of mental illness or disease. Therapy should help persons to function more clearly in the here and now—to have what I call the *freedom to be:* to actualize one's being.

Interviewer: To develop one's potentials more completely?

Shostrom: Yes. So I think, first, the way we can do that is to do what Rogers does: to focus on the *feelings.* Actualizing Therapy more clearly delineates the feelings that I think are important: the feelings of anger, hurt, trust, love, and fear. All of these are feelings that need to be focused on.

I think, secondly, we need to continue to do what Perls says: to focus on the client's awareness in the here and now. We really have to recognize that our own reality is the here and now, so my approach does this.

Finally, I highly respect what Ellis is saying: that therapy is the process of revising our assumptions about life.

If we can create the kind of relationship that Rogers talks about, in Perls' here and now, and examine those assumptions that we have made about ourselves and others, as Ellis suggests, then we can put these into a gestalt—a total whole—and develop the best parts of all three approaches. This is what I attempt to do and what I call *Actualizing Therapy* [see Figure 4].

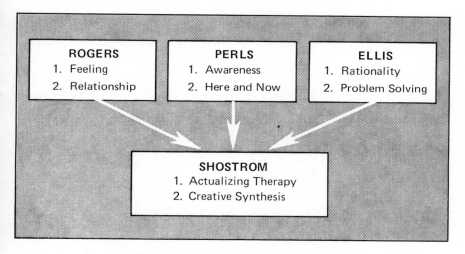

Figure 4. Integration of Three Approaches to Psychotherapy

Interviewer: Many persons seem to have difficulty understanding the concept "actualization."

Shostrom: I use the term "actualiz*ing*" rather than "actualiz*ation*." Actualizing is the freedom to be, which means the ability to experience and express oneself in the here and now. It seems to me that the goal of therapy, if we can define it as such, is the attempt to help a patient or a client or a person get a feeling for what he is feeling inside and then to experience that feeling sufficiently to express it to the leader and to the group.

SUMMARY

In this chapter we have introduced some of the fundamental tenets of Actualizing Therapy. We have shown that Actualizing Therapy emerges from ten parameters of psychotherapy that have their roots in the works of many established leaders in the field. We have also cited the research on these parameters, showing how Rogers, Perls, and Ellis use them in their work. Having shown how Actualizing Therapy attempts to integrate the central dimensions of each of these three approaches, we will now expand on the research roots of Actualizing Therapy and on its relationship to other therapeutic systems.

CHAPTER 2. THE ACTUALIZING ASSESSMENT BATTERY

This chapter deals with a large number of empirical studies and statistics that give scientific credence to Actualizing Therapy. While the research data will be of particular interest to the reader who is interested in the scientific roots of Actualizing Therapy, the critical dimensions that the inventories under discussion measure should be of interest to all readers because they are central to the understanding of the individual.

The technical instruments of Actualizing Therapy are a set of psychological inventories known as the *Actualizing Assessment Battery*. These instruments, discussed more fully below, measure the power or energy involved in *intra*personal and *inter*personal relating. The value of an inventory is that it reveals, in a short time, principles and assumptions people have made about themselves that would otherwise take thousands of hours of interviewing to discover. The recognition of the principles and assumptions a person has made is important in launching Actualizing Therapy and in suggesting directions that the client can take in his journey of actualizing.

Actualizing Therapy is committed to the value of paper-and-pencil questionnaires as measures to assist in therapeutic growth. Moreover, Actualizing Therapy emphasizes the value of the intellect as a form of experience *along with* the emotions and the body. The use of standardized tests is comparable to the use of thermometers, sphygmomanometers, and stethoscopes in medicine. Actualizing Therapy, like medicine, is committed to the whole person: intellectual, emotional, and bodily responses. Just as the physician is interested in the whole person and uses his instruments to clarify his understanding of the person, so we believe that the most valid tests available are useful for the therapist.

One of the principal difficulties in evaluating counseling and psychotherapy has been finding adequate and specific criteria for judging progress.

Many inventories, such as the MMPI, that focus on the measure of pathology rather than health, have limited value for measuring the positive effects of therapy. We believe, however, that the introduction of the Actualizing Assessment Battery is an important step in satisfying the pressing need for research on the positive effects of therapy—such effects as are inherent in the concept of self-actualizing.

THE RHYTHM OF RELATING

Self-actualizing may be seen as an expression of fulfillment in two basic contexts: *intra*personal and *inter*personal. The *Personal Orientation Inventory* (POI) (Shostrom, 1963, 1964), and the *Personal Orientation Dimensions* (POD), the latter currently under development as an extension of the POI, are primarily measures of *intra*personal self-actualizing. Two other inventories, the *Caring Relationship Inventory* (CRI) (Shostrom, 1966), and the *Pair Attraction Inventory* (PAI) (Shostrom, 1970), primarily measure aspects of *inter*personal self-actualizing. These four inventories represent the assessment dimension of Actualizing Therapy and are collectively termed the *Actualizing Assessment Battery* (AAB).

The clinical significance of these experimentally validated instruments is important to understand here. Concepts measured by the POI and the POD emphasize a person's *intra*personal being, which is important because a person needs to be in touch with himself and at peace with himself before he can cope with the world. In Figure 5A, two individuals are shown independently existing in the world in a state of withdrawal or independence without reference to any specific other. But it will be noted that these individuals are still in contact with their inner cores. In effect, they are still in contact with themselves, intrapersonally.

The PAI and the CRI, on the other hand, measure a person's *inter*personal being in reference to a specific other, for, in addition to being in touch with oneself, actualizing involves the capacity to interrelate with others in a rhythmic and harmonious manner. Figure 5B shows two people in intimate contact in a state of confluence or dependence, as would exist in a close sexual relationship or in a situation involving high intimacy, such as mutual empathy or sorrow. Figure 5C presents a third alternative—two people are in a state of contact, or interdependence, where the permeable membranes of their facades are touching, but each is also in contact with his own core, and each is in contact with others at his facade or periphery.

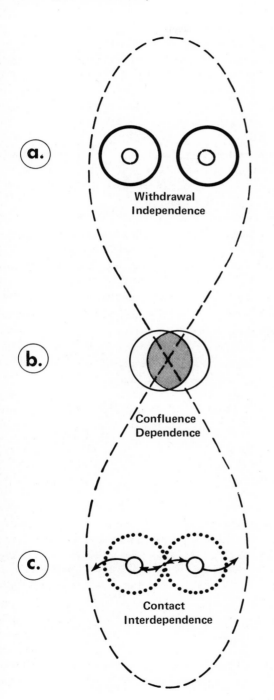

(a.)

Withdrawal
Independence

(b.)

Confluence
Dependence

(c.)

Contact
Interdependence

**Figure 5.
The Rhythm of Relating**

The rhythm of living the actualizing life would be expressed by the *contact* and *withdrawal* that occurs as one moves through phases A, B, and C and back again. A nonactualizing person is one who is stuck at a particular level and is not experiencing the rhythm of his existence. The value of the Actualizing Assessment Battery in this connection is that at any point in one's life we can measure the degree to which contact and withdrawal exists in a relationship.

Thus, Actualizing Therapy is a therapy that focuses on the importance of energizing oneself in relation to one's core, as well as energizing interpersonal relationships. Without intrapersonal and interpersonal energies, deadness, or pathology, is the result.

In the following sections we summarize the primary scales of each of the four inventories in the Actualizing Assessment Battery. For the layman, a reading through of these scales will provide familiarity with what we believe are important considerations in the process of intrapersonal and interpersonal actualizing. In the sections of the chapter relating to validity, the language is somewhat technical. At the conclusion of the chapter, however, we utilize a marital case to demonstrate the *practical application* of the AAB to real-life case histories.

THE PERSONAL ORIENTATION INVENTORY

The Personal Orientation Inventory (POI) was conceptualizied, and the initial scale constructs delineated, by Shostrom (1964) during the summer of 1962, with the consultation of Abraham Maslow. Nine years later, Maslow wrote in his final work, *The Farther Reaches of Human Nature* (1971):

> In studying healthy people, self-actualizing people, etc., there has been a steady move from the openly normative and the frankly personal, step by step, toward more and more descriptive, objective words, to the point where there is today a standardized test of self-actualization. Self-actualization can now be defined quite operationally, as intelligence used to be defined, i.e., self-actualization is what that test tests. It correlates well with external variables of various kinds and keeps on accumulating additional correlational meanings. (p. 28)

One of the purposes of this book is to bring the great accumulation of research with the POI to bear on the creative actualizing ethic and on the implementation of this ethic through the processes of Actualizing Therapy.

The POI's 150 two-choice comparative-value-judgment items reflect significant value judgments as seen by therapists in practice, and are based on the theoretical formulations of several writers in humanistic psychology, including Maslow, Riesman, Rogers, and Perls.

In responding to the POI, the examinee is asked to select the one statement in each pair that is most true of himself. In scoring the inventory, items are logically grouped into two major scales and ten subscales that are used in comparing the examinee's responses to normative samples. One of the major scales (I) is interpreted in terms of a Support ratio, which measures other- versus inner-directedness. The Support ratio defines autonomy by assessing a balance between other-directedness and inner-directedness. The other major scale of the POI (T_C) is interpreted in terms of a Time ratio, which assesses the degree to which one is reality oriented in the present and is able to bring past experiences and future expectations into meaningful continuity. The subsidiary scales are designed to tap values important in the development of the self-actualizing individual: Self-Actualizing Value (SAV), Existentiality (Ex), Feeling Reactivity (Fr), Spontaneity (S), Self-Regard (Sr), Self-Acceptance (Sa), Nature of Man-Constructive (Nc), Synergy (Sy), Acceptance of Aggression (A), and Capacity for Intimate Contact (C).

When used in the clinical setting, the POI provides an objective measure of the client's level of actualizing as well as positive guidelines for growth during therapy. In addition, when used as a variable for the study of the relationship of actualizing to other theoretical constructs, the POI provides an assessment of level of actualizing in terms of its separate conceptual facets—the two major scales and the ten subscales. The polar dimension of anger, for example, may be estimated by means of the Acceptance of Aggression (A) scale score, while the love dimension would be reflected in the Capacity for Intimate Contact (C) scale score. Similarly, strength can be measured by means of the score on the Self-Regard (Sr) scale and weakness through the score on the Self-Acceptance (Sa) scale (reflecting acceptance of oneself in spite of one's weaknesses).

Ratio Scores

Time Competence. The Time Incompetence/Time Competence ratio is a measure of the degree to which one is time competent (T_C), or present oriented, as contrasted with time incompetent (T_I), or living primarily in the past (with guilts, regrets, and resentments) and/or in the future (with idealized goals, plans, expectations, predictions, and fears). The time competent person appears to live more fully in the here and now and is able to tie the past and the future to the present in meaningful continuity. Time competent persons also appear to be less burdened by guilts, regrets, and resentments from the past than are nonactualizing persons, and their aspirations are tied meaningfully to present working goals. The principle of balance still applies, however, in that the self-actualizing person is more *present* and less *past* and *future* oriented but still reflects some of both time competence and time incompetence.

Inner Support. The other/inner support concept defines whether re-activity orientation is basically toward others (O) or toward the self (I). The inner-directed person appears to have incorporated a psychic "gyroscope," which is started by parental influences and is later influenced by other authority figures. The inner-directed person goes through life apparently independent, but still obeying this internal piloting. The source of direction for the individual is "inner" in the sense that he is guided by internal motivations rather than external influences. Other-directed persons *impress* others at a facade level. For them, manipulations, such as pleasing others and insuring constant acceptance, become the primary methods of relating. While the ultimate goal of actualizing is establishing a balance between inner- and other-orientation, for most of us the problem is to become more inner-directed, to increase our capability for expressing the self at a core level from within.

Subscales

The *Self-Actualizing Value* (SAV) scale measures affirmation of primary values of self-actualizing people. Individuals who hold and live by values of self-actualizing people score high on this scale, while those who reject values of self-actualizing people score low. Concepts measured by this scale cut across many characteristics and values.

The *Existentiality* (Ex) scale measures the ability to situationally or existentially react without rigid adherence to principles. Existentiality reflects one's flexibility in applying values or principles to one's life. It is a measure of the ability to use good judgment in applying these general principles. High scores reflect flexibility in application of values, while low scores suggest that values may be so rigidly held that the person is compulsive or dogmatic.

The *Feeling Reactivity* (Fr) scale measures sensitivity of responsiveness to one's own needs and feelings. A high score reflects sensitivity to personal needs and feelings. A low score shows insensitivity to personal needs and feelings.

The *Spontaneity* (S) scale measures freedom to react spontaneously or to be oneself. A high score indicates the ability to express feelings in spontaneous action. A low score indicates that one is fearful of expressing feelings behaviorally.

The *Self-Regard* (Sr) scale measures affirmation of self because of worth or strength. A high score is a sign of the ability to like oneself because of one's strength as a person, while a low score suggests low self-worth.

The *Self-Acceptance* (Sa) scale measures affirmation or acceptance of oneself in spite of one's weaknesses or deficiencies. A low score on this scale would suggest inability to accept one's weakness. It is probably more difficult to achieve self-acceptance than self-regard, though self-actualizing requires both.

The *Nature of Man-Constructive* (Nc) scale measures the degree of one's *constructive* view of the nature of man. One who scores high on this scale sees man as essentially good. He can resolve the good-evil, masculine-feminine, selfish-unselfish, spiritual-sensual, or other extreme dichotomies in the nature of man. A high score, therefore, reflects the self-actualizing ability to be synergistic in one's understanding of human nature. A low score suggests that one sees man as essentially evil or bad.

The *Synergy* (Sy) scale measures the ability to be synergistic—to transcend dichotomies on a broad basis. A high score is an indicator of the ability to see opposites of life as meaningfully related. A low score suggests that one sees opposites of life as antagonistic. The synergistic person sees that work and play are not different; that lust and love, selfishness and unselfishness, and similar "dichotomies" are not really opposites at all.

The *Acceptance of Aggression* (A) scale measures the ability to accept one's natural aggressiveness as opposed to defensiveness, denial, and repression of aggression. A high score reflects the ability to accept anger or aggression within oneself as natural. A low score suggests that one denies having such feelings and avoids expression of them.

The *Capacity for Intimate Contact* (C) scale measures the ability to develop intimate contact-relationships with other human beings, unencumbered by expectations and obligations. A high score reflects the person's ability to develop meaningful, contact-relationships with other human beings. A low score shows that one may have difficulty with warm interpersonal relationships.

Validity of the POI

A measure that is considered to be valid for one purpose may not be valid for another and there are a great many techniques for establishing these validities. Following are a number of studies applying various techniques in validating the POI.

Predictive Validity

When a measuring instrument is used to predict another, perhaps more cumbersome, source of information, the technique is referred to as establishing predictive validity. It was this method that was first employed to demonstrate the validity of the POI. The attempt was to see if the POI actually measures self-actualizing as observed by trained therapists.

In the initial validation study, reported by Shostrom (1964), prominent, doctoral-level psychologists nominated criterion samples of "self-actualizing" and "nonactualizing" persons, who subsequently completed the POI. The participation of these professional clinicians was secured through the cooperation of societies of clinical psychologists. POI scale differences between these nominated samples were statistically significant for the major POI concepts of Time Competence (T_C) and Inner-Direction (I). In addition, nine of the ten POI subscales significantly differentiated these clinically nominated groups. (Profiles for these criterion groups are presented in Figure 6.) Thus comparatively easily obtained inventory scores provided classifications corresponding, for the most part, to observations by highly skilled therapists based on knowledge of behavior gained over long periods of time.

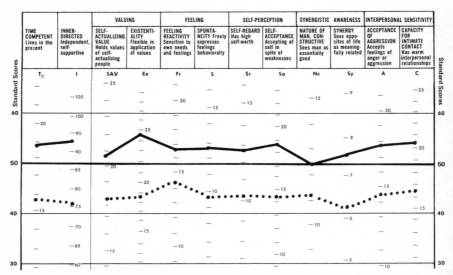

Figure 6. Profiles of Actualizing and Nonactualizing Groups on the POI

Following this evidence of validity, a number of other major studies were conducted to test hypotheses generated from the theory of the self-actualizing person. Pursuing the hypothesis that hospitalized psychiatric patients would represent a nonactualizing population, Fox, Knapp, and Michael (1968) administered the POI to a sample of 100 hospitalized mental patients. The sample scored significantly lower on all POI scales than either the nominated self-actualizing or normal adult samples reported in the earlier study by Shostrom. Further, all differences but one between the hospitalized sample and a clinically nominated nonactualizing but non-hospitalized sample were in the expected direction, but were not so great as the differences between the hospitalized sample and the normals or between the hospitalized sample and the self-actualizing sample. The hospitalized group was characterized by marked other-directedness and distorted orientation in time. The findings indicate that, as a group, the hospitalized population tended to have fewer ego satisfactions, seemed more frustrated, anxious, and tense, and appeared to have less self-esteem than other groups. Since the patients were less reality-oriented and were hidebound, rigid, and other-directed, the ordinary problems of living may have rested more heavily on their shoulders and tended to bring about internal tensions and distress.

While the major scales of Time Competence and Inner-Direction significantly differentiated the hospitalized sample from the clinically nominated nonactualizing sample, there were fewer clearcut differences between these samples on some of the subscales. The nonhospitalized sample was composed of individuals who were relatively more time competent and more inner-directed, were able to react more existentially—without rigid adherence to principles (higher Ex)—and were more responsive to their own needs and feelings (higher Fr). In addition to being more aware of the essential goodness of man (higher Nc) and more able to accept aggressive tendencies within themselves (higher A), the nonhospitalized sample showed greater ability to develop intimate relationships with other human beings (higher C). The hospitalized group was more similar to the nominated non-actualizing group yet displayed some clinically important differences. However, *all* POI scales substantially distinguished between the hospitalized and normal populations, and between the hospitalized and self-actualizing samples.

In relating changes in POI scores to stages of Actualizing Therapy, Shostrom and Knapp (1966) found that all POI scales significantly differentiated a sample of outpatients beginning therapy from those in advanced stages of psychotherapeutic progress. Results from these and other samples in therapy are considered in greater detail in Chapters 6 and 7.

Another form of predictive validity involves the *concurrent* collection of data from instruments reflecting concepts espoused by different personality theorists.

Among the early applications of the POI bearing on confirmation of Maslow's theory was a study by Knapp (1965) in which self-actualizing, as measured by the POI, was shown to be negatively related to the concept of neuroticism as measured by the *Eysenck Personality Inventory* (EPI) (Eysenck & Eysenck, 1963). The EPI dimension of Neuroticism-Stability was negatively correlated with all POI scales, the correlation of highest magnitude being –.57 against the POI scale of Time Competence, the scale measuring orientation to the present as contrasted with orientations of the "past" (guilts) or "future" (anxiety). Negative correlations between measures of self-actualizing and the neuroticism construct, as noted by Hilgard and Atkinson (1967), "would support Maslow's contention that he was describing mentally healthy people." POI correlations against the EPI Extraversion scale were generally positive, but of a much lower magnitude, ranging up to a significant .39 against the POI Spontaneity scale.

To examine the relationship of self-actualizing to major personality constructs defined through factor analysis, Knapp and Comrey (1973) administered the POI and the *Comrey Personality Scales* (CPS) (Comrey, 1970), a measure of major dimensions of personality, to a sample of eighty-four volunteer undergraduate students. Previous findings that concepts of self-actualizing are related to emotional health were reconfirmed, and certain theoretical concepts of actualizing measured by the POI were shown to be meaningfully related to factorial dimensions defined in Comrey's classification of personality. In particular, significant correlations of the POI Time Competence (T_C) and Inner-Direction (I) scales to the CPS Emotional Stability scale supported the hypothesis that self-actualizing is positively related to stability. The negative relationship between self-actualizing concepts, particularly Existentiality (Ex), and the CPS Social Confirmity scale was confirmed, as was the positive correlation between the POI Nature of Man-Constructive (Nc) scale and the CPS Trust versus Defensiveness (T) scale, similarly defined as measuring a basic belief and trust in the goodness and worth of human nature.

In a study relating POI variables to the *Guilford-Zimmerman Temperament Survey* (G-Z) (1949) and to the *Sixteen Personality Factor Questionnaire* (16PF) (Cattell & Eber, 1957), Meredith (1967) reported correlations ranging in magnitude up to .48 between the G-Z Sociability (S) and the POI Self-Regard (Sr) scale. Correlations with the 16PF ranged in magnitude up to .44 between Venturesome (H) and Self-Regard. Considering the major POI scale of Inner-Direction, impressive similarities to the 16PF scales depict the self-actualizing individual as relatively more assertive, happy-go-lucky, expedient, venturesome, and self-assured. Correlations against G-Z factors depict self-actualizing students as active, ascendant, sociable, emotionally stable, and objective. Correlations between the other major POI scale, Time Competence, and G-Z and 16PF temperament scales suggest that those whose primary orientation is in the present would be described from the 16PF as assertive, happy-go-lucky, venturesome, trusting, and self-assured, and from the G-Z as relaxed, active, ascendant, sociable, emotionally stable, objective, and tolerant. The relatively low magnitude of correlations between these instruments and the POI indicates that they are measuring somewhat different aspects of personality.

A widely used instrument based on clinical classifications is the Minnesota Multiphasic Personality Inventory (MMPI) (Hathaway & McKinley, 1951). In general, the MMPI is a measure of pathology and its results would be expected to complement POI results among nonactualizing or disturbed individuals. Shostrom and Knapp (1966) have reported such results, relating POI and MMPI scales among a sample of persons in various stages of Actualizing Therapy. Highest relationships between the POI and MMPI clinical scales were obtained between POI Time Competence and MMPI Psychasthenia, a measure of phobias and obsessive-compulsive concerns, and between POI Inner-Direction scale and the MMPI Depression scale, a measure of retroflectiveness or intropunitiveness.

Examination of scale descriptions for the two instruments suggested the following complementary combinations. The healthy counterpart to MMPI Depression on the POI might be the Acceptance of Aggression (A) scale. Highly significant correlations between these scales for the beginning therapy sample support this hypothesis. The healthy complement to MMPI Psychasthenia on the POI might best be represented by the Spontaneity (S) scale. Correlations in this case, however, were of rather low magnitude, lending little support to this hypothesis. Social Introversion on the MMPI is a measure of social alienation and withdrawal. On the POI, the healthy complement to this characteristic is perhaps best measured by the Feeling Reactivity (Fr), Acceptance of Aggression (A), and Capacity for Intimate Contact (C) scales. Significant correlations of these scales in the beginning therapy group lend support to these hypothesized relationships.

It is interesting to note that more significant relationships were obtained for POI scales against the Social Introversion (Si) scale than any other MMPI scale. The MMPI authors (Hathaway & McKinley, 1951) have presented the Si scale not as a clinical scale "in the strict sense of being chiefly for use with hospitalized patients" but have found it to be "widely used in counseling and guidance work" (p. 8). For example, it has been successful in distinguishing college populations who engage in many extracurricular activities from those not so inclined. The obtained correlations appear to support the notion that the POI is measuring attributes that are also important in developing harmonious interpersonal relationships among "normal" populations.

In general, examination of correlations between the instruments suggests that, although complementary, POI scales are measuring areas somewhat different than those measured by the MMPI. The highest relationships accounted for an estimated 42 percent of the total variance.

A theoretical consideration raised from this study is whether self-actualizing means something more than simply lack of mental illness. Although the conclusion that self-actualizing increases as mental illness goes down may be warranted, it may also be assumed that something is necessary to replace the patient's pathology. Freud is understood to have said that the purpose of therapy is simply to eliminate the symptoms of the patient. In many therapies there is little doubt that this goal is the only necessary one. The work of Eysenck and Rachman (1965) and Wolpe (1958) has demonstrated the effectiveness of the more recently explored behavior therapies in effecting such symptom cures. The distinction between such an approach and that of Actualizing Therapy might be best stated as "cure" versus "growth." Other therapists, such as Rogers and Maslow, say that therapy must do more than eliminate symptoms and that therefore psychotherapy should assist the patient in developing a workable value system. We assume that such a value system is nonpathologic and non-denominational—in a psychotherapeutic sense—and that such values are akin to those measured by the POI. Whether practicing therapists like it or not, they must accept the fact that many therapies do teach values, and the only question is whether such values should be made explicit or implicit. Typically, correlations in this study were markedly greater in the beginning therapy sample. This would appear to support the assumption that the two instruments would be complementary among nonactualizing samples. As growth occurs, new nonpathological dimensions come into play.

Construct Validity

The *construct validity* of a test can be defined as the degree to which the test successfully measures what it purports to measure. In the case of the POI, the concepts measured are those relating to self-actualizing.

The self-actualizing person has been described as possessing qualities of "autonomy," "calmness," "creativity," "joy," "zest in living," and "resistance to enculturation." As Maslow (1970) has stated, "Self-actualizing people are not well adjusted (in the naive sense of approval of and identification with the culture). They get along with the culture in various ways but of all of it may be said that in a certain profound and meaningful sense they resist enculturation" (p. 171). The assertion that self-actualizing individuals resist enculturation was studied by Hekmat and Theiss (1971) through a social conditioning technique. The experimenters started with the assumption that therapy was a form of enculturation and hypothesized that persons with low POI scores would respond more to reflection of feeling as a reinforcer for affective self-disclosures than those with moderate or high scores. (Thus, highly self-actualizing persons were expected *not* to respond to comments by the therapist with emotionally laden disclosures.) The POI was administered to sixty subjects who were assigned, on the basis of their scores, to four groups: high self-actualizing, moderate self-actualizing, low self-actualizing, and stratified control. Conditioning consisted of reflective statements by the experimenter to every self-disclosure comment made by each subject during an interview. An example of affective self-disclosures made by subjects in the experiment and the therapist's reinforcement is provided in the following exchange:

Subject: "I feel frightened by that man" [affective self-disclosure].

Therapist: "That man in the picture frightens you" [reflection].

The results indicated that prior to conditioning the high self-actualizing individuals displayed a significantly higher rate of affective self-disclosures than the moderate or low self-actualizing groups. During conditioning, however, the high self-actualizing individuals showed a substantially lower degree of responsiveness to social reinforcement (represented by reflective statements by the experimenter) when compared to the low and moderate self-actualizers. Analysis of adjusted scores indicated that the low self-actualizing group had the highest rate of conditioning, whereas the high self-actualizing individuals showed a nonsignificant gain in the rate of affective self-disclosures during conditioning. The results thus provided empirical support for Maslow's assertion that high self-actualizing individuals are resistant to enculturation.

One goal of therapy may be to help the client achieve "intrinsic" learning ("becoming") through reflection. Research results suggest that as an individual moves toward greater self-actualizing, the locus of effective reinforcement may move from the external to the internal source, and a traditional therapeutic technique will thus become less effective. It may be that the highly self-actualizing individual responds more to the therapist as a *model,* rather than as a dispenser, of reinforcement. Therapists with high levels of genuineness, authenticity, and self-disclosure may achieve the most effective behavior modification with highly actualizing clients. These conclusions add to previous findings concerning the relationship of self-actualizing behavior to counseling effectiveness.

Maslow's (1970) conjecture that conformity would be negatively related to actualizing received experimental support from a study by Crosson and Schwendiman (1972). POI Inner-Direction scale scores were measured by a Crutchfield apparatus employing perceptual discrimination judgments, consisting of matching the lengths of lines and choosing the largest relative area of geometrical figures. The design of the study represents an important extension of the construct validity of the POI to objective, behavioral predictions and adds to the number of verifications of the nomological network extending from the self-actualizing model. Conformity behavior in a group setting is of theoretical importance to the concept of self-actualizing, since Maslow has described the actualizing person as one who would feel no constraint to yield to social influences. This independence from social pressures should hold for pressure to conform to the expectations of the group and for reliance on other's responses as information. Thus, it was hypothesized that relatively self-actualizing individuals would exhibit independent behavior in a conformity situation. The obtained correlation of -.28 between Inner-Direction scale scores and the conformity behavioral score was significant and was accepted as supporting the hypothesis of a negative relationship between self-actualizing and conformity. Although significant, the obtained correlation is low, which may be due to restriction in range of the POI scores. Subjects in this study were introductory psychology students, a population of individuals who are unlikely to have realized a high level of actualizing, a fact further supported in this study by the observation that the distribution of the Inner-Direction scores had a slight negative distortion, with most subjects falling in the nonactualizing range.

Faking Actualizing

As long as there are tests, people, for a wide variety of reasons, will try to "beat" them. Perhaps a simple ego trip is involved, or the need to present what one feels is his best possible profile. Neurotic patients, because of the very nature of their conditions, fake answers, as do felons, who quite naturally are anxious to impress custodial personnel and parole boards. However, the POI has proved to be remarkably resistant to attempts at deliberate distortion of its conclusions in a favorable (actualizing) direction.

Studies of the effects of attempts to fake favorable responses to the POI have disclosed some interesting implications involving our theory of self-actualizing. In the earliest of these studies, Knapp (1966) administered the POI to a college sample under standard instructions and then to another similar sample under instructions to "fake good." "Faking" instructions were to "answer the questionnaire as though you wanted to make a good impression of yourself. You should answer as though you were applying for a job and wanted to make the most favorable impression." Contrary to what might be expected, the greatest discrepancies were not in the direction of the appearance of greater self-actualizing; in fact, under the faking instructions the major Inner-Direction scale, plus seven of the subscale means, moved in the direction of nonactualizing, as shown in Figure 7.

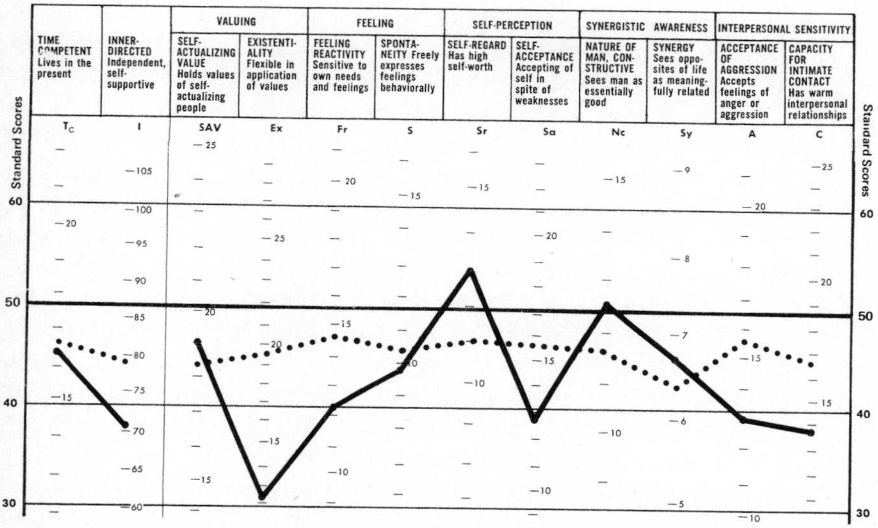

Figure 7. **Comparison of Students Responding to POI Under Normal Instructions with Students Instructed to "Make a Good Impression"**

It will be noted in examining the profiles that the Existentiality (Ex) scale in particular is distorted in the direction of emphasizing rigid adherence to traditional values—away from the values espoused by self-actualizing persons. Perhaps the individual who follows society's rules and principles, compulsively nullifying all objections, might appear to be a good organization man, thus explaining the responses of the "fake good" sample instructed to respond as though applying for employment. Several other scales showed wide discrepancies under the two testing instructions, leading to the conclusion that deliberate distortion does not produce a profile characteristic of self-actualizing individuals.

A number of other studies both substantiated and expanded the theoretical implications of these findings. Fisher (1973), using much the same design as the Knapp study, asked a sample of 120 felons committed to a California Department of Corrections facility to respond to the POI under standard instructions and again under instructions to create a favorable impression on members of the Adult Authority, who would make major decisions concerning them. Again much the same results were obtained, with nine of ten significant changes being toward *lower* self-actualizing under the simulation instructions.

Following a series of studies into the "fakability" of the POI (Braun, 1966, 1969) that resulted in profiles similar to those obtained in the studies described above, Braun and LaFaro (1969) concluded that the lower scores resulting from attempts to make a good impression or to appear well-adjusted on the POI demonstrate an "unexpected resistance to faking," making the instrument "unique among self-report instruments."

In a study by Braun and LaFaro (1969) the POI was administered to four college student groups under standard instructions followed by readministration with instructions either to "make a good impression" or to appear "well-adjusted." In addition, two other groups received special instruction on what self-actualizing is supposed to entail. Faked administration scores for the four groups were consistently *less* favorable than under standard instructions, while the two groups receiving information about the concept of actualizing achieved considerably *more* favorable scores. Braun and LaFaro concluded that unless subjects have special information about the POI and self-actualization and are motivated to fake, the inventory shows an unexpected resistance to faking.

Based on clinical experience with the POI, Shostrom (1973) observed:

> From a clinical standpoint, the POI has a "lie score profile" which can be identified easily. Since "actualizing" persons score between T standard scores of 50 and 60, those with excessively high profiles (all T scores of 60-70) may be interpreted as "over-enthusiastic" attempts to take the test in accordance with "rightness" from reading Maslow and other humanistic literature. Even Maslow, himself, scored between the 50-60 T score range! (p. 480)

At this point the interested reader may well be searching for the reason behind this discrepancy between actual responses of self-actualizing persons and the distorted responses of those *attempting* to present themselves as actualizing.

Many personality scales are keyed in the direction of generally accepted cultural standards. Development of the POI, however, was based on logical keying supported by an empirical demonstration of validity. Keying of the POI is based on the direction of the self-actualizing model of personality, rather than on cultural norms. To the extent that values and behaviors defining the self-actualizing person differ from those of currently accepted cultural standards, POI scores may be expected to deviate under extreme motivational conditions.

An earlier study by Grater (1968) and the study by Braun and LaFaro (1969) described above suggest that knowledge of the characteristics of self-actualizing persons as defined by the POI, in addition to the motivation to make a good impression, is necessary in order for individuals to distort their POI responses appreciably in the direction of self-actualizing. Warehime and Foulds (1973) have presented data supporting this hypothesis. In their study, POI scale scores were correlated with scores from a scale developed to measure the tendency to give socially desirable responses. Their results indicated that individuals who would tend to be successful in dissimulating scores in other evaluation situations were not successful in obtaining higher POI scores. The magnitudes of correlations were interpreted as indicating those concepts wherein the model of the self-actualizing person and cultural standards are most widely at variance.

Particularly high relationships were obtained against the Acceptance of Aggression (A) scale. Cultural standards regarding recognition and verbal expression of aggressive feelings ("play it cool") were interpreted as being quite different from behavior sanctioned by self-actualizing individuals. Other significant relationships were obtained against the Existentiality scale, which measures flexibility in the application of values and reduced compulsiveness and dogmatism as well as increased ability to react without blind or rigid adherence to principles.

Results of a study by Knapp and Comrey (1973) corroborate these findings. When correlated against the Response Bias (R) scale of the Comrey Personality Scales (CPS) (Comrey, 1970), a measure of tendency to answer in a socially acceptable way, POI scales of Inner-Direction (I), Existentiality (Ex), Feeling Reactivity (Fr), Self-Acceptance (Sa), Acceptance of Aggression (A) and Capacity for Intimate Contact (C) were all significantly and negatively correlated.

Thus the person who truly accepts and lives by such statements as "I do not always tell the truth," "I do not always need to live by the rules and standards of society," and "I do not feel obligated when a stranger does me a favor" may, in fact, be more self-actualizing, but, when asked to give the favorable answer, might respond, "I feel I must always tell the truth," "I live by the rules and standards of society," and, "I feel obligated when a stranger does me a favor." To conclude, the self-actualizing person is one who is aware of both his strengths and weaknesses. The person who is trying to fake the POI and attempts only to "fake good," giving only expressions of his strength, will not do well on the other concepts measured by this instrument. Thus, built into the POI is a "lie profile" exhibited by naive subjects that is easily detected by those who are trained in evaluation of this instrument. We believe this "lie profile" is a more significant measure of fakability than a "lie score," as used in other instruments.

THE CARING RELATIONSHIP INVENTORY

Although the POI has been a very useful measure of positive personal growth in therapy, it is our feeling that other measures are needed. Specifically, what is needed are measures that describe interpersonal changes in the behavior of the client going through therapy. We believe that, ultimately, the effect of therapy, and of group therapy in particular, must be a measure of *interpersonal effectiveness*. Until now, no tests have measured this critical dimension.

Therapists, marriage counselors, religious leaders, and others dealing with the problems of marriage have expressed the need for an objective measure of the nature of the emotional attachment between a man and a woman. Scales in the Caring Relationship Inventory and the Pair Attraction Inventory are designed to meet this need.

The relationship existing between a man and woman, whether they be sweethearts, engaged, or man and wife, is perhaps the most vital and important interpersonal relationship there is, and yet it is the least studied or understood. The investigation of so complex a relationship is dependent upon both an underlying theoretical framework of the structure of such relationships and measures of the specific relationships. Quantified measurement scales are needed to provide tests of hypotheses generated by the theoretical model.

The Caring Relationship Inventory (CRI) is a measure of the essential elements of love or caring in human relationships. The guidelines used in the initial development of this inventory were based, in part, on the theoretical writings of Fromm, Lewis, Maslow, and Perls. The CRI consists of eighty-three items concerning feelings and attitudes of one member of a male and female pair toward the other member.

Responses of either true or false are made to each of the items, first as applied to the other member of the couple (spouse, fiancé, sweetheart) and, second, as applied to an "ideal" mate. Two forms of the CRI are used, one for the male's rating of the female and one for the female's rating of the male. Development of the CRI was based on responses of criterion groups of successfully married or actualizing couples and of nonactualizing couples —troubled couples in counseling and nonactualizing divorced individuals.

Major Scales

Affection, or *agape,* reflects the capacity of a person to feel a sense of unconditional love for others in a manner similar to the way God is said to feel for humankind. It is a charitable, altruistic form of love in which one feels deeply for the other individual as another unique human being. It involves compassion, appreciation, and tolerance and has been defined as caring for the needs of another person as a parent does for a child. The danger, expressed through excessive affection, however, is that parents may begin to feel that they "own" the child. Likewise, in a marriage the same principle holds. One marriage partner never owns the other.

Friendship is a helping, nurturing form of love. It involves unconditional acceptance characterized by the love of another's personhood. Friendship is a love of equals based on an appreciation of the other person's talents and worth. Friendship may become manipulative, however, when one begins to "exploit" or use other people rather than to appreciate them.

Eros is a romantic, or erotic, sexual form of love. It develops in the relationship between mother and child, in which there is much skin contact and feeling on the part of both. Any sexual relationship may become manipulative and be referred to as "seduction." Seduction means using the other person's body physically, without appreciating the total spiritual nature of the other person.

Empathy is a form of love reflecting the capacity of a person to feel for another. It develops as one begins to learn peer and sex roles. In later life empathy becomes a peer love based on appreciation of common interests and respect for each other's equality. Manipulative empathy is called "Pharisaism," in that one says one thing and does another.

Self-love is the ability to accept one's own weaknesses as well as to appreciate one's individual, unique sense of personal worth. It includes the acceptance of one's full range of positive and negative feelings toward one's partner. Self-love may become manipulative when a person treats the self as an object or thing rather than as something to be respected.

Subscales

Being Love (B-Love) is the love of another solely for their being as a person; without conditions or reservations. It is an admiring, respectful love; an end in itself.

Deficiency Love (D-Love) is the love of another for what they can do for one. It is an exploiting, manipulating love of another as a means to an end.

In describing the CRI and contrasting it with earlier work, Kelley (1974) has stated:

> A more promising approach is found in the Caring Relationship Inventory developed by Everett L. Shostrom. . . . Shostrom's careful work may well lay the foundation for a more accurate measurement and understanding of the elusive quality of love. . . . With such a test, we can begin to answer the question of what love means and how stable and lasting it is. (pp. 220-221)

Validity of the CRI

In an investigation of the validity of the CRI (Shostrom, 1966) the inventory was administered to samples of actualizing couples, troubled couples, and divorced individuals. The seventy-five actualizing couples had been married at least five years and indicated that they had worked through any marital difficulties they might have had. The fifty troubled couples were receiving marital counseling. The divorced sample consisted of 108 individuals who responded to the CRI in terms of their divorced spouse. Profiles for these samples plotted against the CRI norms based on successfully married couples are shown in Figure 8.

Mean differences between the successfully married sample and samples of troubled or divorced individuals were significant for all CRI scales. The greatest differences were obtained on the CRI Friendship scale. Thus it might appear from results of the CRI that faltering marriages reflect a lack of appreciation of common interests rather than a lack of romantic, sexual, or other aspects of love.

Clinically, it had been felt that the one form of loving divorcees most desire from a second mate is that of friendship. Results from the CRI support this contention. In particular, divorcees seem to want a buddy, not just a sweetheart.

Bustanoby (1974) has recommended the use of the CRI as a device for measuring caring in pair relationships, especially for evaluation in "marriage enrichment programs." Travis and Travis (1975) have presented results from the application of the CRI in a program of this kind (the "Pairing Enrichment Program") showing that such programs result in significant positive changes on the CRI from pre- to post-testing. In the preliminary analysis, data showed that *all* scales were significantly increased

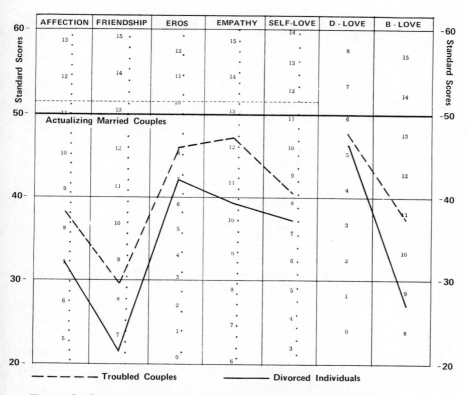

Figure 8. Comparison of Actualizing Couples, Troubled Couples, and Divorced Individuals on the CRI

between pre- and post-administration of the CRI. We believe that the new emphasis on such programs of enrichment will benefit from research utilizing an instrument like the CRI, which measures caring dimensions. Although the CRI is being widely used in a number of other similar settings, the data are just now becoming available.

THE PAIR ATTRACTION INVENTORY

The psychological determinants of lover and mate selection pose problems of both theoretical and practical concern to marriage counselors and therapists. In his pioneering book, *Mate Selection* (1958), Winch postulates that men and women are attracted to one another because of *complementary needs*. It is the *differences* that are attractive, each partner complementing the difference perceived in the other. However, the more recent research of

Lederer and Jackson (1968) and Watzlawric, Beavin, and Jackson (1967) argues the opposite hypothesis: that men and women are attracted to each other because of *symmetry* of interests and of personality.

The emergence of such apparently contradictory points of view and the consequent need for an operationally defined statement of the variables underlying mate selection led to the development of the *Pair Attraction Inventory* (PAI) (Shostrom, 1970), which is designed to measure both complementarity and symmetry in pair relationships. Research upon which the PAI is based has suggested that these two apparently contradictory concepts are compatible, and, indeed, research with the PAI has indicated that *actualizing couples* are, in a rhythmical manner, *both complementary and symmetrical.*

The theory upon which the PAI is based is derived in part from research conducted at the Institute of Personality Assessment at Berkeley by Leary, Barron, MacKinnon and Coffey (Leary, 1957), and others described earlier, in which the scores representing a large sampling of personality characteristics aligned on two basic polarities: anger-love and strength-weakness. The theories of Winch (1958) fit the same scheme.

Recent research with the PAI (Shostrom, 1970) compares scores from divorced spouses, as opposed to lovers. The data collected thus far suggest that with the divorced person the tendency is to select a complementary partner when the original mate is symmetrical, and vice versa. This finding may have implications for a study of unfaithfulness in marriage. Boredom, or routine, is perhaps an important cause of this problem, and this boredom is temporarily alleviated by the choice of a "different" kind of lover, inside or outside of marriage.

The theory underlying the development of the PAI suggests that there are six basic kinds of unconscious mate choices that operate in selecting a marriage partner:

1. The nurturing relationship: *the mother-son pattern.* This unconscious choice is suggested in the writings of Freud. The mother-son relationship permits a man to remain a child and to behave much as he did at home while growing up. It permits a woman simply to imitate the role that her own mother played and requires no creative adjustment to mature adulthood. The weak sonlike husband has unconsciously chosen his opposite, the strong motherlike woman.

2. The supporting relationship: *the daddy-doll (father-daughter) pattern.* The writings of Henrik Ibsen, especially in *A Doll's House,* suggest the presence of this pattern in our culture. The father-daughter relationship is the reverse of the mother-son relationship: The man plays the role of

strength and the woman that of weakness. Each represents a kind of cultural distortion of masculinity and femininity. The man appears to be strong, and the woman plays a childlike role in response to him.

3. The challenging relationship: *the bitch-nice guy (shrew-nice guy) pattern.* The writings of James Thurber have cleverly lampooned this pattern, and this has become a kind of prototype of the unhappy American marriage. The shrewlike woman has exaggerated her expression of anger, and denies her vulnerability. The nice guy has exaggerated his expression of love, and denies his assertiveness. This pattern is often referred to as a "matriarchal" marriage.

4. The educating relationship: *the master-servant (tyrant-nice gal) pattern.* The tyrant-nice gal relationship is immortalized in Shaw's *Pygmalion,* wherein Professor Henry Higgins transforms a servant girl into a lady. In this pattern a strong husband educates and trains a weak, servile wife. The nice gal lacks identity and projects her powers onto the tyranical master in idolatrous love.

5. The confronting relationship: *the "hawks" pattern.* This relationship is illustrated in Edward Albee's play, *Who's Afraid of Virginia Woolf?* It is often called "competitive marriage" and occurs when a top dog marries another top dog, with each geared for battle. Competition replaces love in this power-play relationship. The overt hostility is, in reality, a muffled and unacknowledged cry of deep pain.

6. The accommodating relationship: *the "doves" pattern.* C. S. Lewis, in his classic *Screwtape Letters,* writes tellingly of the dove relationship, insisting that a young couple need only be convinced that they should spend a lifetime struggling to please each other. We call this the nothing-nothing relationship: two underdogs with no substance or identity. Doves are passive manipulators and use guilt as their primary weapon to control one another.

7. The actualizing relationship: *the rhythmic pattern.* In contrast to each of the above, the rhythmic relationship is like the ebb and flow of the tides or the revolving motion of the seasons. Actualizing couples are able to be strong and weak, angry and loving, and to respond with freedom and creative rhythm. Rather than an institution rigidified in roles, the actualizing relationship is a workshop for growth. The actualizing relationship synthesizes, *in rhythm,* all of the relationships above.

A detailed analysis of each of the above relationships is presented in *Between Man and Woman* (Shostrom & Kavanaugh, 1971). The rhythmic relationship is discussed further in this volume in Chapter 10.

Validity of the PAI

A recent study conducted by F. Larry Shostrom (1973) compared predictions of trained therapists, based on their knowledge through client
interviews, with results on the PAI for the same subjects. The thirty therapists participating in the study were drawn from the fields of marriage and
family counseling, psychiatry, psychiatric social work, pastoral counseling,
and psychology. Each therapist selected two or more clients. Altogether 150
clients were rated. After familiarization with the PAI categories, each
therapist selected the one scale that best described each client and the
client's relationship to his partner. The administration of the PAI followed
the therapist's diagnosis. Client profiles were plotted for each of the seven
PAI scales and compared to the judgment of the therapist. Analysis of the
data yielded a high correlation between therapist diagnosis and client score
on the PAI for five of the seven PAI categories, although two categories,
Accommodating Relationship and Supporting Relationship, failed to
achieve significant correlations. The five categories that correlated significantly with the judgments of trained therapists in this study suggest that the
PAI is a valid therapeutic tool and the results seem to show that the PAI
facilitates identification of problem areas in interpersonal relationships. It
appears that the PAI might be successfully utilized in nontherapeutic settings, such as premarital counseling, and presents an interesting opportunity
for long-term research along these lines.

As with the CRI, the PAI is currently being used in a number of research
studies, but the data are just becoming available. Because both the CRI
and PAI are *inter*personal instruments that have been more recently
devised, data are less available than on the POI, which has a longer history
and is a measure of *intra*personal actualizing.

A CLINICAL APPLICATION OF THE ACTUALIZING
ASSESSMENT BATTERY

Recent research by Diana Sjostrom (1975) suggests the clinical value of
analyzing the inventories that make up the AAB. This Battery is shown to
be especially helpful in cases involving marital or relationship problems
between a man and a woman.

The following clinical report is a blind analysis, done for a clinical
psychologist, of a couple in marital therapy. The researcher, Diana

Sjostrom, composed this case study from the profiles of the inventories comprising the *Actualizing Assessment Battery* and had no other information or contact with this couple. The reader will find it helpful to study the summaries presented and, in particular, to examine the inventory profile data—in the right-hand columns—showing how these conclusions were reached. Figure 9 presents an AAB profile sheet for this report.

Clinical Report

NAMES: Mary and Bill
YEARS IN RELATIONSHIP: Eight

Overall Profile Analysis
Bill: "pseudoactualizing" profile on POI: Time Ratio 1:10.5
Support Ratio 1:4
Mary: unusually high expectations on CRI for "Ideal," may indicate unrealistic goals

Diagnostic Patterns

Bill is a perfectionistic person who is somewhat impulsive. He is able to function in the present without regretting the past or worrying about the future; he is not dependent on the support of others. Sometimes this independence is taken to an extreme and he may appear to be aloof.

POI: High Sr
Low Sa

High S
Low Fr

High Time/Ratio
High Support/Ratio

Bill assumes a passive-dependent and son-like position to Mary. He uses his weakness and passivity to gain nurturing attention from her. He is locked into a relationship with a mother-provider, which keeps him infantile and dependent in areas where he must express his strength if he is to be fulfilled. He wants more affection and his boyishness is his fierce way of demanding it. His helpless posture is in a way contrived to get him the results of love. He is saying, "I will be a boy so that you will love me without making demands on me." He is afraid to take the risk to love.

PAI: High Mother/Son

CRI: Low "Other" Affection

Mary, on the other hand, sees herself as a subordinate-helpmate to Bill. Her whole existence centers around a man who gives her artificial strength and meaning to her life. In this role of "servant" she can give in to her passivity

PAI; High Tyrant/Nice Gal

POI: Low A
PAI: High Tyrant/Nice Gal
POI: Low Support/Ratio

and is not required to face her insecurity. Mary does not know how to express her anger. She has been taught to know her place and she spends time serving her man and denying many of her needs. Mary would prefer to overlook a problem than to confront Bill openly and directly with any depth. She lacks identity and projects her powers onto the master (Bill) in idolatrous love. She must learn to express her anger so that her love will not be fawning and servile.

PAI: High Doves

POI: Low A
PAI: Tyrant/Nice Gal

Bill perhaps sees her servile and helping posture as nurturing and mothering, but he is also demanding more dominance and support than she is able to give him. He feels fulfilled in this relationship, except in the area of affection; he would like more affectional caring and stroking from Mary.

(M) PAI: Mother/Son
(F) PAI: Tyrant/Nice Gal
            Doves

CRI: "Ideal" and "Other" profiles close
      Gap on Affection

Mary has difficulty functioning in the present and she seeks the support of others. The approval, opinions, and acceptance of others is important to her. Her self-image is negatively affected by this relationship. She has difficulty accepting and loving Bill for himself, she sees him as a means to an end, rather than a unique separate individual. She feels a lack of trust and respect for Bill and finds it difficult to share intimately and feel a comradeship together. She too feels a lack of affectionate caring and she feels that Bill does not understand or feel her personal needs and feelings.

POI: Low Time/Ratio
      Low Support/Ratio

CRI: Low "Other" Self-Love
      High D-Love
      Low B-Love

      Gap on Friendship
      Scale

      Gap on Affection
      Scale

      Gap on Empathy
      Scale

A follow-up interview was done to obtain information held by the psychologist before he received the report. The purpose was to assess the effects of the AAB on therapeutic procedure and to measure growth that might have resulted from the information provided by the report.

The psychologist provided the following information on this couple:

Mary and Bill had never experienced a fulfilling relationship together, and within the last two years they decided that if they couldn't express more affection to one another that they would discontinue the relationship.

Mary had been in therapy for ten months and Bill for five months at the time the therapist received the report. Mary had come to therapy first, with the presenting problem that there was a lack of affection in their relationship. Bill was reluctant to come for therapy and he had difficulty continuing because he insistently wanted to solve his problems for himself.

The therapist decided to share the report with Mary and Bill. Mary was able to clarify insights gained from her therapy prior to this report since the report provided *objective support* for these discoveries. Mary's ability to identify and talk about these insights with her therapist was extremely reinforcing to her.

The therapist had recognized that Bill had two contradictory styles of life. He functioned as a very dominant and independent person at his job and in society as contrasted with his being a very passive and dependent person with Mary at home. The therapist was experiencing difficulty getting Bill to recognize his two different systems of relating. Upon reviewing the report, Bill was able to consider the possibility of this split and later he tentatively accepted its validity. He was also able to recognize that he attempted to pseudoactualize on the POI as a defense against his insecurity and dependence.

The therapist had previously used the POI, CRI, and PAI independently of one another. The approach of using them as a battery with a clinical report provided him with significantly more knowledge than using them as separate tools. He felt the report provided him with information that would have taken many hours of therapy to produce. The therapist commented: (1) the report is direct and unequivocal, not laden with ambiguities; (2) the clients came in with various degrees of confusion as to their individual contributions to marital problems; (3) the clinical report effectively reduced this confusion and pointed each toward their own responsibilities in the situation; and (4) the clinical report provided specific information that supports the profiles, enabling the clients to trust the validity of the profiles.

He felt that, in the future, it would be extremely helpful to administer the AAB and have the clinical report at hand the second time that he sees a couple for therapy. This would provide immediate insight into the complexity of discovering the interpersonal dynamics present in a relationship and would stimulate immediate progress, especially when one member of a couple is the "uncomplaining" partner, who not is only difficult to bring in for therapy, but denies that there is anything wrong with their marriage. The clinical report provides an objective measure that not only stimulates immediate insight, but encourages the "uncomplaining" partner to recognize and admit that there is a problem. This procedure can also alleviate feelings of guilt or responsibility and strengthen the self-esteem of the other partner who assumes that it is "all my fault."

The therapist plans to have the battery administered again after a period of positive growth. This will show the couple directions in which they have moved and allow for consideration of whether "actualizing" goals have been achieved.

In conclusion, it was felt that the use of a battery of interpersonal and intrapersonal inventories without the use of pathology terminology is a most useful tool to be employed in an actualizing approach to therapy. These instruments may be used along with other traditional tests, such as the MMPI and Rorschach, or may be used alone, since they provide a non-pathological diagnosis that can be easily shared with clients in therapy.

Diagnostic Patterns

The following are some diagnostic patterns from the AAB, that have been found valid in research by D. Sjostrom (1975). They are indicated in the right hand side of the preceeding clinical report as sources for the generalizations made in the report.

POI Patterns

Impulsive behavior.	High S
	Low Fr
Dichotomy between an individual's belief system and actual living. Person cannot put accepted value system into practice.	High SAV
	Low Ex
Perfectionistic behavior.	High Sr
	Low Sa
Explosive behavior.	High Fr
	High A
Person exaggerates weakness to control people; or may indicate religious humility—"don't be proud," "don't be vain," etc.	High Sa
	Low Sr
Rigidity, inflexibility, conservatism; often indicates fundamentalist Christian attitudes.	Low Nc
	Low Sy
Person is unable to express physical warmth and caring.	Low S
	Low C
Person pleases and placates for control; exaggerates caring. Love is fawning and manipulative.	Low A
	High C
Depressed and withdrawn individual.	Low C
	Low Sa
	Low S

Person is insensitive to his feelings and needs, but is unable to express himself to others.

High Fr
Low S

Person uses hostility to control others and denies his vulnerability.

High A
Low C

Person appears aloof and pseudo-independent. Operates on assumption that he doesn't need anyone.

Support/Ratio
Above 0:1 = 3

POI and PAI Patterns

Husband controls weak, servile wife with demanding hostility and has difficulty expressing direct, open warmth to her.

(M) PAI: High Tyrant/Nice Gal
(M) POI: High A
Low C

Husband exaggerates strength to control by remaining aloof and tends to be perfectionistic. Relates to wife in a protective fatherly manner: controlled, moralistic, and little spontaneity.

(M) PAI: High Daddy/Doll
(M) POI: High Sr
Low Sa
Low S

Wife controls husband and avoids authentic intimate contact by using her hostility. Has difficulty feeling and expressing her vulnerability.

(F) PAI: Shrew/Nice Guy
(F) POI: High A
Low C

Wife uses strength to control by dominating and mothering a passive-dependent male. She has difficulty feeling her needs and expressing her weakness; often perfectionistic and compulsive person.

(F) PAI: High Mother/Son
(F) POI: High Sr
Low Sa

Husband has high needs to be liked and accepted. He is indirect with hostility. He placates his wife's irritability; his niceness is his way of fighting by refusing to get involved.

(M) PAI: High Shrew/Nice Guy
(M) POI: High C
Low A

Husband assumes passive-dependent posture to control wife, and demands nurturing. Uses his weakness to get attention and has difficulty expressing his strength. He is locked into a relationship with a mother-provider who allows him to be passive and secure.

(M) PAI: High Mother/Son
(M) POI: High Sa
Low Sr

Wife uses pseudo-feminine helplessness to get protection and fatherly attention from her husband. Often manipulates with her sexuality and she has difficulty expressing her strength. She is a helpless child to her protective-dominant husband.

(F) PAI: High Father/Daughter
(F) POI: High Sa
Low Sr

Wife is weak and servile. Centers her existence around her husband. Her love is fawning and servile and she uses this pseudoloving to control him. She has difficulty being assertive and showing anger.

(F) PAI: High Tyrant/Nice Gal
POI: High C
Low A
Low S

PAI and CRI Patterns

Wife controls husband with sexuality. She tends to be jealous, possessive, and demanding.

(F) PAI: High Shrew/Nice Guy
(F) CRI: High Eros
High D-Love
"Other" profile over "Ideal" profile

Wife uses a false caring, understanding, and affection to control her husband. This makes her love fawning.

(F) PAI: High Tyrant/Nice Gal
CRI: Affection and Empathy
"Other" over "Ideal"

Wife often does not find sex to be important to her and she has denied much of her sexuality feelings and needs.

(F) PAI: High Tyrant/Nice Gal
or High Father/Daughter
(F) CRI: Low Eros

This couple avoid each other. There is little person-to-person relating and sexual expression is minimal.

(M or F) PAI: High Doves
CRI: Low Eros

There is constant confrontation between husband and wife. There is a quality of high emotionality. Sexual relationship is active and sexual expression is open and direct.

(M or F) PAI: High Hawks
CRI: High Eros

Husband has difficulty expressing warmth. Does not give much physical stroking or affectionate caring.

(M) PAI: High Tyrant/Nice Gal
(M) CRI: Low Affection
Low Friendship

CONCLUSIONS

In the past, diagnostic instruments have provided the therapist with an accurate estimate of the client's pathology and have provided a *negative* rather than a positive approach to the therapeutic process. Many therapists, including the authors, have felt the need for diagnostic instruments whose validity can be verified and that give the new client a measure of his current level of self-actualizing. The POI, CRI, and PAI now provide a "launching pad" for a process of therapy that suggests directions for growth toward health.*

---

*Readers interested in ongoing research on actualizing as measured by the Actualizing Assessment Battery should contact EdITS, Box 7234, San Diego, California 92107.

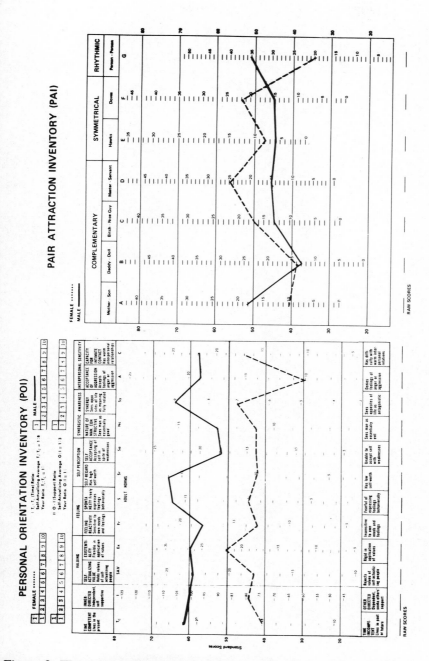

Figure 9. The Actualizing Assessment Battery, an Example (continued)

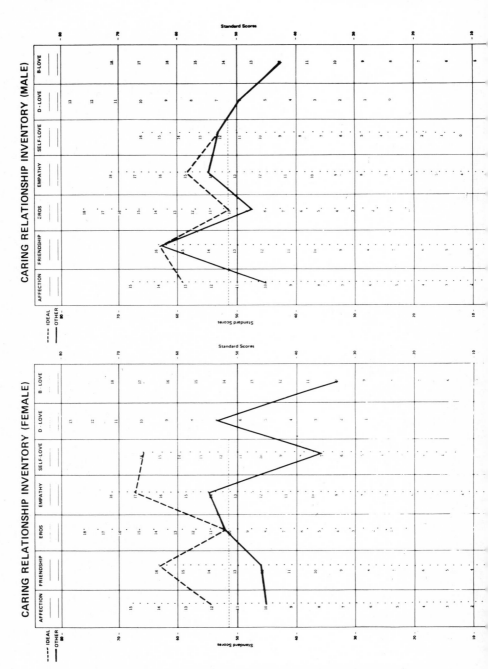

Figure 9. The Actualizing Assessment Battery, an Example

The Personal Orientation Dimensions

In an effort to look to the future, we have introduced a new research instrument called the Personal Orientation Dimensions (POD) (Shostrom, 1974). The POD differs from the POI in that it is a refinement and extension of dimensions of actualizing reflected in the POI. The extensive research with the POI has given impetus to the development of a more comprehensive measure of concepts of actualizing which the POD now fulfills. It contains more items than the POI and includes some concepts of actualizing not previously measured. Following are the dimensions of actualizing measured by the POD.

Orientation

1. *Time Orientation:* the capacity to live primarily in the present with full feeling-reactivity rather than blaming one's past or depending on future plans.

2. *Core Centeredness:* the tendency to trust one's feelings within as a criterion for behavior, as balanced against looking to "shoulds" or "oughts" from authorities outside oneself; the willingness to trust one's own "inner Supreme Court."

Polarities

3. *Strength:* the capacity to experience and express a personal sense of power, security, worth, adequacy, or competence.

4. *Weakness:* the capacity to experience and express one's humanness, vulnerability, hurt, or helplessness; accepting one's occasional impotence and inadequacy to cope with life.

5. *Anger:* the capacity to experience and express one's feelings of anger in mild or in more intense ways, as appropriate to the situation or in accordance with one's reactions to a situation.

6. *Love:* the capacity to experience and express feelings of warmth, tenderness, or affection to different persons in different ways.

Integration

7. *Synergistic Integration:* the understanding that commonly held opposites, or polarities (strength-weakness, anger-love), are not really opposites, but rather are mutually complementary; realization that their power as a whole exceeds their summated power as parts (as the strength of an alloy exceeds the strengths of component metals).

8. *Potentiation:* the understanding that no one principle, such as honesty or fairness, can control one's life. Additional principles, such as humanness and being oneself, can augment, amplify, and empower one's philosophy (as the power of an ambassador is augmented by the power of the group that he represents).

Awareness

9. *Being:* an orientation to life that includes the willingness to be or express whatever one feels, thinks, or senses within (such as joy, sorrow, helplessness, or boredom), as opposed to a "doing" orientation, which seeks to impress others by striving and pleasing.

10. *Trust in Humanity:* the ability to constructively view the nature of man as trustworthy and essentially good, as opposed to seeing human nature as essentially evil.

11. *Creative Living:* the capacity to be effective and innovative and become excited about decisions, judgments, or tasks; the utilization of unique or individual ways of problem solving.

12. *Mission:* a sense of dedication to a life task or mission; a belief in the importance of developing one's highest potentialities.

13. *Manipulation Awareness:* the capacity to recognize common manipulative, or controlling, patterns in others and also to admit that one has a tendency, as do others, to mainpulate from time to time.

Results from preliminary research with the POD are very encouraging. Results have been obtained from a wide variety of populations including samples taken from college students, church congregations, delinquents, alcoholics, teachers, hospitalized psychotics, and nominated actualizing persons.

CHAPTER 3. PERSONALITY CHANGE IN ACTUALIZING THERAPY

Every therapist has a model, implicit or explicit, of what happens in psychotherapy. The Actualizing Therapy model is based on a personality theory that has its roots in the research discussed in the previous chapter.

Having presented the research base for Actualizing Therapy, in this chapter we attempt to clarify the diverse meanings of actualizing, the three expressions of being that are crucial to personality change, and the relationship of personality change in therapy to the dimensions of personality that are measured by the POI.

Actualizing Therapy maintains that psychotherapy is an *educational* problem, dealing mostly with normal persons who have *problems of living.* In this view, the medical model has little relation to the process of psychotherapy.

Robert White (1973), in fact, has made a telling point regarding the therapist-client relationship. "If we are to maintain our reputation for psychological insight," he writes, "we shall do well to admit that we have probably functioned as unwitting preachers" (p. 4). His reference to recent research showing that the values of a client, as reported in questionnaires, move closer to those of the therapist, is not surprising. It is clear that all therapists communicate values. At long last we are admitting that no therapy is nondirective. The authors have consistently maintained that counselors and therapists do have either an explicit or an implicit value system with which they "teach," "preach," or at least, hopefully, "reach" their clients. According to the *National Observer* (1973), psychiatry and psychology may well be on their way to replacing religion in America. Although we do not totally agree with this statement, we believe that an actualizing psychology provides one with the experience to believe in his organism as a trustable system that may ultimately be described as spiritually valid. The organism will be given a new validity if seen as a trustable system for living life.

It is our contention that counselors and therapists should openly agree that they do have a developing ethic that is transmitted in the therapeutic process. The Personal Orientation Inventory, now with its substantial body of supporting research suggesting its validity as a measure of self-actualizing, provides a beginning framework for such an open ethic.

DEFINITIONS OF ACTUALIZING

"If you wish to converse with me," Voltaire often said, "define your terms." Because we intend to "converse" with the reader, in the classic sense of imparting new information acquired as the result of long association with a subject, it seems only fair to apply Voltaire's proviso. The term "self-actualizing" has been variously defined: *statistically,* as a *process,* as a *state,* as an *ethic,* and as a *model.*

According to a *statistical* definition of self-actualizing, the various forms of psychopathology and actualizing that make up the total population can be presented on a bell-shaped curve, as shown in Figure 10 (adapted from Lewis, 1973). The lower portion of the curve, representing pathology, is shown to have relatively low levels of integration of thinking, feeling, and bodily responses, and of inner-direction. The upper portion of the curve represents actualizing, an active process of being and becoming. The middle portion of the curve represents normalcy, a static process of maintaining. Maslow referred to those in the upper 1 percent of the curve as self-actualiz*ed* people. In this volume, however, we are concerned with what we call self-actualiz*ing* people—those in the upper 50 percent of the curve.

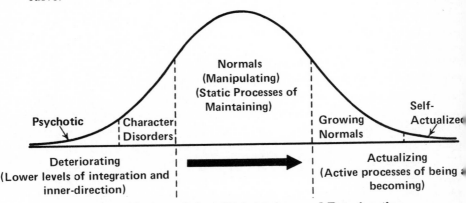

Figure 10. Actualizing, Maintaining, and Deteriorating

Thus, self-actualizing is defined as an active *process* of being and becoming increasingly inner-directed and integrated at the levels of thinking, feeling, and bodily response. It is, therefore, not an *end point*, but a *process* of moving from normal manipulation toward growth, development, and the unfolding of human potential. We assume it occurs in all successful therapy, teaching, and human relations training.

Shostrom (1972, p. 91) defines self-actualizing as a *process* of growing by continuously examining and expanding one's assumptions about life. Self-actualizing cannot be equated with "fun" or "happiness," yet it certainly is not a dour way of living that excludes pleasure. The terms "fun" and "happiness" imply superficiality and evanescence, whereas "pleasure" connotes a state in which one feels the excitement and the adventure of being what he is and of becoming more of what he can be. It involves the zest and challenge of adventure not ordinarily associated with the usual definitions of "happiness." Self-actualizing is continuously discovering a viable ethic for living.

One way in which Maslow (1962) defines self-actualizing is to describe it experientially as a momentary *state* or peak experience. In his own words, it is:

> an episode, or a spurt in which the powers of the person come together in a particularly efficient and intensely enjoyable way, and in which he is more integrated and less split, more open for experience, more idiosyncratic, more perfectly expressive or spontaneous, or fully functioning, more creative, more humorous, more ego-transcending, more independent of his lower needs. He becomes in these episodes more truly himself, more perfectly actualizing in his potentialities, *closer to the core of his Being,* more fully human. (p. 91)

Julian Huxley, in *The Challenge of Philosophy* (Fink, 1965), has set forth some basic assumptions for defining self-actualizing as an *ethic*. These assumptions, adapted by the authors, are that an actualizing ethic:

1. defines good and evil in terms of whether one is fulfilled—whether he is expressing desirable (actualizing) or undesirable (manipulative) dimensions of his personality.

2. places high value on the scientific method for the validation of one's philosophy of life.

3. assigns creative imagination a high place in the discovery of one's life philosophy.

4. emphasizes the experiencing and expressing of one's potentials as an essential aim of living.

5. sees man-within and man-and-society as not in conflict but rather as cooperatively interrelated when actualizing is taking place.

6. differs from most religious ethics in that it centers its long-term aims not on the next world but on this one.

These assumptions, along with others, have been amplified and refined through theoretical and empirical experience to formulate the basic assumptions of Actualizing Therapy as presented in Chapter 1.

Actualizing as an *educational model* is fast replacing the medical model for most counselors and therapists. The medical model stresses movement from "illness" to "normalcy," whereas self-actualizing stresses ways by which normal (well) people can become "weller"—how dog-paddlers can become Australian crawlers. The switch to an educational model, such as actualizing, shifts the central problem of the medical model—that of responsibility. When the "patient" is "sick," the therapist has to take the responsibility for effecting a "cure"; when actualizing is the focus, the responsibility lies with the client to develop "response-ability"—the ability to respond to life's problems. The concepts of self-actualizing developed herein are universal—combining the wisdom of both East and West—and representing a value system that persons of all backgrounds and persuasions may embrace.

Among the major concepts introduced in this chapter, and held to be of paramount importance in understanding and applying principles of Actualizing Therapy, are the *three aspects of being* and the *self-concept.*

THE THREE ASPECTS OF BEING

In theoretical terms, human behavior is reflected in activities involving three expressions of being: thinking, feeling, and bodily expression. A university professor, to give an example, usually uses more *thinking* energy than an athlete who expends much *bodily* energy running for a touchdown. A soldier in combat also shows extreme *body activity*—his adrenalin is flowing, his heart beats fast, and his breathing becomes deep as he fights for life. When he *thinks* about the enemy, he is at one level; when he *feels* about the enemy, he functions at still another level; and when he is actually *bodily* fighting, he is at yet a third level of energy expenditure. Thinking, feeling, and bodily activity are all expressions of the self, or of one's being in the world.

Thinking and feeling, which have usually been contrasted, are accepted as aspects of being in our culture. The distinction often made in psychology is that thinking refers to cortical activities, such as planning and reflection, whereas feelings are more tied to the body and are a means by which we make contact with other people. In this volume we give special emphasis to the integration of bodily expression with thinking and feeling. The importance of the body is expressed in various manifestations of one's basic needs. One does not need to think, for example, in order to be able to eat and sleep—his body tells him to do so. Furthermore, the body reacts more quickly than thought in emergencies. When confronted with the possibility of an accident, a driver does not think about putting his foot on the brake—his body does it automatically. In emphasizing the bodily aspect we do not mean that thinking should be excluded from a therapist's consideration, but we *are* convinced that, in our culture, thinking has been given precedence over feeling and bodily response. In Actualizing Therapy, thinking, feeling, and bodily response are all given equal value.

Utilization of all three of these expressive modes creates a synergistic approach to being, wherein the individual is seen by others as having a sense of unity or purpose. When this situation occurs, the individual is integrated and is expressing his *total* being. In contrast, persons who express only one aspect of their being are limited or partial in their expression. Experiencing one's total being is being totally *there,* listening to the total being, and utilizing all of one's energies conjointly. The actualizing person has "put it all together." Of course, he doesn't always express all three aspects of being, but he has the potential to, as the situation demands. These ideas are shown in Figure 11.

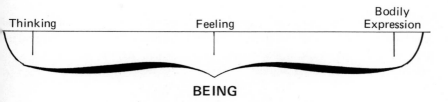

Thinking   Feeling   Bodily Expression

BEING

Figure 11. Three Expressions of Being

The gestalt diagram shown in Chapter 1 (Figure 3) may be divided into these three aspects. At any one moment, one of the three expressions of being is in focus and the others are background. The actualizing person is aware of which aspect of his being is in focus and is able to express it clearly. Moreover, the potential to utilize each aspect provides a balancing force to give him a natural control. The term "actualizing conscience" refers to this ability to use all three aspects in tandem in making decisions.

The average person seems to overvalue thinking to the exclusion of body and emotional expression. This is largely because he has been falsely taught early in life (through imperatives such as "Think!" "Don't get so emotional!" and "Use your head!") that thinking is primary to living. The head has been virtually worshipped as the seat of God, while the body has been seen as the province of the devil. In observing people from the viewpoint of the three aspects of being, it often seems that there is a line separating the head from the body, a notion aptly illustrated by cartoonist Jules Feiffer in Figure 12. Actualizing Therapy, in contrast, sees the body as a total unity rather than as split into warring factions.

The head (thinking) does not have to make all the decisions, as it does in Freudian analysis or Transactional Analysis. As Pascal said, "The heart has reasons the head will never know." The awareness of each aspect of one's being provides data for the expression of what is "right" for the individual at the moment. The organism thus becomes its own valuing system. These ideas are illustrated in Figures 13, 14, and 15 by means of sample comments made by actualizing persons—persons aware of which expression of their being is currently in focus.

These concepts provide a new way of defining conscience without the traditional moralistic admonitions. In actualizing terminology, when all three expressions of being are congruent, then one knows in every sense that he is "right" in terms of his own being.

THE SELF

The *self* is a construct rooted in Gestalt and phenomenological psychology and is typically defined as "the individual's dynamic organization of concepts, values, goals and ideals which determine the ways in which the person should behave" (Brammer & Shostrom, 1968, p. 46). The concept of self is a learned attribute. The various terms that are used to define the self-concept all reflect what individuals speak of as "I" or "me." The main sources of these personal evaluations are direct experience and the values and concepts of parents and important "others," which are incorporated as if directly experienced.

Epstein (1973) has recently noted the importance of the self-concept:

> There are a number of behavioral scientists, representing a variety
> of schools of thought, who believe that the self-concept is not only
> a useful explanatory construct, but a necessary one. Included

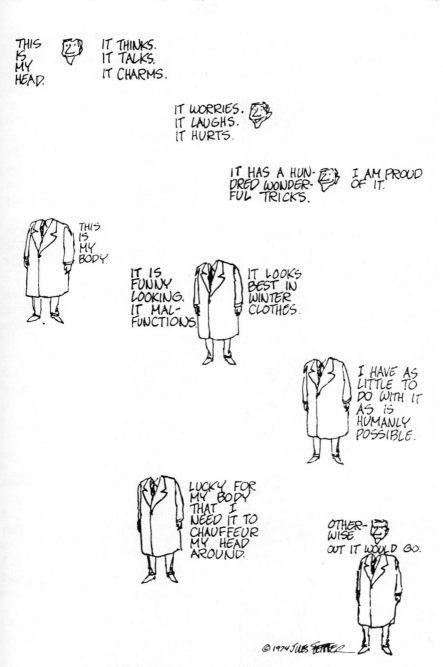

Figure 12. Separation of Head and Body

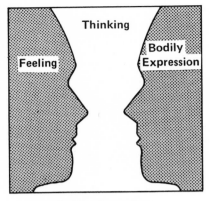

Figure 13. Thinking Primacy

Examples of Thinking Primacy:
I. Positive
    1. I think that will really work.
    2. Aha! I see what you mean.
    3. I think that's significant.

II. Negative
    1. That just doesn't fit.
    2. I just can't buy that.
    3. I don't think that's significant.

III. Problem Solving
    1. What decision should I make?
    2. What are the alternatives?
    3. What are the consequences?

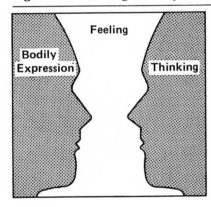

Figure 14. Feeling Primacy

Examples of Feeling Primacy:
I. Positive
    1. I'm real happy about that.
    2. I feel very warmly toward you.
    3. I feel so alive!

II. Negative
    1. Something doesn't feel quite right about that.
    2. I'm fed up with that.
    3. That's too heavy for me.

III. Problem Solving
    1. What do I really want?
    2. What do I really prefer?
    3. What do I really wish?

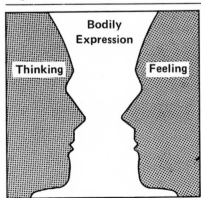

Figure 15. Body Primacy

Examples of Body Primacy:
I. Positive
    1. I feel like I'm flying.
    2. My heart feels light.
    3. I'm so excited I have goose-pimples all over my body.

II. Negative
    1. That gives me a pain in the neck.
    2. My stomach feels queasy about that.
    3. Get off my back!

III. Problem Solving
    1. What does my gut feel?
    2. Can I stand that?
    3. Do I have the heart for it?

among these are James, Cooley, Mead, Lecky, Sullivan, Hilgard, Snygg, Combs, and Rogers. To make matters more interesting, those self-theorists identified as phenomenologists consider the self-concept to be the most central concept in all of psychology, as it provides the only perspective from which an individual's behavior can be understood. (p. 404)

As shown in Figure 16, the self includes two aspects, *core* and *facade*. By "core" we mean that essential nature of each person that is individual and

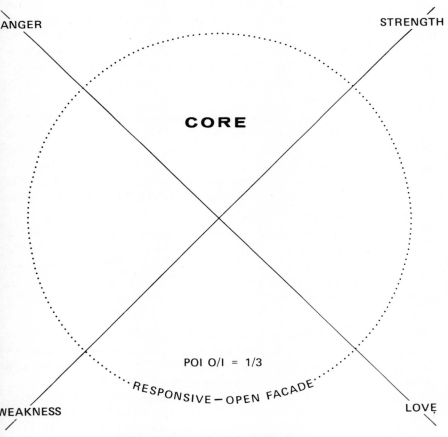

ANGER

STRENGTH

CORE

POI O/I = 1/3

RESPONSIVE — OPEN FACADE

WEAKNESS

LOVE

Figure 16. The Actualizing Level

unique and is the center of one's existence. The core is a *private* self that is concerned primarily with *personal expression*. By "facade" we mean the programmed responses in which we are heavily involved for survival—for making a *public impression.* In Figures 16 through 19, the differences in thickness and intensity of the lines representing the facade at the four levels of growth (actualizing, manipulative, character styles, and psychotic) are illustrative of an important principle. The actualizing person's facade and core self (Figure 16) are *congruent*—the facade, or *public* self, does not materially differ from the core, or *private* self. On the manipulative, the character styles, and the psychotic levels, however, there is a marked difference between the public and private selves.

An actualizing person's behavior at a crowded cocktail party would not essentially differ from his behavior when he is with an intimate group of friends at home. The typical manipulative person, on the other hand, worries about what other people think and would therefore put on a front that did not accurately reflect his private feelings. Similarly, the psychotic often holds himself together to make a public appearance and then falls apart when he gets home.

The *actualizing person* is one who has learned to trust the world, thus Figure 16 shows that he has developed a permeable and flexible facade, or persona, that is described as *responsive* and *open.* Like the amoeba, experiences cause him to expand or contract as he contacts others. (It should be stressed that we use facade here in a positive sense rather than in a negative sense, as it is sometimes used. A building, for example, can have a beautiful rather than an ugly facade.)

In everyday language, a "thin-skinned" person is too sensitive and a "thick-skinned" person is insensitive. The "skin," or the facade, of the actualizing person is neither too thin nor too thick but rather is permeable. The actualizing person is able to contact others empathically in order to feel as they feel, but he does not feel substantially more or less than what the other person feels.

The normal, or *manipulative,* level of growth, however, is characterized by greater *rigidity* and *control,* and thus in Figure 17 the walls are relatively more rigid and nonfunctional. There is now less flow and less growth and contact with the world, except through manipulative mechanisms, which have safety and survival as their basic motivations. The words "reticent" and "controlled" characterize the more programmed behavior of the manipulative level of being. Note also the *reduced* size of the core, indicating greater *constriction* as one becomes manipulative and controlled. The person who feels he is manipulating can be made aware of his manipulating by the degree to which he feels a sense of tightness and control in his body. His body is rebelling against the pressure of his

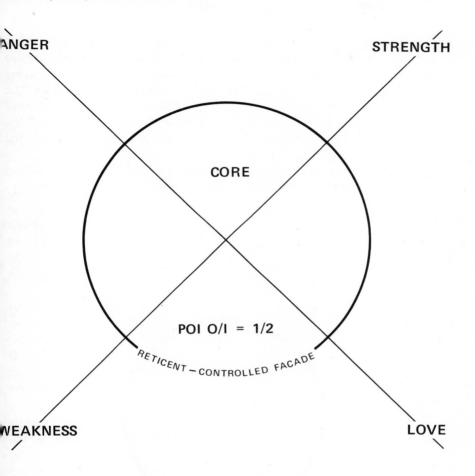

Figure 17. The Manipulative Level

manipulation because he is trying to *im*press rather than *ex*press. He is literally pressing against himself (in-pressing).

The manipulative person is insensitive to others but, because of the increased thickness of his external armor, is often unaware of this. Such a person is like the woman who is unaware of dragging her heels across the threshold of a new car because she is not aware that her heels are part of her. Once the woman is cautioned to be aware of her extended heels, she is less likely to be destructive. Similarly, when the effects of his behavior are called to the attention of the manipulative person, the increased awareness helps him to see how he can reduce his destructiveness. For example, the therapist may say, "Are you aware that your need to defend yourself sometimes hurts people and blocks their caring for you?" Hopefully, increasing awareness in this manner will create change in the manipulating person.

The *character styles* level of functioning is shown in Figure 18. Note that the walls are even thicker and more rigid—the neurotic is characterized as

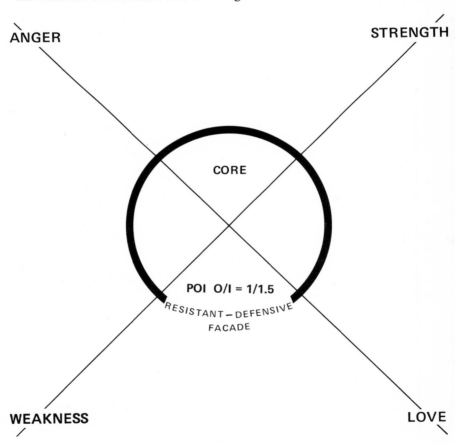

Figure 18. The Character Level

more *resistant* and *defensive,* with a further reduced core. The manipulative process has rigidified even further in the character style and the subject has now lost some of the awareness of manipulating. The manipulative processes have become a part of his general style of living. The character style has rigidified to the point where aspects of the subject's being are now controlled by the defensiveness of his personality structure rather than by an awareness of his own thoughts, feelings, and bodily expressions at the moment.

Wilhelm Reich has described a person who has constructed character defenses as one who has developed a coat of armor, much like the knights of old. His armor is so thick and heavy that he has lost most of his mobility and therefore is unable to cope with life effectively. He is stuck with the illusion that he must, for survival, wear his coat of armor while, in actuality, he is severely impairing his ability to cope with life.

Figure 19 illustrates the *psychotic level*—the level opposite from actualizing. As shown, the psychotic person has a broken but rather heavy wall, indicating that, at the *chronic* stage, he is strongly under control and closed to growth and contact with others. At the *acute* stage, however, the psychotic becomes fragile and disintegrative, and the broken wall suggests the chaotic flow from within. Differentiation of self from others is lacking and the self is fragilely defended.

Research by Rothstein and Boblitt (1970), using Wolpe and Lang's *Fear Survey Schedule* (1969) with psychotics, has shown that the most frequently expressed fear among this group is the fear of losing control. This research supports the conceptualization of the psychotic as one who is chronically under strong control or who becomes disintegrative and fragmented in the acute phase. It is as if the psychotic wears a coat of heavy armor in the chronic phase but in the acute phase the armor becomes so heavy that when he moves he "comes apart at the seams."

OTHER- VERSUS INNER-DIRECTEDNESS

As shown in Figures 16 through 19, a key score on the POI is the O/I, or other-directedness versus inner-directedness, ratio. Previously presented by David Riesman (1950), this concept relates to the self in that the other-directed person is more *facade*-oriented, whereas the inner-directed person is more *core*-oriented. Dependence on the views of others is characteristic of the other-directed person. The inner-directed person, on the other hand, is much more independent and appears to have incorporated an "inner gyroscope," whose internal piloting he obeys. The source of direction for

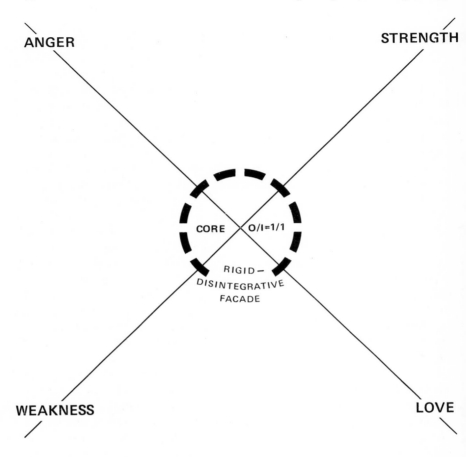

Figure 19. The Psychotic Level

energy investment is inside out in the sense that guidance is by internal or core motivations rather than by external influences.

Examination of research with the POI on the O/I ratio (also termed the Support ratio), bears out the theories illustrated in Figures 16 through 19. Each of these shows the O/I ratio that corresponds to the illustrated level of personality expression. Figure 20 shows these ratios graphically. The actualizing person scores an O/I ratio of 1/3, other to inner. Thus actualizing persons may be thought of as relying upon their own inner being three times more than they rely on others. The manipulative person, on the other hand, shows an O/I ratio of 1/2. A manipulative person looks to others more

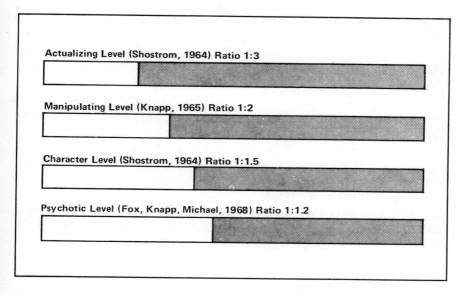

Actualizing Level (Shostrom, 1964) Ratio 1:3

Manipulating Level (Knapp, 1965) Ratio 1:2

Character Level (Shostrom, 1964) Ratio 1:1.5

Psychotic Level (Fox, Knapp, Michael, 1968) Ratio 1:1.2

Figure 20. Comparison of Actualizing, Manipulative, Character, and Psychotic Groups on the POI Support Ratio

than does the actualizing person in making decisions in life. The character style shows an O/I ratio of 1/1.5, indicating even greater other-directedness. Finally, the psychotic scores 1/1 on the O/I ratio. Still greater distrust of one's inner being can result, and the psychotic state reflects this indecision and deadness. Not knowing whether to trust oneself or other people leads, in many cases, to trusting neither.

It is important to note that each of these varying ratios was empirically determined in a series of research studies. The actualizing ratios were found by Shostrom (1964) and the "normal" manipulative and the neurotic (or character style) ratios were found by Shostrom and confirmed by Knapp (1965) in his study with average, or non-neurotic, college students. The psychotic ratios were found in a study of hospitalized psychiatric patients conducted by Fox, Knapp, and Michael (1968).

The research of Satir (1966) and of Leary (1957) and his associates, based on the large-scale analysis of personality structure, supports the hypothesis that self-expression may be categorized along major polarities having strength-weakness and anger-love as their dimensions.

In support of the emphasis on the dimensions of the polarities presented in Figures 16 through 19, it should be noted that Abraham Maslow (1954), in his classic research on well-functioning people, found them able to express "righteous indignation," or *anger*, yet at the same time able to express tenderness and *love*. He found them very competent and *strong*, yet they had an acute awareness of their own personal *weaknesses*. Thus, self-actualizing persons are what is defined as "rhythmic" in their orientation. That is, they are able to swing back and forth freely on the polarities of strength-weakness and anger-love. The actualizing person has a naturally rhythmic, spontaneous response to life. Like the ebb and flow of the tides and the revolving motion of the seasons, his very being reflects this natural rhythm. But in the life of the average person, rigidity takes place. Our natural rhythmic expression is affected by those parents and teachers who take control of our lives and say "yes" to some of our responses and "no" to others. They teach us to see through *their* eyes, to hear through *their* ears, and to respond through *their* own personal fears. For most children life becomes simplistically good and bad, right and wrong, acceptable and unacceptable. They give adults and even siblings the right to judge their worth, to determine their merit, and to manipulate their love. Such children no longer permit themselves freedom to be—they give in to the "shoulds" and "have tos" and lose their personal rhythm.

TIME INCOMPETENCE VERSUS TIME COMPETENCE

Another fundamental score on the POI (the T_I/T_C ratio) has to do with *time orientation*. As shown in Figure 21, a nonactualizing person is *time incompetent*. He lives in the past—with guilts, regrets, or resentments—and/or in the future—with idealized goals, plans, expectations, predictions, and fears. In contrast, the actualizing person lives from the core of awareness of his own body and feelings and from the ability to experience and express these feelings fully to others. Such persons are primarily *time competent*, appearing to live more fully in the here and now. They are able to tie the past and the future to the present in meaningful continuity. They appear to be less burdened by guilts, regrets, and resentments from the past than the nonactualizing person and their aspirations are tied meaningfully to present working goals. They are characterized by faith in the future without rigid or overidealistic goals. This is a common existential value, agreed upon by most Existential and Gestalt Therapists. It is a fundamental ethical assumption about the "way to be."

Figure 22 compares self-actualizing, normal, and nonactualizing persons on the Time Orientation scale. These figures show that the T_I/T_C ratio for self-actualizing persons is, on the average, 1/8 (Shostrom, 1964). The

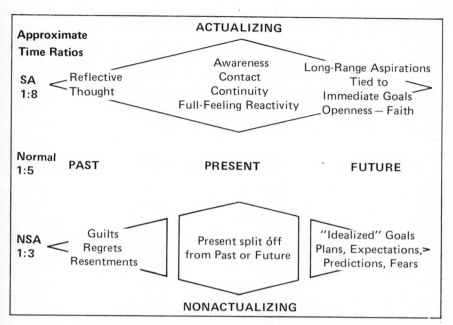

Figure 21. Actualizing and Nonactualizing Time Orientation

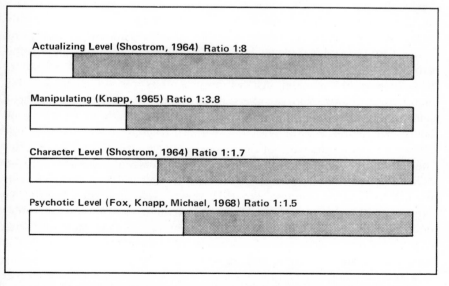

Figure 22. Comparison of Actualizing, Manipulative, Character, and
Psychotic Groups on the POI Time Ratio

manipulative person's average is 1/3 (Knapp, 1965; Shostrom, 1964), the character level score is 1/2 (Knapp, 1965), and the psychotic's average is 1/1.5 (Fox, Knapp, & Michael, 1968). These ratios, like the Support ratios, show a gradual decline in the ability of manipulative, character level, and psychotic persons to live in the here and now, and a greater tendency to live in the past or in the future. These individuals simply have never learned to live in contact with their present feelings and awareness.

MEASUREMENT OF EXPRESSIONS OF BEING

A major supposition of Actualizing Therapy is that the behavior of the human organism can be seen as a series of activities involving varying degrees of energy *investment* in three areas of expression: thinking, feeling, and bodily movement. In rating activities (as shown in Figure 11) thinking, emoting, and bodily activity all are expressions of the same thing: being in the world.

The POI measures constructs that are fundamental to an actualizing self at the core level. Thus the implications for the POI as a measure of one's personal ethic for living become more visible. Paper-and-pencil tests have often been criticized because they simply reflect what one is "thinking" about himself at the moment. They do not reflect "experiencing" oneself, as one feels emotion or as one experiences his body at the moment. On the other hand, if thinking, feeling, and bodily expression are simply expressions of the same continuum of energy or being, then the POI, taken, for instance, at the beginning of any therapeutic experience, gives the therapist a "fix" on what the person "says," or thinks, he is *being* at the moment. As therapy progresses and the client feels his emotions in relationship to others in a group, or as he becomes more sensitized to his body, he can compare his thoughts with his emotional or bodily experiences. Feedback from a therapist or group members gives him a chance to verify the truth of this being, and this "truth" may have to be sharply revised as growth continues. Thus, therapeutic growth may be defined as increased awareness of self on the dimensions of being. Taken toward the end of therapy, the POI should reflect greater honesty in expressing this increased awareness. In Actualizing Therapy, however, measures obtained from the POI are regarded as serving several functions, only one of which is to provide measures of changed awareness within a particular person in a therapeutic relationship. The POI is, in fact, useful as a research instrument to measure change in *all* forms of therapeutic interaction, including therapies based on different schools of thought and on such different training techniques as transcendental meditation and analysis in group experience. For example, encounter groups employing widely varying techniques appear to produce changes that are reflected in POI scores. Another function of the POI is the use of scale scores and responses to individual items as heuristic devices in the therapeutic situation to stimulate further personal inquiry.

CONCLUSIONS

An important tenet of Actualizing Therapy is that actualizing must take shape *from within* the core. Litt (1973) says, "As Goethe observed, man is like a plant, he grows. He is not a sculpture, made from the outside" (p. 72). Behavior Modification is shaping up, or molding, from the outside. This attempts to reverse the natural organismic flow of energy, which naturally grows from the core out to the periphery. Actualizing Therapy focuses on growth, like that of a mustard seed, *from within.* It is not imposed, like a mustard plaster, *from without.*

In *Freedom To Be* (Shostrom, 1972), the actualizing person is described as one motivated by core *subjective needs:* what he *wants, prefers, likes,* and *chooses.* He is not motivated by the feeling that he is an *object* of others; that he *has to, must, can't* or *should.* The latter are familiar *facade inward* approaches to life, motivated by others' needs. In contrast, the actualizing person's primary energy direction is from the *core outward.* Actualizing persons take "response-ability" for themselves and demonstrate the ability to respond or make decisions for themselves. They are not afraid to make decisions for themselves since they trust their own core "inner Supreme Court."

Actualizing Therapy, indeed, assigns high value to scientifically based knowledge. Research data from the Personal Orientation Inventory are used as the basis for the ideas that must be made explicit if psychology is going to press forward to become the means by which the individual can actualize his full potential for living.

CHAPTER 4. THE EXISTENTIAL CHOICE: FACADE LIVING OR CORE BEING

All people have been affected by life both positively and negatively. In the process of growing up, each person has been both helped and hurt to some degree by the teachings and manipulations of parents, teachers, and friends. Most persons must admit to having become both actualizing *and* manipulative in their orientation. In some respects they are "running smoothly" in an actualizing way, but in other respects they are "limping" at the manipulative and character levels of functioning. A few must even admit to having been "disabled" at the psychotic level of functioning. This hypothesis is illustrated by the levels of functioning as shown in Figure 23. The circles in this figure should be viewed as disks stacked one upon the other. As one descends from level to level, the change in mode of functioning can be described as a "process of deterioration." At the actualizing level, the person learns to express feelings from an expansive core of being, for at this level core does not differ substantially from facade (as described in Chapter 3). The process of deterioration progresses as we move toward more constricted levels of functioning. At the manipulative, character style, and psychotic levels, there is less core to draw from, and facade living becomes paramount. Nonactualizing people are content to remain at constricted, facade levels of living rather than to expand themselves intellectually, emotionally, and bodily. Chapter 6 will describe how one can move out of this constricted mode of living, through the process of growth, or actualizing, which basically involves expansion of one's being from one's core.

The best way for an individual to become involved therapeutically is to examine the manipulative level and to decide which of the four forms of manipulating he has become most prone to use (everyone manipulates to some degree). He may further decide which of the polar dimensions he has been least likely to express. At this point, the alternatives are clear. The individual can either continue to move toward the center, in the direction of

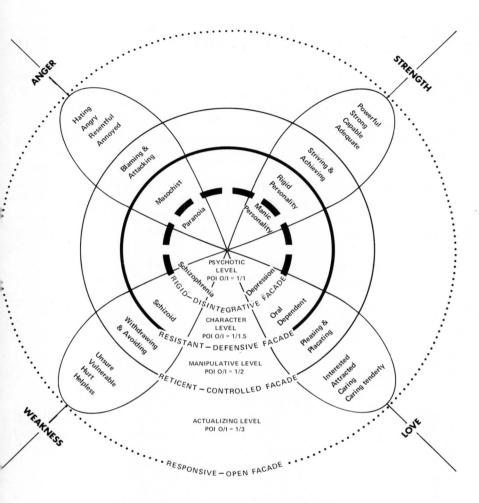

Figure 23. The Process of Deterioration

lesser functioning, or can move outward, in the direction of greater actualizing. Paradoxically, however, moving in the direction of actualizing also
requires admitting to the losses one has suffered in his experiences of
growing up with manipulative people. But herein lies the hope of Actualizing Therapy. One need not spend three to nine years minutely analyzing his
pathology, as in psychoanalysis. Rather one can begin quickly to actualize
his potential, as long as he has faced his losses.

Albee (1970a, 1970b) has severely criticized use of the medical model in
the attempt to understand human behavior. Indeed, many have criticized

psychiatry for starting from mental illness or psychoses and then attempting to "cure," moving from understanding of the psychosis to average functioning.

This chapter expands the suggestion that actualizing, or full-functioning, behavior might be a better starting point. Through understanding exceptionally healthy behavior one can reason back to see how manipulation ("normal neuroses"), neurotic (character style) behavior, and finally psychotic behavior may also reflect actualizing efforts. By starting from "comparative wellestness," as suggested by Maslow (1970), and reasoning back to the pathological, rather than starting with sickness and reasoning to averageness, we propose an exciting alternative to the medical model. Albee (1970a) has stated that "the most compelling reason . . . for persistence of the disease model has been the absence of a satisfactory alternative" (p. 42). In this book we attempt to present one, albeit incomplete, alternative view.

THE RELATIONSHIP OF CORE EXPRESSION, THE POLARITIES, AND THE THREE ASPECTS OF BEING

Popeye's phrase, "I am what I am," is an actualizing credo. In general, the actualizing person is committed to himself—to his core. That is, he is committed to the expression of his essential or unique self. In order to express his core behavior he has to separate out the dimensions to which he will give expression.

According to Maslow, the most important thing he learned from his Professor Wertheimer was the Oriental concept of the difference between *being* and *doing*. Most people try to avoid being. Being is not acting or doing, such as coming home and eating or watching television or talking. Instead it is the *developing* of *awareness* of what is going on inside of our being.* This awareness consists of three forms of expression: the *thoughts* we have as we deliberate about the problems of living, the *feelings* we have that flow as we make warm or angry contact with others, and the *body tension* that we experience relative to our feelings and thoughts.

---

*Although many psychologists have doubts about the value of meditation as a primary technique for actualizing, the recent popularity of meditation techniques from the East has led to studies showing that meditators score better on the POI than nonmeditators. Seeman, Nidich, and Banta (1972), for example, found that the practice of transcendental meditation resulted in increased scores on POI scales. A replication of the study by Nidich, Seeman, and Dreskin (1973) provided equal evidence of the positive influence of meditation. Perhaps theories about the effects of meditation on actualizing can explain the concept of "being versus doing" by simply pointing out that meditation is more of a being technique than a doing technique.

The following outline will illustrate the manner in which the actualizing person uses these three aspects of being with respect to the polar dimensions of anger, love, strength, and weakness (see Figure 24).

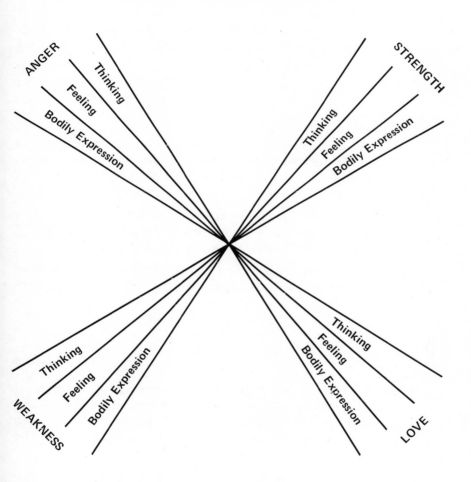

Figure 24. The Relationship of the Three Aspects of Being to the Polarities

I. Anger
    A. *Intellectually,* the actualizing person is committed first to the principle of a here-and-now *verbal* expression of anger, and, second, to the principle of not permitting his anger to build, which may result in a violent behavioral expression of repressed feeling.

B. *Emotionally*, the actualizing person's awareness of his anger comes from being aware of the flow of, and definition of, his emotions in relation to others in interpersonal interactions.

C. *Bodily*, anger is experienced by heavy breathing and by tension in the muscle structure—a need to strike or hit. Anger is especially manifested by clenched fists and tightness in the neck, shoulders and jaw.

II. Love

A. *Intellectually*, the actualizing person is committed to the principle or idea of a here-and-now expression of love, and to the principle that both giving and receiving love in all its forms is necessary for human contact.

B. *Emotionally*, the actualizing person is committed to the expression of love that stems from awareness of a need for *interaction* with the loved one, and by feelings of openness and lightness.

C. *Bodily*, love is experienced by a sense of fullness around the heart and by a relaxed muscle state that involves a feeling of *reaching* to the object of our love.

III. Strength

A. *Intellectually*, the actualizing person is committed to the principle or idea that to experience, or to be, the feeling of strength is commendable and is not an expression of conceit. The actualizing person is not afraid to be the feelings of security, adequacy, and worth.

B. *Emotionally*, the actualizing person is committed to the expression of inner-strength, not as an attempt to experience *power* over others, but rather as an expression of the potency of his own being. The actualizing person does not believe in false modesty or in "playing humble."

C. *Bodily*, strength is experienced by a sense of being able to stand on one's own two feet, and by the ability to reach out and *ask* for what one wants.

IV. Weakness

A. *Intellectually,* the actualizing person is committed to the principle of a here-and-now expression of weakness as a natural aspect of being human. Vulnerability is regarded as desirable—not as something to be avoided in human interaction.

B. *Emotionally,* the actualizing person is committed to experiencing feelings of hurt, tears, and helplessness with others. He assumes that these feelings make contact rather than break contact.

C. *Bodily,* an awareness of weakness is experienced as a sense of emptiness and impotence. It is also experienced as a sense of immaturity, as when a child needs the breast for sustenance.

ACTUALIZING FEELINGS

In speaking of the levels of functioning, life can be likened to a hand-weaving process. One can make the weaving into a net, woven into meshes to entrap himself and others by manipulation; or he can weave a pattern of personality that becomes fixed and deeply ingrained; or he can impair his functioning to a level of psychosis, in which case the weaving process becomes so confused that he cannot tell a real tapestry from a "picture" of the tapestry. One's ability to weave a beautiful tapestry for oneself is parallel to the self-actualizing process.

All tapestry, being handmade, is imperfect, as all human lives are imperfect. But the imperfections of human making create a kind of beauty that machines cannot produce. As Virginia Satir (1973) has said, people are all "people makers," creators of themselves, and in interaction with the environment each person is made into a unique tapestry of individuality.

The tapestry of actualizing begins with the "colors" of feelings on the polarities of anger-love and strength-weakness. All individuals have the potential to express the "fiery red" shades of anger and the "true-blue" shades of love. Each experiences the "mellow yellow" shades of weakness and the various "vital greens" of strength. Understanding the possibilities of behavioral expression, people can sometimes move into the deep colors of a "maxiswing" to points of *intense* feeling at the very ends of the polarities. Other times, when feeling colors are *mild,* timorous pastels, they will move in "miniswings" near the center of the polarities. These shades of feeling are illustrated on the dust jacket of this volume.

Bleuler (1940) has said that schizophrenia is the inability to modulate affect. Actualizing Therapy holds that actualizing includes the *ability* to modulate affect freely. If schizophrenia is the major mental disorder, and it allegedly accounts for 90 percent of the people in mental hospitals, then it is logical to define actualizing as the opposite of schizophrenia. Indeed the data of Fox, Knapp, and Michael (1968), based on the POI, demonstrate that hospitalized schizophrenics are extremely low on all scales of actualizing. If the schizophrenic is unable to modulate affect, then it follows that *the actualizing person must be able to modulate his affect freely.* When one has learned the ability to freely modulate his affect, he has developed the capacity for a "full feeling repertoire."

Fear

The resistance to expressing feelings is manifested by a feeling of fear. It is as if fear exists at the zero-point of the poles in the core, as shown in Figure 25 (page 89). This is the point of indifference, deadness, or apathy, where many people prefer to remain, thus avoiding risking feelings in order to make contact with others.

Actualizing Therapy stresses that people must often begin to express their feelings by expressing their fear, for in the famous words of Franklin Delano Roosevelt, "the only thing we have to fear is fear itself." In expressing their fear of feelings, people paradoxically begin to risk moving out from dead center to the various levels of feeling expressions.

Sam Keen (1970), in a dialogue with his fear, illustrates the importance of facing this feeling:

SK: You demand the most alive part of me. . . . You promise security so long as I surrender my autonomy, my critical ability, my reason, my responsibility for reflecting upon and evaluating my own experience. Your price for comfort is giving up growth. . . . You would refuse me knowledge of my freedom in exchange for comfort, and thus steal my dignity and potency.

Fear: Yes, I speak with the voice of authority. I echo the commands and prohibitions of your parents. . . . My voice is conservative. I would have you love what your fathers loved and hate what they hated. . . . I preserve your energies from being dissipated in folly. . . . Better fear than anxiety, better . . . at the center of your personality the emptiness which is the promise of death, better pain than chaos. The suffering I cause is only . . . enforcing your limits.

SK: Granted, I must have limits or else I would explode into the void of infinite possibility and schizophrenia. However, there is a better way to establish boundaries than you suggest. *Decision* is the alternative to fear. . . . Maturity rather than fate or fear may determine the shape my life will assume. Your presence is not necessary. (pp. 110-112)

Anger

On the first basic polarity, anger-love, the anger dimension is shown in the upper left quadrant (see Figure 25). Here one takes the risk of expressing his feelings of *annoyance, resentment, anger,* and sometimes even *hatred.* To actualize, one must sometimes move out from dead center into feelings that require negative contact with other people.

Many people are afraid of expressions in this polarity, for they fear that if any form of anger is verbalized it may result in destructive behavior. The

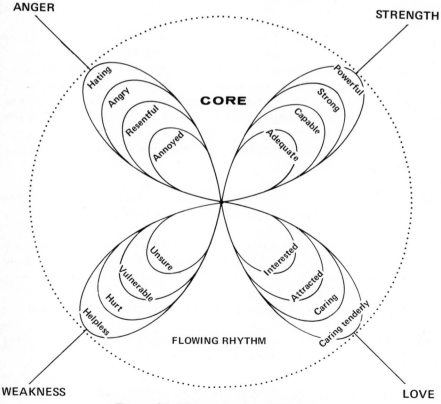

Figure 25. The Actualizing Rhythm

following exercise, again by Keen (1970), illustrates the difficulty most people have with anger:

SK: It has taken me a long time to discover that you are haunting my foot-steps. Like a thief dodging from tree to tree, you hide behind other emotions until it is safe to strike. Now I call you by name—Anger, rage, resentment, hatred. Come out into the open and show yourself.

[*No answer*]

Anger, I know you are there. Only this morning I was ready to scream at Heather and the children with no just cause. I felt your presence also in the way I punished myself with guilt and painful self-conscious-ness. And I know with what frequency I create an enemy in order to have a target for my free-floating rage. So come out of hiding and state your case.

Anger: All right, damn it, I will. Yes, I am here and have been for a long time and it is damn well time you granted me the high honor of diplomatic recognition. Damn generous of you. I was beginning to think you would spend your whole life as a good boy, as a "Christian," as a gentleman, denying my existence. I have been the Red China of your psyche for too long, outlawed, ignored, and cursed. And now you have the gall to pretend to be surprised that I must hide and come out at what you call "inappropriate" moments. How in hell could I emerge at any other moments?

SK: Must you be so profane? I have acknowledged that I have denied you rightful recognition. Can't you state your case calmly?

Anger: You are some damn thin-skinned gentleman! You call me out and you are afraid of the slightest suggestion of violence, even verbal violence. What are you afraid of? Who do you think is going to hear me, God or the Devil? Either take me with my profanity and my raw edges or leave me alone and I will find my own ways of emerging.

SK: All right, I will try to accept you as you are. Could you begin by telling me something about your origins and your aim?

Anger: I would like to begin with clarity and maturity, but I can't. I have been denied so long I am confused about myself. I don't know where I came from or what would satisfy me. I feel like a hurt child and I want to strike out at you and at other people (particularly those you love) to retaliate for all the years you ignored me.

SK: I have already confessed my folly and sorrow in seeking to deny your presence. Let's stop the recriminations and get on with an adult conversation.

Anger: I will try. Let me go back to the beginning. It was not entirely your fault that I was denied a legitimate place in your life. One of the problems of a Christian environment is that it makes aggression and anger shameful. Do you remember, for instance, when you used to fight with your older brother and regularly get beaten up? You were afraid of me. That is why you were defeated. What would have happened if you got angry with your brother? Anger is morally the same as murder, so the New Testament ethic suggests. And do you remember the delicious time when one of your older friends defended you and beat up your brother? Afterward you felt ashamed of being an ally in victory rather than a victim. This seems to be the feeling about life which conservative religion sanctions: better to suffer than rebel. The ideal of love throws anger into question. Turn the other cheek. Be gentle.

SK: Well, what is wrong with gentleness? Certainly it is more rewarding than resentment, hatred, fighting, and killing.

Anger: Now wait a minute! There you go jumping to the conclusion that I either drive people to harbor continual resentment or to commit murder. That is a lie you tell yourself in order not to have to deal with me. I can control myself. When not denied my proper recognition I am a very rational emotion. I can distinguish between appropriate and inappropriate objects. Did you ever consider how valuable I am to you?

SK: In what ways?

Anger: I keep you safe by making your full strength available to you in situations of danger. I help you to identify those enemies that threaten your well-being. I defend the boundaries of the physical, psychological, economic, and social space you need to survive. And, I might say, I add as much spice to life as your highly idealized love. I keep one person from being swallowed up by another and thus preserve the duality which is necessary for love. If you doubt that I am the companion of love, remember the ecstasy of the reconciliation that comes after fighting. After a good expression of clean anger, lovers have established the integrity of their separateness, and they may come together without fearing that either will be eradicated by the act of love. If you can't fight, you can't love.

SK: I agree. I suppose the question I am asking myself is how to maximize the loving and minimize the fighting. I will admit that I would not want to deny you recognition. But you are an exhausting friend to have around. I would like to see you visit less often and on more appropriate occasions.

Anger: Perhaps that is as far as we can go in this conversation. If you will be more sensitive to my comings and goings, I will try to be a more mature and orderly guest.

The person who can give vent to "cash and carry" anger need not fear behavioral expression. On the contrary, the "nice guys" who never get angry often end up as the murderers. All persons need occasional "hostilectomies."

It is the fear of behavioral expressions of anger that causes many persons to assume that feeling expression will automatically lead to hurting or murdering someone. In reality, the expression of strong negative feeling reduces the tendency for behavioral acting out of anger. In reality, one cannot stay angry at someone if he is able to express his anger verbally. Expression of strong negative feeling leads instead to the homeostatic expression of its opposite, as shown in Figure 25. Thus, ability to express anger *fully* to another more often than not leads to warm feelings toward that person. This is an important communication principle.

In handling these feelings it is important to learn to acknowledge the mild forms of each and to avoid letting deeper feelings accumulate. The building up of unexpressed feelings of anger, resentment, and hostility is often referred to as "injustice collecting" or "sandbagging." The experience of irritation, boredom, and annoyance at the lower levels of the anger continuum helps one to avoid building to the feelings of hostility, resentment, or hatred that come from an accumulation of anger.

Love

The love dimension, shown in the lower right quadrant of Figure 25, is expressed verbally by such phrases as "I'm interested," "I'm attracted," "I care," and "I care tenderly." The ability to show caring at various depths is a most important aspect of actualizing one's being. Tenderness, for example, is a need all people have, and yet American culture discourages its expression, as Grace Stuart explains in the following passage from her *Narcissus* (1956):

> It is too seldom mentioned that the baby, being quite small for quite a long time, is a handled creature, handled and held. The touch of hands on the body is one of the first and last of physical experiences and we deeply need that it be tender. We want to touch . . . and a culture that has placed a taboo on tenderness leaves us stroking our dogs and cats when we may not stroke each other. We want to be touched . . . and often we dare not say so. . . . We are starved for the laying on of hands. . . . There is no doubt that Puritanism's long restraint upon the tender touching hand did incalculable damage, as all those will know whose offered caress was in their childhood turned away. . . . [But] our best endeavors to describe an ultimate spiritual well-being say "underneath are the everlasting arms." More perhaps than we have ever realized, our physical handling of each other may make or mar the spiritual state of our civilization.

Strength

Most of us have difficulty in expressing our strengths because we have been enjoined by our parents to "always be humble and modest." We are told, "Don't think too highly of yourself," or "Pride cometh before a fall." All these parental admonitions mitigate against feelings of strength. It is important to remember the admonition of Spinoza that "There is no one as proud as the one who is proud of his humility."

On the strength-weakness polarity one must develop the ability to verbalize *strength feelings* by such phrases as "I am adequate," "I am capable," "I am strong," or "I am powerful," which represent increasing amplitude on this continuum. Herbert Otto (1968) recommends the "strength bombardment" technique to help one member of a group become aware of his strengths: Each group member in turn is asked to state the ways in which he feels strong. The group then tells him how it sees his strengths and suggests ways in which he can improve them.

Maslow (1971) was among the first to catalog the three basic reasons that we shy away from expressing strength. First is the *Jonah complex,* in which the individual decides that it is too dangerous to be great, so he runs from his fate just as Jonah tried in vain to flee from his destiny. This individual deliberately plans to be less than the best he is capable of becoming and evades the reality of his own capacity. An actualizing person, one made aware that he is a victim of this complex, is in constant search for his mission or call in life.

Second is *countervaluing*. In this case the individual tends to counter-value strength in others. He scoffs at the greatness in prominent people because it makes him feel less worthless for not having achieved greatness himself. By contrast, the actualizing person learns to admire and appreciate greatness in others. He learns from them and strives to emulate them.

Maslow's third reason is the *fear of paranoia*—the subject's fear that others will consider him paranoid or arrogant if he openly professes his ambitions. By adopting a posture of mock humility or pseudostupidity, he manipulates his potential tormentors.

Weakness

At the opposite end of this polarity, it is important to get in touch with one's *feelings of weakness*. In American culture, there seems to be a taboo against admitting weakness, especially for men. Phrases such as "I am unsure," "I am vulnerable," "I hurt," or "I feel helpless," represent varia-tions on the weakness continuum. Being able to put into words both feelings of weakness and strength in varying degrees of modulation expands emotional expression and permits actualizing of the full being.

The vital requirement of weakness, or vulnerability, as an actualizing quality is illustrated by Ralph Graves (1972) in his description of Charlie Chaplin:

> He has never lost his little-boy sense of wonder . . . I was struck by the *vulnerability* of the most famous movie actor in the world. The vulnerability, of course, is what made the Little Tramp a figure of more than comedy. This was the greatest experience of my life. I have never been so moved by a man. (p. 3)

Anne Morrow Lindbergh (1973) has also described beautifully the importance of vulnerability in being human:

> Grief is the great leveler. Nor is courage any more than a first step. Stoicism . . . is only a halfway house on the long road. It is a shield, permissible for a short time only. In the end one has to dis-card shields and remain open and vulnerable. Otherwise scar tissue will seal off the wound and no growth will follow. To grow, to be reborn, one must remain vulnerable—open to love but also hideously open to the possibility of more suffering. (p. 215)

Actualizing

The actualizing person needs to develop all four major dimensions: strength, weakness, anger, and love. Werner Von Braun, who made the move from Peenemünde to Houston in one graceful, ideological bound, is an interesting example of successful self-actualizing with particular reference to the anger-love and strength-weakness polarities. Here, it is described by writer Norman Mailer (1969):

> Since he had in contrast to his delivery, a big, burly squared-off bulk of a body, which gave hint of the ponderous deliberation, the methodical ruthlessness of more than one Russian bureaucrat, Von Braun's relatively small voice, darting eyes and semaphoric presentations of lip made it obvious that he was a man of *opposites*. He revealed a confusing aura of *strength* and *vulnerability*, of calm and agitation, *cruelty* and *concern*, phlegm and sensitivity, which would have given fine play to the talents of so virtuoso an actor as Mr. Rod Steiger. Von Braun had, in fact, something of Steiger's soft voice, that play of *force* and *weakness* which speaks of consecration and vanity, dedication and indulgence, steel and fat [emphasis added]. (p. 33)

Keen (1970) has defined *grace* as a willingness to accept one's total self. Many people have been taught as children that all good feelings must be paid for by an equal amount of bad feelings. They learn that they ought not to be too happy and that there is something virtuous and secure about suffering.

Contrariwise, the willingness to risk feelings—to express oneself on all polarities—may be defined as *pleasure*. But even this is difficult because many people have "been more afraid of the angel of happiness than the demons [they] have kept chained in the dark prison of the psyche" (Keen, 1970, p. 138). Graceful freedom is having the courage to be all one's polarities in rhythmic tandem.

Chapter 6 will discuss in detail exercises for the bodily expression of anger, love, strength, and weakness.

MANIPULATIVE RESPONSE FORMS

In general, manipulative expressions are those that are less spontaneous and more constricted than actualizing expressions. This is shown in Figure 26 by the increased rigidity of the facade and the more narrow constriction of rhythm. A manipulative response is less of a *feeling* and more of a *calculating* response.

It must be emphasized that manipulative behavior is defined as "normal neuroses," or behavior that deviates from actualizing behavior in spirit only. It is sometimes difficult to determine, for example, whether a person is genuinely loving or simply pleasing and placating. Two criteria that have been helpful in this differentiation are the evidence of one's own seeing and hearing, and the consensus of therapeutic groups. But the distinctions are sometimes difficult to make. Further understanding of manipulative behavior can be had by reading *Man, the Manipulator* (Shostrom, 1967).

The four basic *manipulative response forms* are shown in the inner circle of Figure 26. The first manipulative process begins when a child learns that

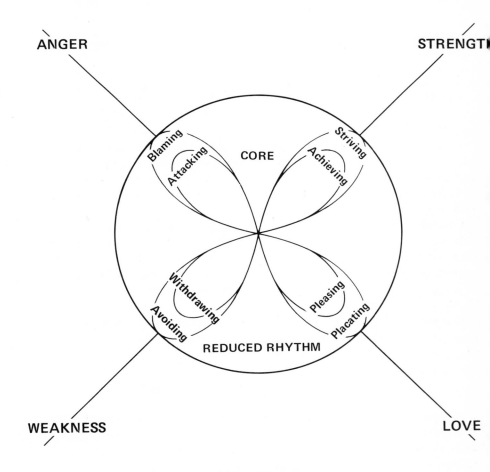

Figure 26. The Manipulative Styles

the alternative to loving is to *please and placate* his parents and others—to please them by erasing himself. This pattern—one of reducing one's own significance—is usually done by either "playing nice guy" or "protecting." The person "playing nice guy" says, "No matter what happens, I'll always be nice to you. I don't count; *you* count." The "protecting" pattern is the stereotype of the Jewish mother: "My *children* count. I'm going to care for you, be good to you, *sacrifice me* for you." These are two forms that the first manipulative pattern takes.

We believe that most "normal" manipulating persons *feel* their behavior to be *creative,* or even "actualizing," at the level of competence that is possible for them. Thus, when the child is "playing nice" he is *denying* his *anger*—the opposite dimension of this polarity. He unconsciously manipulates his body to do this. He tightens the muscles of his neck, shoulders, and jaw to deny his hostility. Rigid jaws, overdeveloped shoulders, and tight neck muscles all attest to this bodily manipulation. Along with this self-manipulation of the body goes the interpersonal manipulation of others.

The second manipulative process that a child learns is the *blaming and attacking* pattern. Instead of being genuinely angry, he chooses to blame and criticize others—it must be someone else's fault. The blamer may be "bullying," trying to strong-arm everyone into admitting he is right, or he may be "judging," preaching to others about what they should be and where they have gone wrong.

As Figure 26 shows, the placating and blaming patterns are opposites. They represent opposite ways of manipulating, one by erasing the self and one by destroying others. Again, however, notice the *creative* dimension. Here the blaming person also makes an opposite choice: he *denies* his *tender* or *loving feelings.* To love is to be hurt, therefore it's better to attack. Once again he manipulates his body: his stomach tightens—he armors his vital organs tightly, ready for attack, and keeps on the offensive. Life becomes a battle for survival.

The third manipulative pattern is the *striving and achieving* process, represented by "calculating" and "dictating." The striving or achieving person has learned that instead of expressing genuine strength the way to survive is to have a plan or scheme for living: "It really doesn't matter what *I* count for or what *you* count for; it's *proving oneself* that is important." The person "dictating," for example, needs to prove his superiority to the group. He will tell others what is good for them and how to achieve it. The "calculating person" is similar but is more obtuse—he proves his worth by getting you to "buy" his ideas. The father who "sells" his kids on going to college and the person who sells cars may both pay little attention to the wishes of the other people involved and care only about achieving their own goals. But, once again, the *creative* solution is apparent. The proving person has learned that he must *deny* the opposite dimension of the polarity of *weakness,* and his "system" keeps this vulnerability carefully hidden. The "puffed chest" of a supersalesperson or a dictatorial parent are physical manifestations of a system of rigid personal as well as interpersonal control.

The fourth process pattern is to manipulate by weakness; by *withdrawing and avoiding* others and also by avoiding problem situations. The person "playing weak" says, "I can't do it—I give up!" The person "clinging" says, "I can't do it—*you* do it," depending on others to think and act for him. The avoiding person has learned to believe that he can't do anything on his own, so he has stopped trying.

But, as in the previous patterns, the *creative* power of the weakness dimension must not be overlooked. The avoiding person has found that by pleading innocent and weak, he can seduce others to do his job. *Strength* has been *denied.* The body reflects this chosen style of coping with life; hearing and seeing defects develop; the person has creatively learned not to look and listen!

THE CHARACTER STYLES

In general, the character style is a personality structure that has rigidified even more than the manipulative patterns. The behaviors of the four primary character structures are stereotyped and *control* of others and one's own feelings is characteristic of all character types.

For example, what begins as genuine love (as an original organismic expression by the child) and later, at the manipulative level, becomes pleasing and placating, is, at the character style level, passive or *oral dependence.* As with the other character structures, the oral dependent person uses *denial* as his chief mechanism. Denying his need for love, he turns this need around and *acts* loving, getting others to seek love from him. His rationalization is that he is *giving in* to others' needs. Thus he does get some nourishment, but his core suffers in that he cannot openly express his energy from within for the satisfaction of his own needs. As shown in Figure 27, the reduced size of his core results in further reduced rhythm.

In a similar manner, the genuine anger of the actualizing person, which had become distorted by the manipulating person as blaming and attacking, becomes *masochism* at the character style level. Again, the mechanism of denial is involved, since the masochist denies his anger (which is evident by the muscular heaviness in his shoulders and neck) and claims to be the "nice guy." He pleads innocence and humility, blocking his spite or resentment within. Thus he blocks his tenderness as well and remains in a "masochistic morass," frozen in his ability to love or feel anger.

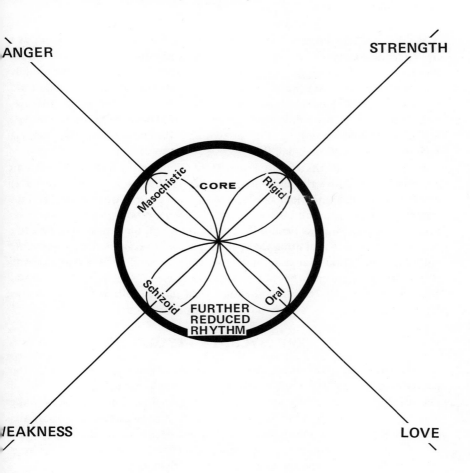

Figure 27. The Character Styles

When genuine strength becomes manipulative it rigidifies into striving and achieving (see Figure 26). At the character style level, it moves to the *rigid personality* (Figure 27). In attempting to appear to be strong and self-confident, the rigid character substitutes achievement for his need for love. To get love, he has become a producer—a doer—and attempts to prove himself by becoming a *workaholic*. Achievement gives him an air of strength, but not genuine strength from within.

Finally, when genuine weakness becomes manipulative, it is characterized by withdrawal and avoidance. At the character style level the individual becomes the *schizoid personality,* who is cold, aloof, and emotionally detached. But he *denies* his detachment and rationalizes that he must hold himself together against a basically hostile world. He then seeks affirmation from others by manipulating them into telling him he is special, talented, or understanding. But he still is constricted and still lacks a feeling of "is-ness," or being.

It appears, then, that genuine anger, love, strength, and weakness can become manipulative through either *distortion* or *deterioration. Distortion* refers to genuine expressions of emotion that are twisted during the developmental phases from childhood onward; *deterioration* means that it is possible for one who has been self-actualizing to fall back into manipulative patterns. One cannot assume that once a person is self-actualizing he or she will *always* maintain that state, any more than one can assume that a person will always be physically healthy in every respect. It is technically accurate, then, to refer to self-actualiz*ing,* rather than self-actualiz*ed* persons. As we have stated previously, self-actualizing is a process—not a fixed state.

THE PSYCHOTIC STYLES

In general, the psychotic is characterized by styles opposite those of the actualizing person (see Figure 28). Whereas the actualizing person has a permeable boundary or facade and has strong feelings from within to make contact with others rhythmically, the psychotic is blasé, weak, and sporadic; his muscular contractions hold him together like a rigid but fragile container; and he is threatened with acute collapse if his repressed feelings from within break through his already shaky rigid facade.

One of the psychotic's chief mechanisms is projection. When the *oral dependent* breaks down, he does so because he feels the "burden" of the demands from others, which he has fabricated. He feels *depressed*—he feels pressed by others. He develops feelings of self-destruction as he continues to deny his own need for support and help. The pseudoactualizing might be expressed as: "Hasn't a person a right to run away from it all?" The ultimate expression of depression is *suicide.*

Similarly, the *masochist's* denial of his own anger flows into psychosis when projection of this anger or spite is developed into *paranoia.* Not only are others guilty of being angry at the paranoiac, but they are *so* mad at him that he rigidly defends himself from a potentially hostile world. The paranoiac's ultimate defense, obviously, is the destruction of others before they destroy him. The pseudoactualizing logic would perhaps be: "Isn't self-protection justifiable?" The ultimate expression of paranoia is *homicide*.

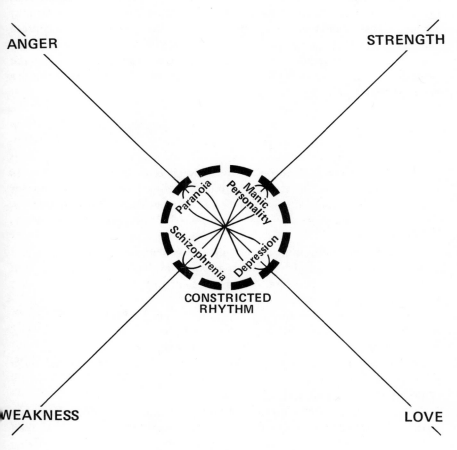

Figure 28. The Psychotic Styles

The *rigid personality,* continuing his denial of the need for love, becomes *manic* as he strives to maintain the image of strength and self-worth by becoming more and more productive. He often becomes a candidate for cardiac failure in his forceful, superproductive attempts to prove himself worthy of love. The pseudoactualizing logic comes from our culture itself: Work is considered virtuous in our Puritanistic culture; thus the manic is even given plaudits in his pseudoattempt at appearing actualizing. But the ultimate expression of rigidity is the self-imposed death by *heart attack.*

Finally, the *schizoid personality* melds into the *schizophrenic* when projection becomes a primary mechanism. When repressed feelings break through from within, the schizophrenic decompensates and retreats into earlier infantile behavior. The schizophrenic totally retreats from contact with the world because he sees others as attempting to annihilate him—as forcing him to be weak and helpless. The ultimate result is catatonic *psychosis:* "Why not quit if life becomes unbearable?" (Even schizophrenia has a pseudoactualizing logic.)

CONCLUSIONS

The schema described above is obviously an *inter*personal as well as an *intra*personal one. It focuses on the individual-in-relation-to-others rather than on the individual alone. It moves away from case history and symptomatic labels and proceeds in the direction of actualizing gains or payoffs found in interaction.

An important assumption underlying this schema is that normality and abnormality can be defined as different points on basic continua. The conceptual terminology, therefore, includes the entire range of human activity. Few other theories do this.

It must be emphasized that only certain character or psychotic behaviors (those most exemplary of behavior on the basic anger-love and strength-weakness continua) are described here. Actualizing theory does not purport to account for all character or psychotic behavior, *but it does explain much pathological behavior as abortive attempts at actualizing:* It joins a theory of function with one of malfunction.

Generally, actualizing may be defined as a sense of relatedness to the world based on genuine interdependence. Psychopathology may be described in terms of limited or distorted attempts to actualize. When the actualizing person can feel that he is separate and autonomous and at the same time rhythmically able to be angry and loving, strong and weak interpersonally, he can avoid the control and rigidification that ends in neuroses or psychoses.

Perhaps psychology needs new therapeutic methods, such as the one presented here, that do not diagnose sickness but that really appreciate the creativity involved in pathological attempts to survive in the world. If, as Skinner (1971) says, positive reinforcement is superior to punishment, we need to congratulate the client on the creativity of attempts to actualize rather than to criticize his pathology. Perhaps therapists need to say, "Man, that was really ingenious," rather than, "Man, you are really sick."

Laing's (1965, 1967) point that we can learn a great deal from the special strategies of psychotic persons, which they invent in order to live in an unlivable world, is relevant here. The therapy process may be seen as a gradual replacing of creative attempts at wellness (survival methods) with behavior that is much more creative (actualizing or expressive behavior).

Another way of stating the problem is that perhaps behavior is coactively motivated by two processes: (1) the need to survive (for example, assuming one must never be angry), and (2) the need to actualize (realizing that mutual growth comes only from creative confrontation). Thus, *survival behavior* is defined as facade-like, narrowly strategic attempts to cope in a world that is felt to be basically unlivable. But this behavior is rigid and fixated, and ultimately relationship-destroying. *Actualizing behavior* is defined as more core-like, expressive behavior that is rhythmic and relationship-enhancing. Therapy is a process that moves a person outward from a basically *survival* frame of reference to a basically *actualizing* frame, but the therapist must appreciate the actualizing involved in all survival behavior.

It would seem that manipulative behavior, character disorders, and psychotic behaviors represent survival forms of pseudoactualizing. They all represent systems or games by which one tries to exist in a world that has been hurtful in some way. They are all desperate attempts to win in a world that is a battleground rather than a world that can be a rhythmic dance of polarities. All systems of survival fear *admission of defeat.* But Actualizing Therapy holds that there is a difference between admission of defeat and *acceptance of losses.* None of us has been spared hurt and losses.

Therapy can be a system of rebirth wherein the individual may reexperience his losses and find the strength from within his core to stand alone in spite of the negative responses of the world.

One good symbol for actualizing, then, would be the phoenix, a bird of Egyptian legend that burned itself on a pyre and from whose ashes another phoenix arose. This legend has served as a metaphor for death and resurrection throughout pagan and Christian literature.

SUMMARY

Figure 23 (page 83) summarizes the processes shown in Figures 16 through 19 and Figures 25 through 28. As one moves from the actualizing level to the psychotic level, several phenomena occur:

1. The *facade* decreases in permeability and openness and increases in rigidity and inflexibility, as illustrated by the change in heaviness of the walls and as expressed by the individual's behavior.

2. The *rhythm* reduces in fluidity and becomes more and more constricted, as illustrated by the maxiswings of the actualizing level and the miniswings of the psychotic level. Behaviorally, this means full expression of feelings versus careful computation of one's response.

3. The size of the *core* reduces in magnitude, indicating that the person who is actualizing is making maximum use of inner resources and that the psychotic is making minimal use of these resources.

4. The *O/I ratios* reduce from 1/3 to 1/1 as we move from actualizing to psychoses. This means that the actualizing person is very inner-directed, while the psychotic is caught in the double bind of not being either inner- or other-directed.

5. The T_I/T_C *ratios* show a gradual change from living in the present, when actualizing, to living more in the past (with regrets and guilts) or in the future (with unfulfillable illusions).

6. The *polar dimensions* show a change as one moves inward to more and more defensive postures, which are increasingly more drastic in their *survival quality*. Manipulative postures are relatively harmless in their effects, but character styles become much more difficult to change. Psychotic postures are last-ditch survival stands that are founded on the fear that one may not survive unless he employs them. The "protection game" becomes self-defeating, however, as one builds harder and thicker armor around himself. The protective shell eventually becomes the problem rather than the solution, and the individual loses contact with his own inner energy as well as with the world.

The purpose of Actualizing Therapy, then, is not to focus on how to *undo* the pathology of the inner shell, but rather to facilitate *experiencing and expressing* of the self at the actualizing, manipulative, and character style levels. Further, the actualizing person's huge *reservoir of core* focuses on the tapping of the energy of his feelings, his thinking, and his bodily response. In the vernacular of today's youth, the actualizing person has "put it all together."

CHAPTER 5. ACTUALIZING AS DEVELOPMENTAL AWARENESS

Sigmund Freud's system of therapy focuses primarily on the past; that is, psychoanalysis sees the past experiences of an individual as primary in determining his present adjustment to life. Fenichel (1945) and Dollard and Miller (1950) reflect this emphasis.

The writings of Adler (in Ansbacher & Ansbacher, 1956), Buhler (1962), Allport (1955), and French (1952) all emphasize the future. Allport's "becoming," French's "hope," and Buhler's "reality principle" are all illustrations of this emphasis.

In recent years, existential therapists have emphasized a here-and-now, or "being," orientation to living and have stressed the here and now as the significant variable for therapeutic work (May et al., 1958).

In contrast to each of these approaches, Actualizing Therapy focuses on all three temporal dimensions of human existence: past, present, and future.

The most significant question that the Actualizing Therapist can ask his client is "Where are you?" as opposed to the more common question, "Why?" "Why" puts the client on a "head trip" in which he attempts to give rational answers that are not rooted in experience. By focusing on the "where" or the "when," the client can easily move from the present to past memories or future goals. An important aspect of this "whereness" is the person's location in terms of specific stages of life. By understanding one's own life history and by seeing the direction one's life is taking, one can gain a greater feeling of support and direction in his present situation. It is for this reason that a developmental analysis of a person's life history is important in therapy. The actualizing orientation embraces the present with the past and the future into an integrated whole that helps give the client's life a sense of meaning. The analysis that follows is a generalized model for helping the individual to achieve such integration.

Understanding one's unique developmental history gives the client a better opportunity to appreciate his actualizing potential as well as to face his personal historical losses. Each person may be said to be stunted in growth of expression on each of the polarities to some degree. An analysis of one's personal emotional education in the therapy process enables him to see how he has been stunted and where he needs further expression. Further, a historical analysis of oneself enables one to determine how he has managed his dependent, independent, and interdependent tasks of living.

For young people, the developmental sequence provides a roadmap of the obstacles and opportunities that lie ahead. For all persons, this analysis suggests compassion and the ability to "forgive" oneself and others for the inevitable mistakes that occur in living.

We have defined the core as one's fundamental nature, from which polarities may be expressed in an actualizing way. In growing up, one develops what we describe as the ego boundary, or facade. The facade consists of programmed responses that arm one for survival. Because of childhood experiences of bombardment by parents and other authorities, most people do not trust their original emotional responses to life. Instead they begin to develop two ways of relating to life: *illusions,* or ideals, and *repression*—the exclusion of unacceptable material from awareness. Instead of being their natural selves on the anger-love, strength-weakness polarities, most people attempt to give the impression of being something they are not, of being "perfect." In addition, people repress expression of these polarities and create a heavily invested ego boundary that keeps them from being genuine and authentic.

The role of Actualizing Therapy, then, is to help such individuals to become aware of their illusions and ideals and of the means by which their feelings are being repressed. For it is illusions and repression that keep the self from being whole. In helping the individual, the therapist focuses on three areas: assumptions, feelings, and the body. The therapist continually refers to these three dimensions of experience to help the client become increasingly aware of the ways in which he is repressing feelings—in which he is restricting his rhythmical expression on the polarities. *Emotional education* may be described as a person's learning of supports, or lack of supports, in these three areas, which, combined, determine his adjustment to living in the present.

In his book *Love and Will* (1969), Rollo May defines "daemonic" as "any natural function which has the power to take over the whole person" (p. 123). In terms of Actualizing Therapy, the natural rhythmic being of a person who has had few developmental traumas does not have a daemonic but rather is living in a rhythmic relationship between natural anger-love and strength-weakness expressions of his feelings. An individual becomes daemonic only when one aspect of either polarity is overemphasized to the exclusion of the other. For example, a person is daemonic when he flies into a rage and becomes excessively angry or when sex takes over his entire being. A person is daemonic when he expresses impotence rather than genuine weakness. Similarly, an abnormal need for power is daemonic.

The interest in the daemonic as exemplified by the popularity of both the book and film versions of *The Exorcist* is relevant here. In the moral sense, Actualizing Therapy holds that a person becomes daemonic when he is not allowed to express a godlike sense but only a raging, lustful devil-like self. Each person is born with a homeostatic tendency—each daemonic has an antidaemonic, which gives a natural balance to one's being. The daemonic results when one aspect or dimension of a polarity "exorcises" the other aspect because the individual has failed to express each counterbalancing dimension in his daily being.

Actualizing Therapy may be thought of as a therapy of effectiveness as opposed to a therapy of illness—of acceptance of the client's homeostatic capacity for expression and control rather than of stress on his limitations and illness. At the same time it is a psychology of *compassion for one's limitations*. In the process of growing and developing, everyone is subjected to ideas that limit his ability to fully experience himself as an actualizing person.

In this chapter we outline the relationship of the basic polarities to growth and development, and we present a theory of developmental actualizing. We hope to provide the reader with a historical appreciation for the complexity of the person who chooses Actualizing Therapy. We then move on to the individual and group methods that treat this complexity.

THE RELATIONSHIP OF STAGES OF CHRONOLOGICAL GROWTH TO THE CARING SEQUENCE

Figure 29 illustrates the *caring sequence* that parallels the various periods of man's development. Buhler and Goldenberg (in Buhler & Massarik, 1968) utilize a similar model in describing the structural aspects of a person's unique history. We present their schematic presentation of an average middle-class life history as an illustration of how our developmental theory may be applied specifically to an individual's life history:

> When presenting a person's life history schematically, one has to make a somewhat arbitrary decision about which data to include and which to omit. The selection usually depends on the purpose.

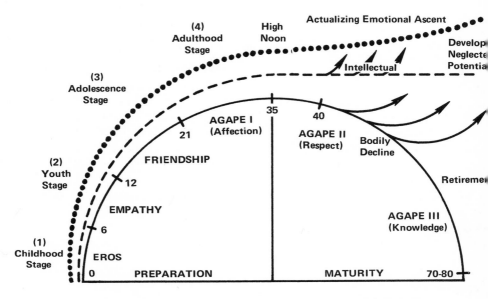

Figure 29. Actualizing or Deteriorating Developmentally

The purpose of this [section] is to show what might be called the most basic data of a person's life history because they reveal the structure of the life cycle. Although one might debate the inclusion of one or another "dimension," as C. Buhler calls these data, the reader probably will agree that most of the dimensions included here are basic. [Figure 30] then is a schematic rendering of Bill Roberts' life, presented to make the basic dimensions of this life history "visible."

Line a refers to Bill's age up to an interview [with the researchers], which took place when he was 67 years old. Lines b to f refer to the main events and activity areas of Bill's life.

The broken line above the data represents the schematic growth and decline curve. . . .

Using [Buhler's] expansion-restriction model, we find a gain in new dimensions until Bill is about 30 and the family acquires its first home. This is followed by a fairly stationary period in which the family grows and Bill's jobs improve. At 46, Bill experiences what he himself considers the peak in his life, when he and the family take a trip through the United States. Bill's serious kidney operation at 49 marks the beginning of his relatively early descent. After a short return to work, he decides he is no longer strong enough to hold a full-time job. He buys a grocery store with the family's savings and works part time, with his wife assisting him. At 64 he retires completely.

Second, using the self-determination model, we find that Bill's period of tentative self-determination starts relatively early, i.e., at 14 when he leaves his parents' home. The phase of his definite self-determination begins with his marriage at age 26, and it unfolds more fully two years later when he settles down in a steady job and at a place where he intends to remain. He then starts his family and buys a home.

The phase of self-assessment and reorientation begins when Bill is 49 and, following his kidney operation, he decides he can no longer cope with his office job and turns to running his own grocery store with his wife's help. But at 64, Bill feels he is not strong enough to share the responsibility of the store and he retires.

Bill Roberts' biography exemplifies the phasic structure of events and activities during a life cycle. (pp. 59-61)

The Caring Relationship Inventory (CRI), described in Chapter 2, measures the forms of love that relate to these stages of development. In this chapter, specific phases relating to each of the different stages of growth will be outlined. Figure 29 illustrates the stages that follow.

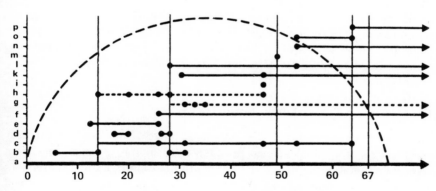

a. Time dimensions in ages
b. Education
c. Career
d. Service in army
e. Dating
f. Marriage
g. Children
h. Changes of domiciles
i. Extended trip

k. Home ownership
l. Church and organizational
   memberships
m. Illness
n. Children on their own
o. Departure from job and
   beginning of own business
p. Retirement
— — — Biological life cycle

Figure 30. Schematic Presentation of a Sample Life History

Childhood (Birth to Six Years)

Childhood may be defined as a period during which the individual is involved in a dependency-*eros* relationship with the parents. When first born, the child is completely dependent upon the mother; if left to its own devices, the child would ultimately die. The child is also in an erotic relationship with the mother—their first contact is through the breast and the feeding process.

In the first parental contacts, the child is expected to behave as the "good" child. Operationally, "good" is understood to be whatever the parents choose; it has nothing to do with any absolute standards of morality. When one thinks of a "good" child, one realizes that there are many different standards imposed by parents, who often depend on their own neurotic or manipulative tendencies.

The child's initial contacts with playmates, relatives, or parents are based essentially on the anger-love polarity. Children are taught to love their neighbor, love their brother, never to feel angry, never to feel hostile but to accept their role as big brother, to accept their role as helper, and generally to behave in a manner that reflects the views of the authorities as to what their proper role should be.

The childhood role is a "dependency role"; until age six, children are very much dependent on authority figures for their understanding of proper behavior. These standards of behavior often lead to emotional and body reactions as the child's developmental growth begins to rigidify.

Youth (Six to Twelve Years)

As the child grows older, the emphasis moves from eros to *empathy* toward peers, from dependence to independence from parents, and from other-direction to inner-direction. The youth now relates more essentially to the strength-weakness polarity and begins to learn peer and sex roles as well as the leader-follower relationship. Subject to school discipline for the first time, the youth begins to focus on personal strengths or weaknesses, asking such questions as: "How intelligent am I?" "How good a player am I?" "How good a friend am I?"

In preadolescence there are rather relentless standards for judging oneself and others. Theodore Lidz (1968), in his developmental study of the person, speaks of the way in which the juvenile develops his or her self-concept: "We have noted that at this age children have rigid standards of what is right and wrong, for they consider ethical values as fixed, rather than suited to the circumstances, and believe individuals should be judged according to egalitarian standards and punished in an expiatory manner" (p. 284). These years are characterized by the youth's excessive preoccupation with personal adequacy and feelings of impotence, and they represent an important second developmental stage.

Adolescence (Twelve to Twenty-one Years)

With adolescence, the individual moves from the empathy stage to a chosen form of loving—the *friendship* stage. The emphasis changes from the dependent and independent stages to a synthesis of both: *interdependence.* The adolescent understands the meaning of a hetero-sexual relationship and becomes preoccupied with relating to the opposite sex through the anger-love and strength-weakness polarities.

The period of adolescence is often referred to as the potentially schizophrenic years because the individual begins to feel the split between the polarities and often experiences difficulty in making the shift from natural-homosexual to natural-heterosexual relationships; has difficulty in selecting and training for a career; and is coming to grips with a new set of rules for relating to the world.

Adulthood (Twenty-one Years and Older)

The focus is now on *agape I*—which is *affection,* or the "brotherhood" form of love—rather than on eros, empathy, or friendship. These adult years represent a second synthesis stage because the adult learns that, as Jung has said, "The rules for the second half of life cannot be the same as the rules for the first half." The adult has to learn what it means to become spouse and parent, and to achieve success or failure in a career.

In the early phases of the second half of life, *agape II,* or *respect,* begins to emerge from agape I. As husband and wife work and grow together, agape II (in the form of full acceptance of the unique individuality of one another) develops.

Finally, as the sunset years approach, it may be necessary to learn what it means to face physical decline. The sunset years are defined in terms of *agape III,* or the *dimension of knowledge.* The love of mature people for one another is described as knowing the very core of each other and loving the totality of each other's beings. As shown in Figure 29, emotional and intellectual growth may continue to accelerate and even reduce the rate of physical decline.

STAGES OF EMOTIONAL EDUCATION

Having outlined how the polarities of actualizing are related to love growth through life, our concern now is to outline more specifically those experiences in the stages of life that are important to an understanding of the person seeking an actualizing way of life. The relationship of various experiences to dependence, independence, and interdependence will be referred to whenever relevant.

Childhood (Birth to Six Years)

The *eros stage* lasts from birth to six years. It is characterized by dependence and defense as the child relates to the mother in a most physical, sexual manner, both through touching her breasts and through being fondled by her in turn.

Much of what the child first learns about human relationships is derived from the feeding process. This is why Freud (1949) called the first year of life the *oral period.* If the mother's attitude is one of warm acceptance combined with prompt alleviation of the child's hunger, the child experiences pleasurable feelings. If the child perceives rejection or distance, the experience becomes one of anxiety and displeasure.

The eating function thus becomes allied to feelings of security, and the child develops a concept of what happens to people who are dependent. These may be lessons in security and love. When fed regularly and with accompanying warmth and affection, and when weaned gradually, the child learns to tolerate frustration.

Child development theory holds that privations should not be too many, too early, or too sudden. When dependency needs of this period are met and handled properly, the way is paved for continued development. Harlow's (1958) studies on deprivation of mothering in primates lends support to the importance of meeting dependency needs.

If the child is frustrated or deprived in the early *oral period,* there may be significant repercussions for *dependence* in later personality development. Erikson (1950) suggests that the child learns to trust or mistrust from early oral experiences. Love at this stage is a primitive *dependency* love that is largely *received* from parents. Dependency needs predominate at the oral stage and problems may develop if these needs are not met.

The lack of capacity to express affection, so often noted in the adult, probably has its roots in this stage. The child who has *received* love generously and unconditionally seems to be able to *give* love later in life with less effort. Children who experience inconsistency and rejection in their early love relationships may be unduly demanding of love, attention, and dependency in later years. Others, fearing rejection of their tender feelings, may ward off dependency and intimacy with others to avoid repetition of unpleasant experiences. Such efforts are frequently unsuccessful and are likely to reflect an impaired capacity both to receive and to give love.

Thus, for the future growth of the child, it is essential that there be a close, warm, loving relationship between mother and child. In psychotherapy of adults, the recollection of early childhood memories or, more commonly, the childhood data as related by parents or friends, may give valuable insights into the origins and purposes of a client's unhealthy attitudes toward dependency and love.

According to Bioenergetic theory, the need to *be* or to *exist* or to be safe in the world is generally established in this first year of the dependency period. Anytime this need is threatened, especially by parents or by parent figures, a *schizoid tendency* may develop. Out of his fear the child contracts and withdraws in an attempt to hold the self together. This happens during the *first* months of existence. If, at later times in life, the need to say, "I am," is seriously threatened, the individual may develop a schizoid tendency.

In this same period, the child needs the security that comes with the support of a nourishing mother. A basic lack of such support results in an *oral tendency,* which is characterized by an exaggerated *dependency* or holding on to others. The oral person still feels "I need you" and feels impotent and weak, even in adulthood.

Independence begins to develop between the ages of two and three, as the child learns to walk and to move things with his or her hands. Not only is the child learning control of his movements but he is also increasing his differentiation of the elements of the environment that are specific to his own personal needs and pleasures. As the sense of power develops the child begins to rebel more directly against restrictions and he wants to make independent decisions about matters.

The period from ages two and one-half to three and one-half can be referred to as the "negative phase"—the *first adolescence.* The child feels a new sense of independence but adults seem to thwart him at every turn. Aggression and its control become a central problem. Charlotte Buhler (1951) sees the negativistic period as one in which the child tests other people's love. She describes the period from eight months to four years as the period of testing relationships. Needs for self-determination are tried out, as are experiments with independence from mother. The child must learn to let mother out of sight and to trust in her ability to return.

This period is called the *anal* phase, because the first real clash in the child's need to be autonomous is associated with parental efforts at toilet training. The first lessons in bladder and bowel training affect the child's relationships with his parents. He soon learns that he can give pleasure or create anxiety by either giving or holding back feces or urine. Thus, in addition to food resistance, the elimination process becomes one of the child's first weapons in dealing with parents. Psychoanalysts point out that harsh bowel or bladder training may cause the child to develop a rigid or strict conscience, while lack of parental assistance in learning these important values may result in the child's not developing a conscience. Psychoanalysis traces an adult's "compulsive giving" to the necessity of conforming, during the anal period, to the parental demands for control of elimination.

Rigidity, or "overcontrol," in adulthood can often be traced to premature teaching of bowel and bladder control. The overcontrolled person is frequently afraid of natural impulses, and this fear often spreads to other areas of the personality. He feels he must always conform, thus reducing his spontaneity.

Compulsive habits about cleanliness, neatness, time, or organization also appear to have roots in severe bowel or bladder training. Persons in whom such habits are entrenched are said to be "overresponsible," having learned early to worry about a function that is "dirty" or that must adhere to a "schedule." There are also people who are overly independent or who cannot delay pleasures, suggesting that their training in this period was without control. Tensions concerning elimination processes are evident when one considers the number of efforts at humor about them. Underlying this humor are feelings of shame and anxiety. The ability of the average child to label his anatomy, excepting the eliminative organs, illustrates the inhibitions and avoidance tendencies that have been learned from parents. The parental problem at this stage, therefore, is one of channeling the child's aggression so that it is not unduly postponed, disguised, or displaced.

The management of aggression becomes a paramount problem in this phase. Fenichel (1945) compares this problem to the management of sexual tensions: "If they cannot find gratification in their original form, they have the capacity to change, to alter their objects or aims, or to submit to repression by the ego and then to make themselves apparent again in various ways and in different disguises" (pp. 55-57).

Because it is as harmful to give the child unlimited freedom as it is to overly restrict him, it is important to remember, as Karen Horney (1939) points out, that it is not the frustrations and deprivations that are crucial in the development of the child, but rather the *manner* in which they are imposed. Actually, the child is able to endure a great deal if he is backed with love and otherwise considerate attitudes.

The preceding viewpoint on the relationship between anal-stage developmental problems and later aggression and frustration difficulties is in line with classical Freudian hypotheses. Newer psychoanalytic approaches introduce more social-learning principles to account for aggressive behavior. Freud used biological terms to describe the consequences of the mishandling of eliminative functions, but he recognized that the social microcosm of the family during these early years provided the bases for later behaviors. The child, for example, learns how to feel safe during the dependency phase even though he is helpless and weak. Similarly, during the anal period the child is concerned with testing the social climate in the family, and eliminative processes are the principal visible aspect of this developmental problem.

Rosensweig (1944) suggests that there are three possible ways to manage aroused aggression: (1) *Extrapunitive.* Here, hostility is directed outward to other people or objects. When this becomes the primary method, the person may be a "chronic criticizer." (2) *Intropunitive.* In this case, direct blame and anger are directed toward oneself in a punishing manner through self-criticism or self-accusation. Intropunitive persons may be overly apologetic and accepting of blame. (3) *Impunitive.* Here, the aggressive elements in a situation are minimized. When this method becomes primary, the person may so minimize his aggressive feelings and actions that he fails to estimate their effects on himself and on others.

Each of these ways of dealing with aggression may be appropriate in certain situations. The parental role is to help the child learn that sometimes others are responsible, sometimes the child himself is responsible, and sometimes his own feelings are exaggerated. The child is then given opportunity to channel his aggressive or angry feelings, as discussed in Chapter 7.

Erikson (1950) refers to this early phase as the "stage of autonomy." The child develops a need to be independent, yet continues to need dependency and support. In terms of the development of the individual's capacity to love, the child needs to learn at this stage that he is loved for his own "dirty little ornery" self. He needs to learn that he is respected for his independence as well as for his dependence.

Many clients in therapy have problems expressing their aggressive feelings because of improper handling by parents during the anal period. Therapy provides an outlet for *verbal* expression of hostility. Psychosomatic reactions as well as submissive or dependent reactions may be alleviated by therapeutic expression. In therapy one can learn to express aggressive feelings in selected circumstances. One can also learn to channel aggression into constructive action.

The need to be free should be developed in this early independence phase. If a parent of the opposite sex opposes this process by seductive methods, making the child pay for the love received, then the child often counters with similar threats to gain power. This often results in a *psychopathic tendency*. The child becomes manipulative in an attempt to control himself and others.

The struggle for independence is also established through self-assertion in the "negative phase," from two and one-half to three and one-half years. The child needs to say, "No." According to Bioenergetic theory, if self-assertion is crushed, the seeds of a *masochistic tendency* are developed. The child learns to hold in aggression and develops an exaggerated submissiveness. But still the feeling persists: "I need to be free." The child feels crushed and burdened.

A need for even greater freedom is experienced between the ages of four and six. Curiosity and exploratory activities expand in many directions, and an interdependence begins to develop whose nature is, in many respects, determined by the manner in which the parents relate to the child.

The child's curiosity about his sexual organs and about differences in sexual roles reaches a peak during this phase. The natural outcomes of this curiosity are the discovery of pleasurable excitement through masturbation and the playing of masculine and feminine roles, for which the parents are the models.

How the parents react to the child's curiosity about sex and masturbation has important implications for the child's self-regard and later feelings about sexual impulses and activities. Parents and teachers should neither overemphasize nor underemphasize the sexual activities of the child. Many fears of punishment and castration, which the psychotherapist has to help clients overcome in later years, can be tied back to being shamed, scolded, or threatened with dire punishment for early innocent sexual activities. If parents understand the natural development of the child's interests and do not themselves relate to the child in either a highly sexualized or overly prudish, intolerant fashion, the child is better able to develop healthy attitudes toward sex and sexual roles.

Interdependence begins to develop when children accept their own sex through a process of identification with the sexually similar parent. Parents provide the models from which children develop notions of "masculinity" and "femininity." The child must emerge with a feeling of value toward, and acceptance of, self.

Normal heterosexual relationships tend to result if, during the interdependent phase, the child's affections are accepted by the parent of the opposite sex. In adolescence, when it is important to establish good heterosexual relationships, the foundations for "liking" members of the opposite sex begin first in relationships to one's parents. During this initial phase of interdependence and extension of initiative, parents need to exert practical controls in order to assist the child in the development of a conscience. Parental controls are internalized as inner controls, or conscience.

Fromm (1947, p. 175) feels that the conflict of this period is not brought about primarily by sexual rivalry but is the result of the child's negative reaction to parental authority. It is a battle between the child's freedom or spontaneity on the one hand, and the expectations, and sometimes irrational authority, of the parents on the other. Parents can assist their children in the development of a conscience through a combination of praise and punishment given with understanding. At this stage the child may learn that love is not always expressed by warmth and loving attention but can be expressed by anger as well. Parents can encourage curiosity, open-mindedness, willingness to try new things, and readiness to see new solutions. They can give the child a positive conscience wherein the child is assured that, within limits, his impulses can be trusted and followed. However, parents can also stifle curiosity, kill initiative, and create a punitive conscience that prevents trusting of one's impulses. The development of conscience is more readily aided by subtlety and indirection than by force. It seems to be most readily facilitated by example—by the kinds of behaviors that the parents model for the child and the way in which they deal with him in everyday family relationships.

Bioenergetic theory holds that a parent-child interdependence begins to develop at this stage. A *rigid tendency,* characterized by exaggerated independence or holding back, may develop. In such a case, the child, rejected by a parent, denies his need for love. The rigid child needs to give up this exaggerated independence, and to give in to the need for love, so that further maturity is not affected.

Polarity aspects of self-actualizing relate to three major developmental problems: (1) the expression of warmth and affection, (2) the handling of hostility and anger, and (3) the management of sexual tensions. Each of these problems has its roots in the first six years of life. Affection can be traced to the dependency phase of the childhood stage, in which the child is given love and security and learns to rely on others. In the independence phase of childhood, the child develops a knowledge both of power and of how to handle first frustrations. The parent who deals wisely with tantrums and aggressions, recognizing them as acceptable developmental expressions, gives the child the means of managing acceptably aggressive tendencies later in life. Finally, in the interdependent phase of childhood, effective relationships should be established with the opposite sex so that satisfying heterosexual relationships later become possible.

The later relevance of the character patterns developed in these first six years will be discussed in Chapter 6.

Youth (Six to Twelve Years)

The *empathy stage of life,* from six to twelve years, is characterized by further sexual development of masculine and feminine roles and by a sense of individuality and separateness. It can be very exciting to observe children learning to empathize and to care for others as much as they do for themselves. Erich Fromm contends that empathy usually does not develop before the age of nine and that sometimes parents ask their children to feel more than they are prepared to feel. In general, however, it is possible to see this empathic feeling develop during the earlier years.

Gesell (1949) has likened development to a spiral similar to the concepts of homeostasis and transtasis shown in Figure 1 (page 6). In the youth stage, the spiral of life "widens" remarkably. In the words of Havighurst (1953), "There is the thrust of the child out of the home and into the peer group, the physical thrust into the world of games and work requiring neuromuscular skills, and the mental thrust into the world of adult concepts, logic, symbolism, and communication" (p. 25).

Children from ages six to twelve enter, for the first time, a world that is not completely dominated by parents and siblings. Dependence on authorities other than parents may create more problems for the parents than for the child. By going to school, the child is thrust into dependence on a peer group to which conformity must be learned and with which cooperation and sharing are demanded. Friends are no longer restricted to the child's immediate neighborhood, and intellectual and cultural interests widen as well.

Young people of both sexes continue their role-playing and tend to be dependent on others of their own sex. The differences in sex roles become more apparent, and young people strongly emulate the behavior of their friends in dress and behavior. This is a time in which they are exploring many more and varied behaviors relative to their sex role.

In the dependency phase of youth, the individual continues to need control combined with freedom of initiative. Parents can provide a rich environment in which the child may learn and may experiment with a wide variety of experiences and human relationships, as well as have a sense of belonging to a wider group than the family. On the other hand, parents, through undue restriction, disinterest, or privation, may force the child into a narrow, frustrating orbit. Balancing of control and freedom is a developmental task of the parent in this period.

From ages ten to thirteen the child's world is shaken up by two major developments: (1) achieving independence from family domination, and (2) the maturing of sexual functions. The youth's behavior is often characterized by irritability, restlessness, moodiness, and backtalk. Frequent threats to run away are symptomatic of efforts to break free of the family. The young person experiences an increase in heterosexual interests. Hopefully, the capacity to love, which hitherto has been qualified by dependency, identification, and narcissism, begins to change in the direction of interdependence. Fromm (1956) described this period as a basic change from narcissism to mature love manifested by a concern for the needs of others.

Another important characteristic of this period is a feeling of uniqueness. Preadolescents become more aware of their identity as persons. Parents must be willing to "give up the child to himself" and to respect this growing freedom. Fears and guilts that parents retain from their own youth make them fearful for their own children, and so hinder the parents from letting go of emotional control.

Adolescence (Twelve to Twenty-one Years)

Childhood ends and adolescence begins with the onset of sexual maturity. The adolescent is faced with physiological and psychological revolutions due to rapid body growth and genital maturation. Because the age of adult interdependence is chronologically approaching, the adolescent becomes subject to increasing pressures and restrictions from others. Early conflicts and experiences are relived in the struggle to find the self.

Growth rates of various aspects of the body such as height, weight, circumference, hands, feet, and neck differ widely, and sex differences in growth create special problems. The findings of Shuttleworth (1939) reveal almost a two-year difference between the maximum physical growth rates of boys and girls. The mean age for maximum growth of girls is 12.6, whereas for boys it is 14.8. Shuttleworth finds that at about age thirteen girls are both heavier and taller than boys. Some boys reach their peak physical growth as early as twelve years, whereas others may not fully mature until the age of seventeen.

In the *friendship stage,* from thirteen to approximately twenty-one years, intimacy and identity emerge. Contrary to the sex-oriented thinking currently in vogue among the more permissive schools of encounter therapy, we strongly suggest that friendship is a more significant part of adolescent growth than is sex because it contributes more to the development of the individual's identity during this crucial period. People develop their identity partly in response to the feelings that others have toward them and the feelings of worth that they receive from those relationships. As Harry Harlow says, the influence of peers is probably even more important than that of parents during the adolescent period.

Teenagers often "go steady" too soon in an attempt to attain the sense of identity that comes from feeling that someone cares. We believe it is better to take the risk of having many friendships at this time in order to learn to feel comfortable in different human relationships. (This, of course, is quite different from advocating indiscriminate sex, or, as it is euphemistically termed, free love.)

Variable growth rates contribute to feelings of uncertainty regarding one's sexual identity. Erikson (1950) has described early adolescence as the "stage of identity," during which doubts about one's sexual and personal identity become a major problem. The feelings of inadequacy resulting from the "awkwardness" of uneven growth are well known. Teenagers are subject to joking remarks from adults and contemporaries, and they view with alarm any asynchronous growth patterns. Adolescents become preoccupied with dress and with behaviors that help them to identify with their group. The youngsters who are late developers often resist activities involving physical display because of feelings of physical inadequacy. Those who cannot compete, or who perform awkwardly in sports, often feel ridiculous and foolish.

Growth rate differences tend to drive the sexes away from interdependence in their own age groups. Junior-high-school girls, for example, usually prefer the companionship of high-school, or older, males because the boys of their same age are still "boys," whereas the girls have developed into young ladies. Successful dating between the ages of twelve and fifteen seems to be the best insurance for assisting youth to cross into interdependent heterosexual relationships. Young people are often thrown into sexual panics in which they feel a threat to their sexual security. This happens especially in situations in which they have been rejected by the opposite sex. Klopfer (1961) estimates that about one-half of all male clients have anxieties about homosexuality. Kinsey's findings (Kinsey, Pomeroy, & Martin, 1948) suggest that about one out of three males has had a homosexual experience. The sexual panic that some adolescents experience in their early teens may be related to anxieties about hetero-sexuality, the need to exhibit sexual prowess and prove oneself through masturbatory activities, and the opportunities for homosexual exploration that come in gangs and sexually separate groups.

Actualizing Therapy can reduce the usual sexual anxieties of this period by verbalizing them and helping the adolescent to realize that they are part of normal development. Developmental problems may be traced to their source in earlier stages to determine the way in which masculinity or femininity has been made unattractive. For example, if the boy's mother was cold or smothering, he may have withdrawn from her. If at the same time, the father showed excessive affection, the son may have withdrawn from normal rivalry with the father. Later, as an adolescent, he may try to get the mother to assume the father's role and to get the father to love him like a mother. A similar, but reverse, situation can occur with girls. The roots of this problem seem to develop in the childhood stage and then appear to be reactivated during adolescence.

As the adolescent approaches the more adult age of interdependence there are increasing demands and restrictions from others that complicate his struggle for self-identification. Western culture places serious demands on adolescents. Some of these pressures are: the selection of one's life work, the securing of an education, the choice of a life mate, and the achievement of true interdependence.

In addition to these tasks, Western culture also places certain difficult restrictions on the adolescent. Parents, for instance, have various forms of legal authority over the adolescent until he reaches the age of eighteen or twenty-one. Young people are in continuous conflict: wanting to be dependent and to have needs cared for, and yet wanting all the privileges that come with independence. Adolescents are concerned about their education. They have a dependence on their parents for financial help to get them through, and they may have difficulty acknowledging this fact even though they know it to be true. In turn, this lack of self-assurance may carry over into their school world and interfere with the interdependence that is the touchstone of self-actualizing. It may sharply decrease their scholastic effectiveness, stifle creativity, and cause them to underachieve and to have doubts about the capacity of their intelligence to see themselves through this difficult period.

Prohibitions against sexual gratification and against alcohol and other drug use also are sources of conflict in this stage of development. Boys of eighteen have reached a peak of sexual interest, whereas girls, because of the profound transformations involved in becoming a woman, tend to be more interested in sex than boys at an earlier, prepubertal, stage (twelve to fourteen years). Masturbation serves as an avenue of tension release for some—its only known adverse effect being the possibility of feelings of guilt developing as a result of real or imagined parental punishment, scolding, or disapproval.

Adolescence is a natural period of rebellion. Young people relive their early psychosexual problems. They have a need to be dependent and to be orally occupied—chewing gum, smoking, and chattering—yet they also have a need to be independent. They are often obstinate, are constantly testing limits of authority, become hoarders, and display an interest in telling "dirty stories." They have strong genital interests: masturbate and pet and are narcissistic and exhibitionistic. Both the parents and the adolescent need reassurance that the development of autonomy must take place if the child is to mature to interdependence. Development may proceed much more smoothly if insight is acquired before serious misunderstandings develop. A great deal of help can be given if parents and other significant persons will take the sting of the "forbidden" away from sexual matters and "dirty stories" by listening, affirming, loving, and avoiding the anticipated "shock" reaction.

A mature capacity to love is within the grasp of those young people who successfully replace their idealized parental images. The idea that one can both love and hate the same person, and that people have faults as well as assets, is learned during this stage. When their dependency and independency needs are in rhythmic balance, adolescents are in a position to look for a mate with whom they can share their life on a realistic interdependent basis.

Adulthood (Twenty-one to Sixty Years)

The final love stage of the human encounter journey, the *agape stage,* begins at about age twenty-one and lasts throughout adulthood. It is characterized by concern for the welfare of others and by knowledge and mutual support. During the agape stage of life a mature person is able to identify with the needs of other people and to care for them in a deeper and broader sense—to love them in the way, perhaps, that Eleanor Roosevelt and Albert Schweitzer did: with all-abiding, universal love for the people of the world.

Ages twenty-one to thirty represent a second probing period, similar to that which occurs between eight months and four years. For the first time, young adults are completely on their own, testing the areas of love and work. Selection of a mate and of one's life work are important decisions, requiring an accumulation of experience to choose wisely. There is often a dependent tendency to make such decisions too quickly. Parents and counselors, utilizing the POI in part, can assist young people in assessing their highest potential level of uniqueness, autonomy, and self-fulfillment. One cause of stress in this early adulthood period is the transition from an age-graded society, as fostered in the educational system, to a social-status-graded society. Selecting a marriage partner is one of the most disquieting tasks in the early part of this period. While now less importance is attached to "settling down" to married life, unmarried persons still must cope with social pressures. Frequently, they are the objects of unnecessary attention and subtle ridicule, as well as of clumsy attempts at match-making. Unless young people have been able to find the right mate in school or college, meeting a potential mate may be difficult.

Havighurst describes developmental tasks as goals toward which earlier education should aim. The final examinations are met later in life. That many fail these examinations is indicated by the great demand for reeducative experiences in psychotherapy.

During this experimental, or young-adult, phase of life, young people go through many significant experiences and life crises. According to Havighurst (1953), "Early adulthood . . . usually contains marriage, the first pregnancy, the first serious full-time job, the first illness of children . . . and the first venturing of the child off to school. If ever people are motivated to learn and to learn quickly, it is at times such as these" (p. 257).

A healthy marital relationship should be one in which there is a fusion of erotic love and mature love. A healthy sexual relationship, climaxing in an orgasm, causes a convulsion-like discharge of tension that, according to Erikson (1950) "breaks the point off the hostilities and potential rages caused by the oppositeness of male and female. . . . Satisfactory sex relations thus make sex less obsessive, overcompensation less necessary, sadistic controls superfluous" (p. 230). Furthermore, Erikson puts sex into a larger framework of love and describes it as: "(1) Mutuality of orgasm; (2) With a loved partner; (3) Of the other sex; (4) With whom one is able and willing to have a mutual trust; (5) And with whom one is able and willing to regulate the cycles of work, procreation and recreation; (6) So as to secure for the offspring, too, a satisfactory development."

Establishing and preserving a healthy marital relationship is a complex problem in which the partners need to recognize that marriage is not a dependent fusion of two lives; each must accept the other's need to maintain a healthy independence. Young married couples must face the merging of career plans with demands of the marriage partnership. Each partner must deal with the conflicting roles of dependent spouse versus independent career person or homemaker.

Threats of divorce frequently affect the lives of young couples during this stage. Often, divorce does not offer a solution but simply treats the symptoms of an unhealthy personal dependence. The divorced person has most of the problems of the unmarried person plus many more; financial insecurity, for instance, can be a major problem, as can sex, particularly in the case of the divorced woman.

Particular importance has been attributed to the age of twenty-nine in our culture. There is much joking, for example, about the fact that women are allowed to stay twenty-nine for ten years. This concern arises, of course, out of the frequent appearance, at this time of life, of signs of physical deterioration: wrinkles, sagging muscles, excess weight, and so on. Yet, according to Kinsey's data (Kinsey, Pomeroy, Martin, & Gebhard, 1953), the peak interest in sexuality in women comes at about this time. Men, furthermore, are often in the maximal years of vocational productivity but, because of this, are not giving women the attention that characterized their earlier courtship years.

Men tend to push themselves to the limit to prove their masculinity. Crampton (1955) has identified four common damaging patterns of health abuse in the average male:

> (1) He hides illnesses. When a man's wife contracts a nasty head cold he will insist that she stay home, keep warm, rest, give her doctor a ring and let her housework go. Yet when he himself is really sick and wretchedly uncomfortable he takes pride in working harder than ever. He props himself up with coffee, aspirin and alcohol. He grouchily insists he is not ill. Then afterward, he boasts he never spent a day in bed.
>
> (2) He denies fatigue. He is just too proud to admit that a "real man" ever gets tired. . . . There are thousands like him. He enjoys people saying "Jim puts in a twelve-hour day at his desk."
>
> (3) He conceals emotion. The ability to choke back tears, to deny fear, to conceal humiliation, disappointment and embarrassment is another of the exreme burdens these men load upon themselves. . . . It is impossible to estimate what enormous damage to nervous and emotional stability is caused by so much grimly repressed feeling.
>
> (4) He ignores injury. So many men who are invalided at 55 with heart or circulatory disturbances admit that they felt the first warning flutters 20 years before. There was shortness of breath, pain, dizziness. "I was scared all right but I made myself forget about it. I figured if there was anything wrong with me, I didn't want to know about it." (pp. 8-12)

The years from age twenty-five to age thirty-five may be a lonely period because many of the most important tasks of life must be accomplished with little attention and support from others. Because of their intense awareness of problems, and because their general education, experience, and social development provide the ability to express their ideas cogently, individuals in this age group seem able to benefit more than others from the continuous growth process implicit in self-actualizing. A person enters the second half of life at about the age of thirty-five. Usually, his or her energies, interests, and values have already taken direction. The average person has attained a vocational goal by the time he reaches his mid-thirties, and he may be beginning to reach financial security. Both mothers and fathers find new freedom as their children begin to reach adolescence. A new state is reached after age thirty-five: the afternoon of life. New values must replace some of the values of the morning of life.

The dread with which some adults anticipate their later years is exemplified in the enduring success of Jack Benny's joke about being "thirty-nine." Men and women at forty often feel that they are "over the hill" and have lost their youth. Many cannot accept this feeling of aging and go through a phase of intensive sexual experimentation or other frenzied attempts to look and act youthful. Jung (1933) suggested that the forties create special problems for the counselor and psychotherapist:

> Let us take, for example, the most ordinary and frequent of questions: What is the meaning of my life, or of life in general? Men today believe that they know only too well what the clergyman will say—or rather, must say—to this. They smile at the very thought of the philosopher's answer, and in general do not expect much of the physician. (p. 267)

But this problem does not let the therapist off the hook. As Jung further states, "That is why we psychotherapists must occupy ourselves with problems which, strictly speaking, belong to the theologian" (p. 278). Thus, although the psychotherapist does not know or give specific answers, he must know the *questions* people are asking themselves and some of the answers they are likely to discover. The emphasis of Rilke (1934)—that we should not seek answers but rather live the questions—is one way of describing Actualizing Therapy. Jung's outstanding work with people in the second half of life suggests the importance of the idea that therapy assists the individual to find a workable philosophy of life. Creative selfhood, one goal of psychotherapy, does not come easily. Jung comments: "It is no easy matter to live a life that is modeled on Christ's, but it is unspeakably harder to live one's own life as truly as Christ lived his" (p. 293).

Agape II, which occurs during the early phases of the second half of life, seems to be best described by the word "respect," meaning the ability to accept fully and completely the individuality of the other person. In marriage, particularly, it means respecting the uniqueness of the marriage partner. It means that each partner is so secure individually that he has his own individuality, his own center, his own life; yet, each is able to relate to the other without dominance or exploitation.

As adults enter the second half of life, energies and values must be recast from *preparation* to *maturity,* as was shown in Figure 29. Jung, perhaps more than other writers, expresses the need for reevaluation to preserve and enhance actualizing for the years to come:

> We see that in this phase of life—between thirty-five and forty—a significant change in the human psyche is in preparation. . . . Just as the childish person shrinks back from the unknown in the world and in human existence, so the grown man shrinks back from the second half of life.
>
> In order to characterize it I must take for comparison the daily course of the sun. In the morning . . . the sun pursues its unforeseen course of the zenith. . . . At the stroke of noon the descent begins. And the descent means the reversal of all the ideals and values that were cherished in the morning.
>
> . . . We cannot live the afternoon of life according to the programme of life's morning—for what was great in the morning will be little at evening, and what in the morning was true will at evening become a lie.
>
> For a young person it is almost a sin—and certainly a danger—to be too much occupied with himself; for the aging person it is a duty and a necessity to give serious attention to himself. After having lavished its light upon the world, the sun withdraws its rays in order to illumine itself. Instead of doing likewise, many old people prefer to be hypochondriacs, niggards, doctrinaires, applauders of the past or eternal adolescents—all lamentable substitutes for the illumination of the self, but inevitable consequences of the delusion that the second half of life must be governed by the principles of the first. (pp. 120-125)

As we have said, the emphasis of Actualizing Therapy in the latter half of life is to stress emotional and intellectual growth in order to slow the accelerating process of bodily decline.

In considering the many competitive social and economic demands made on the middle-aged adult, who often has restricted creative potentials with which to meet them, it is no wonder that some nonactualizing individuals develop the pattern described by O'Kelly and Muckler (1955):

That paranoid ideas of infidelity and discrimination by superiors are so prevalent and that the disorder occurs primarily from age 35 on suggests the validity of ascribing paranoid delusions to this mechanism. It is at middle age that the individual first starts to experience competition, sexually and in his work, with younger people. To face the fact that age brings with it a reduction in some types of adjustmental potential is too bitter a fact for many individuals to face; the easier way is to seek for the causes of inadequacy in circumstances exterior to himself. (pp. 299-300)

Between the ages of forty-five and sixty a type of depression can develop. It often occurs around the menopause, or change of life, in women, and may result in an extreme reaction, such as involutional melancholia. Men often experience depression when they are aware of a decline in virility. This decline is caused not only by endocrine dysfunction, but also by psychological problems associated with the time of life. The menopausal period may be likened to the period of adolescence. In both stages there is a physical and psychological metamorphosis of the individual's code of life, and a consequent period of intense self-evaluation.

At this stage, individuals may feel the passing of their peak productivity and the unattainability of many ambitions, ideals, and goals. Women, especially, feel that their beauty is fading fast, and their inability to bear children tends to make them feel that their life is spent. Old insecurities, successfully repressed during maturity, are often felt again.

This middle-adult period is experienced as a "second adolescence." The individual begins to feel forgotten—taken for granted as a family provider or needed parent. The children have grown to maturity and business or marriage security is threatened by younger competition. The individual worries about health, sexual adequacy, and "success." Adults in this period may defend themselves by projecting the reasons for their dissatisfaction onto their mate. The partner is blamed for the individual's own troubles and is believed to have never been loving or understanding. Often the next step is to find a substitute who will provide the fancied need for under- standing and love.

Today, the middle years are much different from those in past genera- tions. Medical science has added about twenty years to the average life span. In order to avoid spending these years in empty diversion and in order to use post-family freedom constructively, mothers might be en- couraged to return to work or to perform some community service. The number of mothers who go back to work when their children reach second- ary school age has increased enormously since World War II (Mace, 1956, p. 29).

New understandings are assisting persons in the middle years to accept the high rate of divorce that is now prevalent in our culture. Marriage is now on trial, whereas a few years ago, persons who failed at marriage were on trial. Our research on the CRI and PAI shows that many clients now frankly admit that their failure at marriage was a problem of immature choice made prior to mature adulthood. Their choices were, for the most part, based on vague feelings of attraction and were acted on quickly, with little understanding of the dynamics of complementary or symmetrical choices. Today many people find themselves involved in second or third marriages based on an increased wisdom and understanding of the meaning of love and on enlightened choice. We believe that use of the CRI and PAI has helped many people to achieve better marriages and that increased use of these instruments is a reflection of the new orientation toward divorce and remarriage.

Actualizing Therapists see this period as a renewed opportunity to establish approaches to interdependence and personal growth. From a theoretical standpoint, it has been hypothesized that the peaks of actualizing cannot be reached until full maturity is attained. In searching a college campus for self-actualizing persons, Maslow (1970, p. 150) found that the level of actualizing found in his older subjects could not be achieved by young, developing persons in our society. Empirical data based on administration of the POI have supported this contention. Mean scores for adult samples tend to be higher than those based on high-school student samples, advanced college student samples are higher than those of entering college freshmen, and samples from both college groups are higher than high-school-age samples. Data reported from a number of studies support the relationship of increased actualizing in the stages to full maturity in the middle adulthood years (Shostrom, 1974).

Erikson (1950) refers to this period of life as "the stage of generativity," during which adults can meet the many problems they must face by developing an interest in the leadership of young people and by achieving true interdependence. Love at this period of life means being able to give, particularly to one's children. One form of giving that should be avoided, however, is that of projection. Parents during this stage often project the problems that they are reliving from their own adolescence onto their children. The Actualizing Therapist often has opportunities to interpret these ideas to clients and to point the way to actualizing interdependence.

The woman in this middle period of life may actively resume the roles of *wife* and *careerwoman*; roles that may have been of secondary significance during the years of childbearing. She may give renewed attention to her husband as a man, with both spouses meeting each other's needs for affection, understanding, and solitude. Nevertheless, the woman may need to be more concerned about maintaining her own personal interests. Each partner needs to understand the special concerns of this period of change. Such understanding should increase genuine courtesy, attentiveness, and regard. The couple's interdependence will, in this way, become more fully actualizing.

Love at this crucial stage of life can be expressed in a unique way. It is becoming well known that masculine and feminine components exist within each man and each woman. As Fromm (1962) says, "Just as physiologically man and woman each have hormones of the opposite sex, they are bisexual also in the psychological sense" (p. 33).

Recent understanding emanating from the Women's Liberation Movement suggests that psychology has contributed to misunderstanding of humankind. Freud suggested that masculinity was the superior function and that women suffered from penis envy. Jung saw man as operating on the logos principle of wisdom and logic and women as operating on the eros principle of relatedness and feeling. Fromm suggested that the masculine character could be defined as aggressive, penetrating, and active and the female character as receptive, submissive, and passive. Today these definitions are obviously closed and arrogant. The emphasis of Actualizing Therapy is that a *person* is both active and passive, strong and weak, angry and loving. The actualizing person rhythmically expresses all aspects of his being.

When men and women reach the period from ages forty to fifty, a crucial psychological change occurs. Jung (1933) describes this change vividly as follows:

> There are many women who only awake to social responsibility and to social consciousness after their fortieth year. In modern business life—especially in the United States—nervous breakdown in the forties or after is a very common occurrence. If one studies the victims a little closely one sees that the thing which has broken down is the style of life which held the field up to now; what is left is a tender man. Contrariwise, one can observe women in these self-same business spheres who have developed in the second half of life an uncommon incisiveness which pushes the feelings and the heart aside. Very often the reversal is accompanied by all sorts of catastrophes in marriage; for it is not hard to imagine what may happen when the husband discovers his tender feelings, and the wife her sharpness of mind. (p. 124)

It would seem, therefore, that one aspect of love in marriage, at this stage of life, should involve each partner's understanding and encouraging the development of neglected potentials in the other. This would mean the development of respect for the individuality of each. As Fromm (1962) points out, Freud's extreme patriarchalism led to the assumption that sexuality per se is masculine; thus he ignored the values of feminine character components.

Immature love in the involutional phase, therefore, would be criticized in the same way that Freud is criticized by Fromm (1956): "My criticism of Freud's theory is not that he overemphasized sex, but his failure to understand sex deeply enough" (p. 37). The middle-aged revolter can often be helped to regain his love for his spouse when sex is translated and deepened into a characterological and psychological dimension.

After Sixty

According to Erikson (1950), this period of later maturity is one of *integrity* or of *despair,* depending on the individual's adaptation to life. The self-actualizing possessor of integrity is ready to maintain the dignity of personal interdependence. On the other hand, fear of death and the feeling that one's life was spent unwisely can lead to a period of despair and renewed dependence. Erikson relates the period of adult integrity to the first stage of infantile trust by saying that "healthy children will not fear life if their parents have integrity enough not to fear death" (p. 233).

According to Adler (in Ansbacher & Ansbacher, 1956), a major problem of old age is that of not knowing what to do with leisure time. The elderly feel futile and useless, and try to prove their worth again, just as adolescents do. "They interfere and want to show in many different ways that they are not old and will not be overlooked, or else they become disappointed or depressed" (p. 443).

Because most women outlive men, Havighurst (1953) claims that by the late 1960s there were, in the average community, as many widows as there were women living with their husbands. Learning to live alone again, to attend to business matters, can be a difficult task to undertake. The various solutions to this problem generally involve moving into "leisure world" communities, living with children, remarriage, or moving in with relatives.

Even though there is *bodily decline* in this period, the *personality* can continue to grow and mature intellectually and emotionally (as shown in Figure 29) as long as interdependence is established—through finding what it means to be "retired," through identifying with the achievements of offspring, and by evident results of work, play, and community service. It seems, therefore, that old age can be enriched by a healthy, interdependent view of life.

Gilbert (1952) suggests that older people can maintain psychic health if they will "develop neglected potentials." Areas for development might include service, travel, music, arts and crafts, and gardening, as well as developing one's professional competence further.

Fisher (1951) a practicing psychiatrist in his later years, wrote vividly of his feelings about growing old:

> If it is a sad thing to be a psychiatrist because you become uncomfortably aware of your own neurotic tendencies, then, I have discovered in recent years, it is a doubly sad thing to be an aged psychiatrist. For you may sit and watch the encroachment of senility with an abstract and almost professional attitude—like a surgeon watching the mirrored reflection of his own appendectomy.
>
> At least once to every man, I'd imagine, must come the sudden and disconcerting discovery that the corporate cells of his physical body are rapidly approaching insolvency. The sand is running low in the hourglass of time. And the option has already lapsed on a thousand youthful dreams which were never brought to pass. . . .
>
> Youth rides in the cab of the locomotive and jubilantly surveys the track ahead. Age rides in the observation car and gazes back with sweet sorrow, upon the fading scenes of the past. And it requires a certain amount of readjustment.
>
> In my struggle to avoid melancholia and to keep interested in the game, rather than bowing gracefully to Father Time who holds all the trumps, I have striven particularly hard in recent years to keep alive a fading curiosity and hold an open mind capable of admitting new ideas. This, in fact, is why I felt impelled to go traipsing off to Lima, Peru, at eighty-two years of age to study the progress of psychosomatic medicine.
>
> And thus, in my eight-seventh year, I find myself planning, not a trip back to Boston or Vienna, or Zurich, or Paris, or Chicago, or any of the places I have known in the past. Rather, my plans include a visit to Jackson Hole, Wyoming, and after that a trip up the Inside Passage to Alaska—two places where I have never been and both of them which have been described in glowing terms by others.
>
> And these things, I am afraid I would have to recommend to others who might come to me, as a psychiatrist, and ask how best to postpone the eventual encroachment of advancing senility. Don't sit in the observation car, with folded hands, gazing back upon the fading scenes of the past. Force yourself to seek new experiences and to turn your eyes to the track ahead. Spend at least a share of your time peering into the future. (pp. 254-256)

Love between husband and wife during these years can best be expressed by *agape III*—the dimension of knowledge. To love a person completely means, in part, to *know* them—from the very core of personality. Making this a developmental task of later maturity is a way in which the self-actualizing principle may be completed. Before death, persons can therefore discover, partially at least, the "secret of life." One's total being is unique and infinitely complex, but the penetration into the being of a person whom we love most completely expresses, in a very real, interdependent way, the need for self-understanding. Fromm (1962) illustrates this idea of more complete knowledge as follows:

> I may know, for instance, that a person is angry, even if he does not show it overtly; but I may know him more deeply than that; then I know that he is anxious, and worried; that he feels lonely, that he feels guilty. Then I know that his anger is only the manifestation of something deeper, and I see him as anxious and embarrassed, that is, as the suffering person rather than as the angry one. (p. 29)

Couples in the later phases of life who have an actualizing approach to living seem to have mastered the problem of really knowing one another in a way similar to that described above. This mastery seems to give them a certain peace not discernable in others and the *communication* of their knowledge freely to one another makes them a team in the business of living.

Facing death is a significant aspect of old age. The following statement from Bertrand Russell (1951) illustrates a quiet acceptance of death:

> Some old people are oppressed by the fear of death. In the young there is a justification for this feeling. Young men who have reason to fear that they will be killed in battle may justifiably feel bitter in the thought that they have been cheated of the best things that life has to offer. But in an old man who has known human joys and sorrows, and has achieved whatever work it was in him to do, the fear of death is somewhat abject and ignorable. The best way to overcome it—so at least it seems to me—is to make your interests gradually wider and more impersonal, until bit by bit the walls of the ego recede, and your life becomes increasingly merged in the universal life. An individual human existence should be like a river—small at first, narrowly contained within its banks, and rushing passionately past boulders and over waterfalls. Gradually the river grows wider, the banks recede, the waters flow more quietly, and in the end, without any visible break, they become merged in the sea, and painlessly lose their individual being. The man who, in old age, can see his life in this way, will not suffer from the fear of death, since the things he cares for will continue. And if, with the decay of vitality, weariness increases, the thought

of the rest will be not unwelcome. I should wish to die while still at work, knowing that others will carry on what I can no longer do, and content in the thought that what was possible has been done. (pp. 52-53)

The following, from Italian psychologist Roberto Assagioli (in Keen, 1974), spoken just a few weeks before his own death, also illustrates an actualizing attitude toward death:

Death looks to me primarily like a vacation. There are many hypotheses about death and the idea of reincarnation seems the most sensible to me. I have no direct knowledge about reincarnation but my belief puts me in good company with hundreds of millions of Eastern people, with the Buddha and many others in the West. Death is a normal part of a biological cycle. It is my body that dies and not all of me. So I don't care much. I may die this evening but I would willingly accept a few more years in order to do the work I am interested in, which I think may be useful to others. I am, as the French say, *disponable* (available). Also humor helps, and a sense of proportion. I am one individual on a small planet in a little solar system in one of the galaxies. (p. 107)

THE PRINCIPLE OF GENERATIONAL REVERSAL

As one views the life processes described in this chapter, one becomes aware that they are very much the same for every individual, regardless of race, creed, or color.

An orientation to living often seen in therapy is an individual's attempt to reverse the values of his parents. Thus, for such an individual, the truth of living becomes the values of the parents in reverse (see Figure 31). Such a person is simply going from one polarity to its opposite, and truth is never found by opposites. Only by a discovery of a principle of rhythmic living are people able to integrate dependence and independence, manipulation and directness, secretiveness and openness, decisiveness and evasiveness. Otherwise the process of generational reversal continues and the truth of rhythmic living is never discovered.

SUMMARY

In this chapter we have sketchily traced the life history of humankind. Much has been left out, of course, but at each stage we have described some of the significant activities and events that seem to have pronounced psychological effect upon the individual as he travels through life. It is hoped that students of Actualizing Therapy will utilize this chapter as a

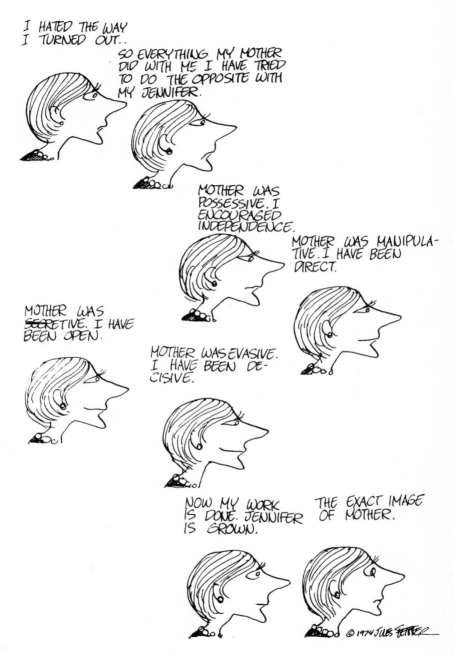

Figure 31. Generational Reversal

beginning in the collection of normative data. Such data can be useful in helping the therapist to understand his clients better as he meets them in various stages of life.

The "golden thread" running through this chapter is that each stage of life may be understood psychologically by relating it to the various forms of love as well as to the three dimensions of being.

CHAPTER 6. THE PROCESS OF ACTUALIZING THERAPY

Chapter 4 discussed the process of deterioration, whereby the manipulative responses and character styles deteriorate into psychotic styles. The purpose of Actualizing Therapy is to reverse this process, as Figure 32 reverses the processes shown earlier in Figure 23 (page 83). An examination of Figure 23 will show that as deterioration develops, the facade and various layers of the personality decrease in permeability and openness and increase in rigidity and in flexibility. The rigidity ultimately ends up at the psychotic level as either a chronically heavy barrier or an acute break in the wall.

In the process of actualizing, the reverse occurs: as actualizing develops, the facade increases in permeability and openness in contact with others, manipulative and character styles reduce, and, instead of psychoses, a core of being develops in which the individual is in contact with the essence of his being and at the same time is in contact with others at the facade level. This rhythmic expression of one's being is shown in Figure 32 by the arrows moving through the various levels of personality, to contact with the core, and then back again, to contact with others at the periphery of the personality.

Actualizing Therapy emphasizes progressive awareness through a *growth process.* To understand this process the reader should begin by looking at the concentric circles in Figure 32, starting at the outside circle and moving inward. These circles represent the four levels of personality:

1. *The actualizing level.* This is the level of freedom of *expression of feeling in contact* with others. This freedom in expression is illustrated by four modular feelings, moving from more passive to more active expression on each of these polarities.

2. *The manipulative level.* This level of expression represents ways of relating to others without having to feel. Instead, systems or "games" are used to manipulate the environment for support.

3. *The character level.* This level of expression consists of essentially negative feelings expressed by muscular rigidity designed to hold back other feelings.
4. *The core level.* This is the center of one's existence, which can be transformed into a "home" of harmony with the world when all levels of feeling in the personality are "worked through."

The process of actualizing begins with working through the manipulative and character levels to the core level and finally reaching the actualizing level, which then interacts coactively with the core, as shown by the arrows in Figure 32. Thus actualizing is both intra- and interpersonal.

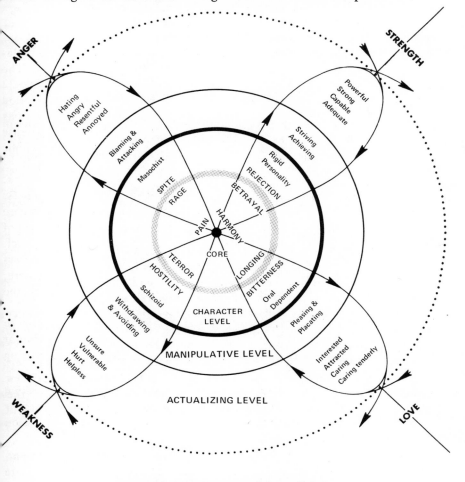

Figure 32. The Process of Actualizing

ANALYZING MANIPULATIVE STYLES

As implied in Chapter 5, the child, at the core level, needs to feel loved and lovable, but life experiences threaten this feeling as he is manipulated by parents and significant others. Through these experiences, he learns to avoid pain and to manipulate for survival. Manipulations are basically patterns of survival by which people adapt to their environment without having to feel. Figure 33 shows the manipulative patterns of the basic polarities broken down into eight specific manipulative styles.

Actualizing Therapy departs from Gestalt Therapy in that there is not a direct frustration or attacking of "phony manipulations" but rather a more gentle process of replacing manipulative and character patterns with actualizing patterns. This process requires the therapist to utilize *manipulation analysis* and the *manipulative dialogue.*

Manipulation Analysis

Description of primary manipulation is the first step in manipulation analysis. As the client talks, the therapist begins to see a pattern emerging in which the individual is utilizing one or two of the basic manipulative patterns shown in Figure 33. For example, the client may continuously resort to the patterns of helplessness and stupidity, characteristic of playing the weakling, or he may utilize the power plays and blackmailing techniques of bullying.

Once the pattern becomes clear, the Actualizing Therapist *describes* to the client what seems to be his primary manipulative game or games. Manipulations are then analyzed from the standpoint of "gains." The active manipulations are seen to have *coercive* controlling value, and the passive manipulations are seen to have *seductive* values. Gains are analyzed from the short-range, as well as from the long-range, viewpoint. The client is asked to state the short-range gains received from the particular manipulation. For example, manipulations are most often used for the control of others, for exploiting others, for avoiding situations, for structuring time, and for seducing others to work for one. From the long-range point of view, however, they can always be shown to be self-defeating, because they alienate the individual from others and keep him immature and dependent, rather than mature and self-supporting.

Restoring inner balance is the second concern in manipulation analysis. The principle of inner balance is illustrated by the rhythmic loops seen in the many figures in this book that show movement between the polarities of anger-love and strength-weakness. At any given time a client might be at

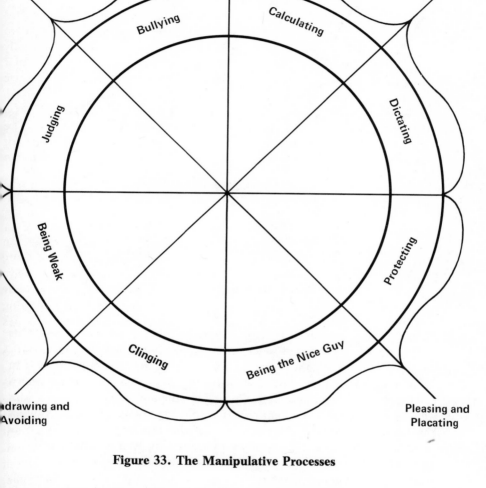

ming and
tacking

Striving and
Achieving

Bullying

Calculating

Judging

Dictating

Being Weak

Protecting

Clinging

Being the Nice Guy

drawing and
Avoiding

Pleasing and
Placating

Figure 33. The Manipulative Processes

any one point on either of these polarities. If, for example, a client is a little bit angry, as shown in Figure 34, the therapist will facilitate his expression in one of two ways: by encouraging *exaggeration* of the expression of anger, or by encouraging *reversal*—the expression of the opposite polar dimension. In the latter case he is likely to encounter some resistance from the client, since this is not where the client is "at" at this moment. Thus it may be wiser for the therapist to encourage the intensification of the feeling of anger (see Figure 34A). The therapist's purpose in asking the client to

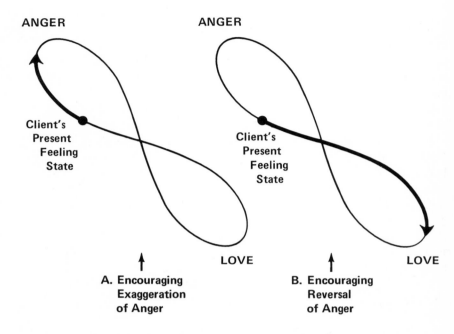

Figure 34. Restoring the Inner Balance

exaggerate the manipulative tendency is to allow him to experience its foolishness when expressed to such an extreme. As shown in Figure 34B, the therapist may ask the client to reverse—to express the opposite pole of the manipulative pattern he is demonstrating. For example, a person who is playing weak may be asked to try to play dictator. The reason for this technique is the fundamental hypothesis that the exaggerated expression of any manipulative pattern is indicative of the repression of the opposite pattern. For example, playing weak by expressing hurt is usually covering up a strong need to dictate and to express the vindictiveness that a dictator might feel. A clinging person, through the expression of dependency, is really covering up a deeper need to control others and to calculate. Playing nice guy, a person may attempt to make others feel guilty for contesting him, and he is often covering up a need to express his hostility. The protecting person, in his need to feel his responsibility for others, is often covering up his need to play judge and to be omnipotent. The therapist, however, must constantly be aware of the principle of resistance and not *demand* the expression of any feeling but rather *encourage* feeling expression.

Integration, the final step in manipulation analysis, involves merging both active and passive dimensions into a unified working whole. In order to do this, the therapist continues to encourage the client to express all of his active and passive potentials, so that he might appreciate that actualizing involves the integration of all his polarities into a unified whole. The actualizing person is like an ice skater who freely skates from one potential to another, creatively employing each in his movement through life.

In this connection, the client must realize that *self-defeating* manipulative behavior may be naturally transformed into self-fulfilling actualizing behavior: Dictating can be transformed into leading, playing weak can be transformed into empathizing, and so on. Any behavior at the manipulative level can be transformed into actualizing alternatives at the actualizing contact level (see Figures 33 and 35).

How manipulative behavior is transformed into actualizing behavior needs further explanation. This is a process of changing one's attitude or set about a behavior. Psychologically, an attitude is a kind of mental set. It represents a predisposition to think, and feel, and act in certain ways. Referring to Figure 36, an attitude can be seen as a frame of reference. How a frame of reference can change one's view of himself as manipulating or actualizing is illustrated by this diagram, in which the interpretation of the inner figure depends on the outer frame. In 36A and 36B, the inner figures are the same, yet one appears as a diamond and the other as a square. In 36C and 36D, the situation is reversed. The same figure can be either a diamond or a square, depending on how it is framed.

If one thinks of the inner figure as himself, the diamond as actualizing, and the square as manipulating, then it follows that one's opinion of himself depends on his frame of reference. This frame of reference is one's attitude toward himself. Therapy deals with "twisting" the frame of reference through experiences. It means developing an *awareness* of one's worth by understanding that his manipulative behavior was an attempt to survive in a world that has manipulated him, and that actualizing is transforming this self-defeating pattern into a self-fulfilling pattern at the core level.

The Manipulative Dialogue

The manipulative dialogue is a variation of Perls' "hot seat" empty-chair technique. The hot seat is the chair the client sits in and the "empty chair" faces the client. The empty chair represents the many "selves" within, as shown in Figure 33. Moreover, the empty chair may also represent a physical *symptom*, an *object* in a dream, or *other persons* in the client's

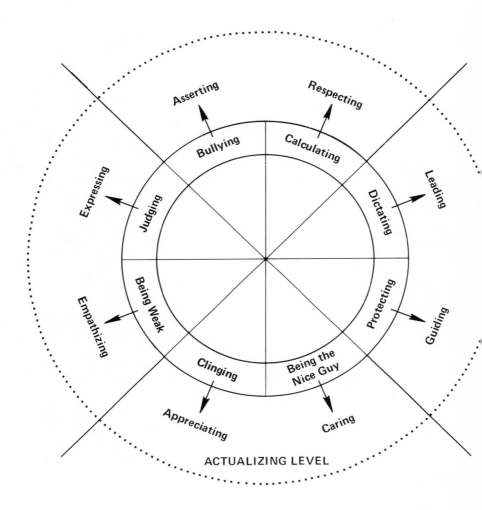

Figure 35. Actualizing Alternatives to Manipulating

life. A person whose personality is fragmented by polarization operates in an either/or manner. He plays nice guy or bully; he is strong or weak. In Actualizing Therapy, one learns to play both ends of his polarities.

The therapist asks the client to switch chairs, playing the role of nice guy in one chair and bully in the other, alternately. When sufficient switching takes place, each side of the dialogue can "appreciate" the other, and integration is taking place. The tendency for most people is to *reject* one side of themselves, rather than to accept and integrate. The integration is

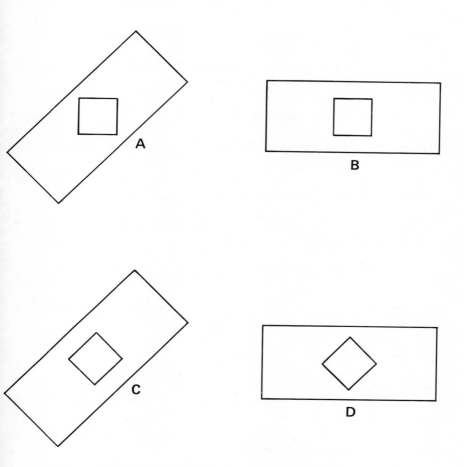

The inner geometrical figures in A and B are the same, yet they are seen as a diamond and a square, respectively, because they are framed differently. The same two frames applied to the small figures in C and D make them appear as a square and diamond, respectively. Just as the frame gives specific meaning to the inner figure, so an attitude determines an opinion. A change in attitude may radically change opinions. (After Koffka, 1935.)

Figure 36. The Influence of a Frame of Reference

similar to seeing that it is basically one's attitude toward oneself that makes one worthy or not.

Perhaps the most important thing to understand is that an individual may be compared to a two-party system in politics, to a battery with positive and negative poles. The actualizing person is developed from the integration of manipulative poles. A simple example illustrates:

Therapist: Be your top-dog self.

Client [as top dog]: I run this show, Marian. I think you're worthless. You have no value. You're too damn nice!

Therapist: Now, be the underdog and answer.

Client [as underdog]: I think I have value. What makes you think you're so damn smart?

Therapist: Change roles again.

Client [as top dog]: You just smile: you're trying to act worthwhile, but you aren't. Without me you'd be lost!

Therapist: What does she answer?

Client [as underdog]: But I do care for people! You always try to push them around.

Therapist: Give her hell!

Client [as underdog]: You're such a big shot that I'm not going to waste my time with you. I don't care what you think, I'm the one that really cares about people!

Therapist: How do you feel now?

Client: I feel better. Together.

This exchange shows an individual *listening* to both sides of herself, both "weak" (underdog) and "strong" (top dog). Through the conflict, antagonistic poles become complementary.

A further step in the process of integration comes when both top dog and underdog learn to appreciate one another. The following sequence illustrates this process:

Therapist: Be the top dog and tell the underdog what you appreciate about her.

Client [as top dog]: Well, I guess without you I wouldn't have my friends. You're the one who expresses tenderness toward others.

Therapist: Now be the underdog and answer.

Client [*as underdog*]: That's right. Why haven't you appreciated that before?

Therapist: Now continue being the underdog and tell the top dog what you appreciate about her.

Client [*as underdog*]: Well, sometimes I think you're just a bigmouth, but I guess without you people would push me around a lot. I appreciate your aggressiveness.

Therapist: Answer as top dog.

Client [*as top dog*]: Well, why the hell don't we work together?

Therapist: Be the underdog.

Client [*as underdog*]: Yes, that's a good idea.

A final step in such an internal dialogue could focus on the *need* of the top dog and underdog for each other:

Therapist: Be the top dog and tell the underdog how much you need her.

Client [*as top dog*]: I really need you to balance my insensitivity.

Therapist: Be the underdog and answer.

Client [*as underdog*]: Yes, but I need you to balance my passivity.

Therapist: Be the top dog and answer.

Client [*as top dog*]: I guess we're really facing how much we need each other.

Therapist: Be the underdog and answer.

Client [*as underdog*]: Finally!

Appreciation and acceptance of both sides of oneself leads to the power of integration.

THE CHARACTER LEVEL

Character styles, which are complex systems of negative muscular defenses, have their roots in early manipulations by parents and significant others. Thus, we cross over the "Iron Curtain" in Figure 32 to the new game of character styles. The relationship between manipulative and character patterns is as follows:

1. Pleasing and placating is often transformed into the *oral character.* The oral person needs *love,* but he feels abandoned by parents or significant others. He feels dependent and fears isolation.

2. Blaming and attacking often turns into the *masochistic character,* who has been crushed by parents or others and needs *freedom.* He feels burdened by their demands, but fears expressing anger, because he fears losing others.

3. Striving and achieving having failed, the *rigid character* develops. He needs to *love others,* but having been rejected as a child, his strength and independence have become a substitute for his real need to love—to give his heart to someone.

4. Withdrawing and avoiding not having worked, the *schizoid character* has contracted further and seeks solace in his illusion that his being is his *mind.* He avoids relationships. But he still needs to *exist.*

As the therapist and client discuss the client's present and past relationships, manipulative and character styles are discovered and exposed. The client has to become aware of his primary manipulative patterns and learn to understand the muscular character blocks that reinforce his manipulative patterns. His body expresses the feelings of distrust and hostility in three ways, according to Kirsh (1973):

1. *Holding.* Tight, spastic muscles bind feelings inside the body.

2. *Flacidity.* Flacid, unusually flexible muscles also bind affect.

3. *Hyperactivity.* Muscles become hypermotile so there is an inability to maintain feelings.

The levels of the personality each have significant feelings associated with them, and these feelings become the focus of psychotherapy. It should be noted that, at the level of manipulation, feelings are *avoided* whereas they become *defensive* or *hostile* at the character level. Finally, at the core, these feelings merge into feelings of pain and hurt.

Character Feelings

When clients begin to work with the body (see Figure 32), the *feelings* expressed (shown at the *character* level) are deep historical feelings that are lodged in the muscle structure as *masochistic spite, oral bitterness, schizoid hostility,* or *rigid rejection.* All these basically hostile feelings develop early in the growth years in response to parental, and other authorities', rejections of one's behavior.

The Character Dialogue

Earlier in this chapter we referred to the manipulative dialogue, which is a variation of Perls' "hot seat" technique. When working with the client at the character level, we refer to the "hot bed" technique. In this approach, derived from the work of Lowen and used either in group or individual therapy, the client lies on a couch, mattress, or pad, and assumes the more passive role characteristic of a child in a crib.

Because everyone has elements of each of the four character styles in his personality, the therapist may express all four varieties of parental rejection toward the client. Most clients will respond to all of them, but they will respond in particular to the ones that seem most characteristic of those they experienced as children with their parents. Once the therapist hears that certain parental admonitions create deeper responses, he tends to zero in on them.

The therapist, through the technique of *character dialogue*, "plays" the role of parents and significant others, expressing the negativity, abandonment, and rejection that they used to manipulate the client earlier in life. This causes angry and rageful feeling, *character feelings*, to be loosened openly. The client traditionally lies on the couch, kicks his legs, pounds his hands, and screams "No!" many times in a tantrumlike refutation of such parental patterns:

Schizoid Client: I AM! [core need: to feel his *existence*].

Therapist [leaning over the client on the "hot bed" and expressing the original parental response]: You are nothing! [*or*] We don't want you! [*or*] I wish you weren't here! [*or*] I wish you were never born!

Schizoid Client: No! No! No! I hate you!

Oral Client: I NEED! [core need: to feel *wanted*].

Therapist: Your needs don't matter! [*or*] There are other people around here besides you! [*or*] Forget it, you're not important!

Oral Client: No! No! No! I don't need you!

Masochistic Client: I WANT TO BE FREE! [core need: to feel *free*].

Therapist: We understand. [*or*] Don't worry about us. [*or*] Just remember all we've done for you. [*or*] Respect your father.

Masochistic Client: No! No! No! Get off my back!

Rigid Client: I WANT YOUR LOVE! [core need: to feel *love*].

Therapist: Of course, you know I love you. [*or*] Stop pestering me! [*or*] Don't sit so close! [*or*] Don't touch yourself there.

Rigid Client: No! No! No! I don't need your love!

THE CORE LEVEL

Once the client has expressed responses to both manipulative and character patterns within, the awareness that results from this expression will lead to the core level of his being. This is in contrast to the processes of deterioration, described in Chapter 4, in which no awareness develops and in which character and manipulative patterns may, instead, deteriorate into psychoses. It must be remembered that the process of Actualizing Therapy is never clearly advancing from one level of personality expression to another, but rather, is a continuous process of reaching the client in multiple ways at all levels of expression. Ultimately, however, the actualizing person becomes more in touch with his core feelings.

At the deepest level of the core, there is an expressed hurt or pain that reflects the experiences of childhood: "Why wasn't I loved, given freedom to be, the right to exist?" All people, to some degree, feel the core pain shown in Figure 32. *Core pain* may be defined as the reaction of the individual to the suppression of his basic right to exist in the world. Sometimes release of these feelings, through the exercises and techniques presented in detail in Chapter 7, causes recall of specific events that led to those feelings. At other times, the recollection of specific childhood experiences is *not* necessary, since the breaking down of body blocks to expression is sufficient for release and working through.

The most important method for opening up the core is *affect release*—expressing the *feelings* shown in Figure 32 at the *core level*. Such expression will lead to the release of the core pain, which manifests itself in the following forms:

1. *Rage.* The masochistic person has deep feelings of murder and rage from parental suppression of growth and expression.

2. *Longing.* The oral dependent person feels deep sadness and longing for the parent, for closeness, for touch and nourishment.

3. *Terror.* The schizoid person has deep feelings of fear of annihilation by parental rage and hatred. Usually these fears are reactions to threat in the first six months of life.

4. *Betrayal.* The rigid person has deep feelings of betrayal because of rejection by his parents, often related to erotic genital needs.

All people have, deep within their cores, all these feelings to some extent. Through individual therapy, working with the body, they must all ultimately be expressed. Specific methods are discussed in Chapter 7.

The *process of growth* in Actualizing Therapy interrupts the deterioration process and instead reverses manipulative patterns and character defenses to create a new center of being for the individual: the *core. When one experiences his core feelings, the pain he has experienced in living is replaced by a feeling of harmony with the world and with himself.* When harmony exists in the core, there is a relaxation of inner and outer conflicts. This relaxation is experienced as a liberation of previously bound-up energy. The person is free to actualize his being because he now has the *energy* previously used to bind conflicts. *A basic theorem of Actualizing Therapy is that the release of conflict equals actualizing energy.*

An important principle of Actualizing Therapy is that one cannot reach the feeling of harmony within the core without experiencing the layer of pain within the core. As Lowen has suggested, when a hand is frozen the process by which it becomes unfrozen is painful, but the result is to move from deadness to aliveness—from immobility to freedom.

Integration and Acceptance of Losses

When a person can give in to his spontaneous body movement expressing his original core needs, integration of body and feeling takes place. This process takes time, however, and therapy repeats it many times.

After integration of body and feeling, realistic acceptance of losses takes place. At the character level the *oral* person accepts that his longing will never be fully filled. The *masochist* gives up his feelings of hostility and spite and accepts his limited freedom. The *rigid* person accepts his betrayal and accepts his heartbreak and his need for love. The *schizoid* person accepts his aloneness and his reality of existence. All become more lovable and loving in spite of their hurt or losses.

It should be stressed at this point that each person can be thought of as having a kind of profile of each of the character types described above. Each person is oral to some degree, masochistic to some degree, schizoid to some degree, and rigid to some degree. When one becomes integrated in therapy, he has to accept the losses in each of these four character profiles, but he also comes to accept the strength that comes from his greater understanding of his historical analysis and from his deeper understanding of how his thoughts, feelings, and body work together. In his acceptance of his losses as well as his strengths, he finds a new *harmony* within himself.

The Involuntary Nature of the Core

An understanding of the core is essential to actualizing. Coming home to one's core is a form of surrender to self, the center of one's existence. It means giving in to the fact that one no longer needs his defensive postures, because he has found his "God within"; the power within the core.

The myth of modern living that has been ingrained in most people is that one's core being cannot be trusted. People have been taught that they must look without for direction from authorities—that they must look to the 1001 commandments for living provided by our society. Typical comments are "If I really trust my anger, I will ultimately kill someone." "If I really let people know that I care, they will take advantage of me." "If I really let people know how strong I feel, they will think I am conceited." "If I really let people know how weak I am, they will defeat me."

The psychology of core being contradicts all of these statements. It is a difficult, but *viable,* philosophy of life.

The *core* is defined as the involuntary energy center for the individual, from which one gets feelings of love for oneself. Trusting one's core is finding the energy within to love oneself. In this context we define actualizing as equivalent to tapping one's core, as opposed to living defensively at a manipulative or character level. The key problem, however, is that living from the core means living *involuntarily* rather than *voluntarily.* It has to be *effortless* instead of *effortful*; it means letting go; it means trusting your own core. It means learning to live without trying, or without effort, and this is contrary to what we, in Western culture, have been taught as children—that we have to try harder.

Suzuki (1953) says, "As soon as we reflect, deliberate, or conceptualize, the original unconscious [core] is lost" (p. 11). Similarly, when Maslow describes peak experiences, he speaks of experiencing effortlessness, freedom from blocks, here-and-nowness, nonstriving, and isness.

Most people's problems come from the fact that they have been taught to evaluate their own behavior as good or bad, right or wrong. When one enters this evaluative way of thinking, he tries harder to avoid badness or wrongness and to repeat goodness. But in each case he ends up trying harder, tightening his muscles and creating internal tension. The alternative to the good-bad bind is simply to trust the isness of one's core, and to avoid the self-judgments that create tension and tightness. An example comes from common gardening. When we plant a seed in the ground, we don't judge it as bad if it doesn't grow immediately. We simply wait for its inner potential to emerge. So the process of trusting one's core is a natural learning process that involves behavior above criticism or compliments from the outside. As Gallwey (1974) says, "Compliments are criticisms in disguise! Both are used to manipulate behavior" (p. 43).

In contrast to the manipulative or character levels, which are voluntary aspects of being, the core may be seen as an *involuntary* reservoir of universal wisdom. The ability to feel one's own core involves a quality of *surrender* to one's own involuntary reservoir of wisdom, rather than a willing or voluntary effort.

Living has to do with willing versus surrendering. Being one's core is a surrender to the reality of life. The best example is trying to get someone to love you. The more you try, the less you succeed. You can never *make* anyone love you; you can only be yourself openly and hope that someone may choose to love you. But many people spend their lives effortfully trying to make people love them through their achievements or manipulations. An example is the father who works day and night to provide well for his family through his work achievements. But love is never given to the achievement; it comes only in the experience of being with another in a relationship. By keeping away from his family in order to "earn" their love, the father is actually losing it. So, paradoxically, to be loved is to stop trying to be loved.

Thus the problem of being one's core involves *efforless effort.* The paradox is that in one sense the harder one tries, the more one fails. This idea is evident in such activities as swimming, in which the more one tries to float, the more one sinks. However, in actualizing, as in swimming, there are certain principles one can learn that will facilitate the process. One of these principles, for example, is synergy. If for every truth there is an equal and opposite counter-truth, then actualizing implies that trying to be any one virtue will be self-destructive. Actualizing requires an awareness of certain principles that provide a backdrop for being, but not a demand or expectation for any specific form of being. Thus, being is simply a surrender.

Relation of Core to the AAB

We believe that the Actualizing Assessment Battery reflects certain principles that will effectively help the person to be oneself more easily, both intrapersonally and interpersonally. These instruments do not have a demand quality but simply suggest principles to more effectively play the game of life. In taking the Battery, one expresses oneself involuntarily in a voluntary way. Thus, the use of the POI, the POD, the PAI, and the CRI becomes a very important therapeutic method.

Another way of describing the core has to do with the POI Inner- and Other-Directedness score. If one believes that his core is like a super self-directing computer within, a sophisticated and competent expression of his being, he simply lets it control him like an inner thermostat. But letting go is different from controlling. It is permitting oneself to be, without contracting and tightening one's muscles. It is discovering that all the potential for being comes from within, without effortful work.

The core is the essence of one's being, but, paradoxically, one's being cannot be expressed on demand. It has to be expressed almost involuntarily. The more you try, the more you fail. Getting to the deepest meaning of what inner-direction means, which is the goal of self-actualizing, is getting to the core of the theory of this book and the core of the theory of the POI.

The lack of trust of one's own being makes one become a taskmaster of oneself, a believer of rules instead of a believer in one's inner thermostat. Living from the core is *believing* that there *is* an inner thermostat. And actualizing is trusting that one's thermostat naturally works. If one is time competent (as measured by the POI), one is in the here and now and trusts that the past and the future will take care of themselves. Some people spend their lives in the past and future, and grow old never having lived in the present.

All the inventories in the Actualizing Assessment Battery are intellectual instruments because one is required to *think* about oneself. But the more one tries to think only about how to be actualizing on the inventories, the more one tends to fail, because there is a tendency to deny one's humanness, as shown by many students instructed to "make a good impression" on the POI (see Chapter 2). Those who try this on the POI fail because inherent in the inventory is a concept of the synergy of human strengths and weaknesses. Most unsophisticated students do not understand this. The implications for living are even greater in that trying to understand inner-direction means listening to the core of one's being rather than imagining being good in terms of some external criterion.

Maslow described the core *intellectually* as trusting one's own "inner Supreme Court." Zen Buddhists describe the core *bodily* as listening to the sensations in and around the solar plexus. Rogers described the core as trusting one's own deepest *feelings*. From the frame of reference of the POI, actualizing means a bringing-together of inner-direction and here-and-nowness. One is not actualizing if he is living primarily in the past; one is not actualizing if he is living primarily in the future. Being in the core means being primarily in the now and attending to what one deeply feels in the moment. Thus, awareness is not only awareness of one's body and inner being, but an awareness of being in the moment.

Perls uses the illustration of cutting a record. Each person's life is like the cutting of a record from moment to moment. Being able to express the feelings of the current cutting edge of one's being comes closest to expressing what one's core being is. Thus, being in the moment, with an awareness of a present situation and a feeling of oneself and others about one, and then being able to express the essence of one's being in the moment, is being one's core.

Relation of Core to Group Therapy

In any actualizing interpersonal relationship, such as in a group setting, the pressures of interpersonal interaction often create an *imploding* process, as shown in Figure 37. Ultimately, this results in the principal participant's *exploding* with his feelings, resisting others with rage, betrayal, terror, and longing, characteristic of the polarities. This leads to the third step, *oozing*, in which individual members tend to meld together in their creative awareness of the humanness of all beings. It is this three-stage process that characterizes the various movements in the symphony of verbal interaction called group therapy. We use the word *oozing* because the psychotic tends to sputter between imploding and exploding, whereas the actualizing person comfortably pulsates between the polarities in terms of his awareness of his needs in the moment.

Core Living

Understanding core living makes the old-fashioned concept of the pursuit of happiness completely untenable. Core living means the ability to

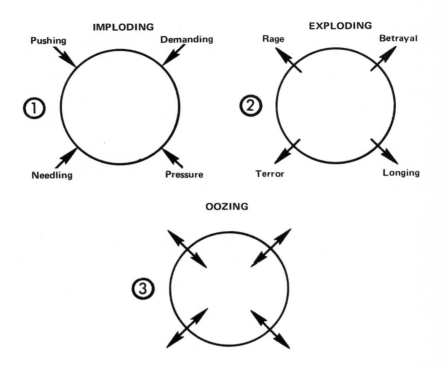

Figure 37. Actualizing Interpersonally

experience the peaks and valleys of life intensely. It means experiencing the periods of ecstasy and joy with feelings of fullness in the moment, but it also requires feeling the nadirs, or valleys, of life with equal intensity. Happiness is a unipolar concept rather than a synergistic one, and is therefore limited.

The analogy of one's core being as a kind of inner thermostat helps us to understand the difference between a person operating at an ego-defensive, or manipulative, level as opposed to an inner level of core being. The person at the manipulative or charcter levels of living, has no concept of an inner thermostat. Rather, he lives at a level of control. He must have his hand on the manual control of his own feelings at all times.

When one has come to terms with his core, he knows that he cannot fully live in the world by control or effortful striving. Rather, he must surrender to the fact that he cannot cope by striving; that to exist in the world, he must give in to a deeper principle within. In *religion* this is called surrender to God. In *biology* it is surrender to one's own nature. In *poetry* it is described as a discovery of what the poet Galway Kinnell (1971) calls "tenderness toward existence" (p. 29). In *psychology* it is surrender to one's core.

THE ACTUALIZING LEVEL

The ultimate step in Actualizing Therapy is learning to come home to the core of one's being. Having learned to move out interpersonally in the group and to become free with the expression of deep character feelings, the client now gets a feeling of "coming home." Replacing the *core pain* is a feeling of harmony with the world and a feeling of having the right to exist. The client feels that others can no longer control him; that there are no more parents in the world whom the client will permit to control him. He has become his own "inner Supreme Court." He can be his adult feelings and his child feelings. He can ask for what he wants, and he manipulates minimally. He has the right to be human, with all the accompanying privileges.

Actualizing means returning to permeable openness and a lack of defensive structures. It means returning to the full rhythm of the original core expression of anger-love and strength-weakness. It is a return to a belief in *inner-directedness* and a reduction in the other-directedness of trusting one's life to others. Life now is the growth of the new child that has been reborn within. Contact with others in the environment becomes free and expressive, and one's own existence is felt to be in tune with the rhythm expressed from within the core.

To be in touch with one's core means to be in touch with life itself. In place of defensive and manipulative living is the feeling of loss of boundary while still retaining identity. This is illustrated by the permeable wall of the core in Figure 32. The self is no longer a constantly constricting fortress for protection from a hostile environment, but rather, like the human heart, is in a state of constant full-feeling expansion and contraction without fear.

Contrasting Figure 23, "The Process of Deterioration," with Figure 32, "The Process of Actualizing," the following is evident:

1. As actualizing develops, the facades increase in permeability and openness and decrease in rigidity and inflexibility. This is illustrated by the reduction in heaviness of the walls in Figure 32 and is expressed by spontaneous, as opposed to calculated, behavior.

2. In the process of actualizing, the rhythm increases in fluidity and results in more and more freedom of expression of one's behavior, as illustrated by the arrows in Figure 32 showing movement between the environment and the core.

3. The core of the rigidification process ends up in psychosis, with either a chronically heavy barrier or an acute break in the wall, while the core of the actualizing person is permeable and flexible.

4. In the process of deterioration, the polarities reflect more defensive postures and have a constricted quality, whereas in actualizing, the polarities are rhythmic and expressive.

Thus the actualizing person freely experiences and expresses himself at the actualizing level but is aware of his manipulation at the manipulative and character levels. He is also aware of his huge reservoir of core where he now has tapped the energy of his thinking, feeling, and bodily responses. The paradox, then, of actualizing comes from the individual's awareness that he has, within himself, the possibility for deterioration into psychosis as well as the possiblity for growing into actualizing. This very awareness spurs the actualizing person into creative thinking, feeling, and bodily response. And it is the awareness of his own freedom to move either way that gives him the limits of his potentials for deterioration, as well as for growth. Robert Frost has said, "Freedom moves most easily in harness." Adler has said, "The possibility of inferiority leads to growth." Both are right. It is the potentiality for either psychosis or actualizing that makes the living of each day a creative act.

A Personal Illustration

Rock musician Stevie Wonder was born blind and therefore has had the "advantage" of not seeing as most people do. He has related to others not on the basis of their external facade but rather in terms of what he calls their "inner face." He does not have to deal with that portion of people's external facade that is contributed by physical appearance, so he is better able to read them in terms of their inner "core" of being.

When one contrasts the facade with the core, or the outer face with the inner face, three alternatives seem to occur:

1. The outer face may be beautiful and the inner face ugly. An example of such a person would be a model who only smiles to try to impress others but does not feel the warmth within.

2. The outer face may be ugly and the inner face beautiful. An example would be a waitress whose personal appearance is not beautiful but whose manner expresses warmth and kindness.

3. The outer face and the inner face may both be beautiful (or ugly). This is what Rogers (1951) refers to as "congruence," in which inner and outer are in alignment with each other. In this case, the actualizing person would be aware of, or be *experiencing,* his own core needs and feelings, and would also be willing to risk *expressing* those feelings in contact with others. A nonactualizing manipulation would be characterized by the unverbalized demand that the other person sense one's feelings without one's openly expressing them.

In current vogue is the trend among certain young people to see only the inner face and to disregard the facade or outer appearance. They look only for "beautiful people." From an actualizing point of view, the inner and the outer face, or the core and the facade, should be in relative alignment so that one can "read" the other person's inner state of being from his outer state of being. This is an ideal, however, that few people achieve completely.

EXPERIENCING THE CORE

Therapy consists primarily of working through the *hostility, bitterness, spite,* and *rejection;* the *terror, longing, betrayal,* and *rage* that has developed from the pain in one's interpersonal relationships with others who have hurt him in the process of growing up. Once one has worked through these deep feelings of pain, he then becomes free to experience the true core of his being, which results in feelings of harmony rather than pain.

The core is a concept that has been discussed extensively in the preceding pages but that needs to be *experienced* and not simply talked about. Therapy can be viewed as having two dimensions: the *inter*personal and the *intra*personal. The interpersonal dimension can be seen as horizontal—it has to do with interpersonal relationships with others on a horizontal plane. The three aspects of being, however, can be seen in the intrapersonal context—existing on a vertical as well as horizontal dimension. The following exercise may be helpful in experiencing the vertical dimension, or what we have come to call the "psychic elevator":

> Your three aspects of being can be viewed vertically, beginning with your head. Imagine a laser beam of energy that focuses intensely, first on your brain or intellect. Imagine the energy surrounding your thought processes.
> But thinking is not enough. Continue with the vertical beam of light energy and let it go down through your throat and into the region of your heart, merging your thinking with your feelings of warmth or tenderness. Let the laser beam fully embrace this part of your being.

Now let the laser energy move into the region of your solar plexus, the place where ancient Oriental psychologists have defined the center of your being, or your core. This is where your "inner Supreme Court" is located. This is where you "come home" to yourself. See if you can feel your laser energy embracing the center of your identity.

Finally, let the laser spread down into your legs and into the earth so that you feel your body fully grounded.

Now see if you can experience all three aspects of your being: your thinking at the top, your feelings in the center, around your heart and solar plexus, and your body being grounded—completing your feeling of totally being in the now. Harmony now prevails among the three aspects of being and there is a feeling of wholeness.

We have found this exercise helpful in presenting, as a physiological experience, the three aspects of being that we discuss theoretically throughout this volume. Its utilization can be helpful in making the theory of this book a practical and real experience.

CONCLUSION

We would like to end this chapter with an eloquent statement from our colleague Alan Levy. Written from the point of view of the client, it is illustrative of the processes described here, and we hope it will provide the reader with a more personal view of the therapeutic experience.

I'm the patient and you're the therapist. I hire you for your attention, your awareness, and your guidance on the most significant and perilous journey of my life: a journey to the center of me.

Please be there, with me and for me, like a wise and loving parent to my inner child. I dare to trust that you'll be straight with me, that you won't spare me the truth about how you feel me and observe me. I need to know that you will touch me when and in a way that I am moved to grow from your message. And I expect the most powerful meanings to come from under the words.

As my need is intense, I demand that you be good to yourself so that you can care for me, and not abandon me as I search.

I want to experience the reality of my life; in accepting that, as painful as it is, I hope to know the pleasure of my life.

But I warn you, I won't give in to the truth without a fight. The stakes are too high. I have invested too heavily in protecting my ego illusions to surrender them easily. The inner battles between my hunger for security and my need for freedom are too intense for me to open up without fear. My fragile sense of self-esteem does not take kindly to opening the Pandora's box of my deepest feelings: the rage, the hunger, the terror within. No, I really don't trust that much of me. It is as if the movement inside were a kind of enemy. And I will not surrender to it until I can wholeheartedly believe that my aliveness will not destroy me but, ultimately, will bring me more joy in living. I need you as a bridge to that faith.

So here I am, facing you with a mixed bag of hope and despair, helplessness and resistance, ambivalently prepared to invest an unknown and unforeseeable amount of time, money, and energy in a quest for what I only vaguely know as "wanting to feel better."

Why?

What do I want?

I want more of my life . . . and I'm afraid of living it.

I want your help . . . and I want to stay in charge.

I want you with me . . . while I push you away.

I want to face reality . . . and find Santa Claus.

I want to love . . . without opening my heart to more hurt.

I want to give up the fruitless struggle to recover what I've lost . . . yet I refuse to acknowledge that I *have* lost.

I want your support . . . Leave me alone! I can do it myself!

Insight is not enough. Analytic answers, will power, rational thinking, and self-control programs all fall short of what a person needs to grow on. I need to be *moved* to change. Instead of proving or improving myself, I need to experience the pleasure of unified contact with myself and others, the shift in my energy from holding and unfeeling activity to self-expression. I need less of my will-exercising and goal-bound determination and more of my irrationality. My heart needs to open. My body needs to know.

As I allow the child-within to play in the light, expressing what is there, regardless of how trivial, foolish, or "ugly" it may be, I will breathe more easily. As I breathe, I will feel more. As I feel, I will know more, experience more of the real world, and act out less of my need-clouded imaginary world. As I surrender to that reality, I have more of me and more to give.

Maybe, if you're gentle and straight with me, I can learn how I stand in my own sunshine, how and why I split away from my richest life experiences, and resist reaching for and taking in pleasure. Maybe I can understand how I've come to hold out against the very love and strength of the nourishing parent that I've needed and needed to be all along.

That is what I bring to you today. And I face you in shyness. Immediately, something stirs inside, and it's not under my control. I grin, almost grimly; my breathing stops. And the grin says:

"I'm embarrassed . . . and I'm fighting my vulnerability by pretending I'm really in charge.

"I'm having such a fun time . . . yet angry enough to kill and scared to death.

"I'm not at all resisting you; see what a nice cooperator I am?
. . . I resent being this exposed.

"Don't hurt me. I'm needy and sad . . . and I'd rather die than
admit it."

And each time I encounter you, I am reminded that those
inadmissible, uncomfortable feelings are real parts of me, and it
becomes a little easier for me to trust me and you and what
happens between us. A faith is building in me: the struggle, the
mutual honesty, the contact that I'm too shy to ask for directly,
but somehow comes anyway . . . the life in me . . . all will lead
me home.

Home is my core. It is where I live, love, and die.

CHAPTER 7. THE TECHNIQUES OF INDIVIDUAL ACTUALIZING THERAPY

Therapy is as much an art as it is a science. The artistic dimension comes into play most prominently in the therapist's ability to accurately sense whether to respond to the client's thoughts, his feelings, or his bodily expressions. As in the Gestalt model, it is almost as if, at certain times, one of them becomes figure and the other two become ground.

As a general guide, the following principles may be helpful:

1. If a client maintains his focus on thinking only, then the therapist would do well to transfer to the level of feeling or bodily response. For example, he may say, "I want to hear what you feel about that," or "I want to focus on how your body is responding, and not simply continue to focus on your thoughts."

2. If the client is responding only at the level of feeling, the therapist may say, "There seems to be a thread running through the feelings you are expressing. Do you see what it is?"

3. If the therapist has been working with the client at the body level only, the therapist might say, "I think that's enough work on the body today. Let's sit up now and talk about the meaning of what we have been doing."

In other words, a textbook cannot specifically tell the reader *when* to do what, but it can offer suggestions for transferring from one aspect of being to another. A corollary to this principle is that any one session might focus on one aspect of being only. For example, we may work with the body for a total session, and the next session we may focus intellectually on the meanings that the former session had. The important principle in Actualizing Therapy is to maintain *flexibility* and not to hold rigidly to simply one aspect of being.

FEELING TECHNIQUES

The following sections discuss particular techniques the therapist might use when focusing on the feeling aspect of being.

Reflection of Feeling

Reflection of feeling is the reexpression, in *fresh* words, of the essential *attitudes* (not so much the content) expressed by the client. The therapist mirrors the client's feelings to increase his self-understanding and to show him that he is being understood. The word "fresh" is emphasized because perhaps the most glaring reflection error of the novice therapist is to mirror exactly the words already used by the client. The Actualizing Therapist should use sufficiently different words in a personalized response.

The word "feeling" is emphasized in the definition to make the therapist aware that he must be able to grasp the underlying *feeling* about what is being said, not just the *content*. Verbal expression is often likened to a river, with the ripples on the surface corresponding to the content. But more important are the undercurrents—the underlying feelings. Considerable skill is necessary to develop the sensitivity necessary to identify these feelings immediately and to mirror them back.

Actualizing Therapy goes beyond Client-Centered Therapy in that the reflection of feeling would seem to involve a more critical dimension than simply the feelings expressed by the client. In the film *Target Five* (1964), Virginia Satir and Everett Shostrom talk about reflection as a technique that requires an analysis by the therapist as to whether he is responding to the client's *self*-feeling(s), to the client's feelings for some *other* person(s), or to the *situation*(s) in which the client finds himself. Therefore, self/other/situation must be kept in mind when responding to the feelings of the client.

Here is an example: If the client says to the therapist, "I am really angry at the situation at home with my father," the therapist can respond in three ways: He can focus on the *situation* of the father at home by saying "The situation with your father really seems to be deteriorating"; or he can respond in terms of the *"other,"* which is really the father: "You are really bothered by your father's attitudes in this situation"; or he may respond to the client's concern about him*self* in the situation: "You are really upset by the situation at home with your father."

Each of these responses reflects different dimensions of the total gestalt of the client's situation. They require an understanding that the reflector of feelings needs to have a clear comprehension of what is being said and an appropriate response to it. All three dimensions help make the client feel understood, and, of course, this is the first requirement of individual therapy.

Two other forms of reflection in Actualizing Therapy are those of reflection of experience and sharing of the therapist's feelings.

Reflection of Experience

A form of reflection in Actualizing Therapy that goes beyond the Rogerian reflection of feeling technique is reflection of experience. This is a technique in which the therapist observes the posture, gesture, tone of voice, and eyes of the client. The therapist reflects back to him not just his intended *feelings,* but also his *observed nonverbal behavior.* The Actualizing Therapy view states that much of a person's expressive potential is projected in his posture, movement, and voice. Actualizing Therapy assists the individual to discover and directly use the energy that otherwise is expended in these projections.

Reflection of experience technique focuses on the contradiction of what the client *says he feels* and what the therapist *sees or observes his total organism saying.* For example, the therapist may make such observations as: "You say that you are angry, but your mouth is smiling. An angry person does not smile." "You say that you hate me, but I seem to hear caring in your voice. Do you hear your anger-love polarity?" or "You say that you care, but every time you talk about her your voice is hostile."

The Actualizing Therapist must have the courage to reflect his own percepts of the client, as well as to state the client's intended or stated feelings. This requires confidence in one's ability to observe what is going on in the here and now of the situation.

Sharing of the Therapist's Feelings

Actualizing Therapy holds that the relationship between client and therapist is the central dimension of the therapeutic process. This relationship may be thought of as being expressed on a *continuum of personal responsiveness* with *reflection of feeling* at one end, *reflection of experience* in the center, and *sharing of the therapist's feelings* at the opposite end. Sharing of the therapist's feelings means the honest effort of the therapist to respond with his own experience in the moment with the client. Sharing of the therapist's feelings, therefore, goes to the deepest level of sharing on the part of the therapist—it is "modeling" for the client in the Behavior Therapy frame of reference. The therapist is modeling how to be a person and is not simply a technician mirroring the client's verbalizations. This requires risking and a willingness to share with the client the therapist's personal feelings at the moment. Utilizing this technique, a therapist might make such statements as: "I'm angry at you for letting her get to you like that." "You *always* hurt and never let yourself feel any other feelings. I'm upset about your limiting your repertoire of feelings." or "You are boring me now."

As with reflection of experience, sharing of the therapist's feelings is a unique dimension of Actualizing Therapy.

INTELLECTUAL INTERPRETATION TECHNIQUES

"Interpretation" has been defined as an attempt by the therapist to impart meaning to the client. We prefer a less directive definition: *Interpretation* means presenting the client with a *hypothesis* about *relationships* or *meanings* for the client's consideration. Interpretation merely brings a fresh look at the behavior, a new frame of reference, or a revised theoretical outlook. The Actualizing Therapist has a tentative tone in regard to interpretation, rather than the air of one who is an oracle from Mt. Olympus. The ultimate criterion of interpretive effectiveness is whether it facilitates behavior change in the desired direction.

The intellectual approach to counseling techniques has been defined as the problem-solving process and is exemplified by Brammer and Shostrom (1968) and Krumboltz and Thoreson (1969). The steps in problem solving as they apply to counseling or therapy have been further clarified by Brammer (1973):

1. Establish a *relationship* and get the helpee *involved*. Helpee must be interested in the process and have hope that they have the power to make decisions that will influence their lives profoundly.

2. State and clarify the *problem* and determine *goals*. This step is a special application of the goal-setting process described in the preceding section.

3. Determine and explore *alternatives* to the mere apparent solutions.

4. Gather relevant *information*. This may take the form of active seeking and reading by the helpee, statements of fact by the helper, simulation games, films, or tests.

5. Explore *implications* of information and *consequences* of the alternatives.

6. Clarify *values* that underlie personal choices. Helpees must know what they desire and the order in which they value those

desires. The helper leads the helpee into exploration of his interests, competencies, family circumstances, social expectations, and realities.

7. *Reexamine* the goals, alternative choices, risks, and consequences. A final check on understanding the information and implications is made before the final decision.

8. Decide on one of the alternatives and formulate a *plan* for or course of action implementing that decision.

9. *Generalize* the process to new life situations.

10. *Try out* the plan for implementing the decision with periodic *reevaluation* in light of new information and changing circumstances. (p. 143)

Albert Ellis has evolved an intellectual point of view for psychotherapy that he calls Rational-Emotive Psychotherapy. This system has value for certain types of clients, particularly those who are bright and flexible in their thinking.

Rational-Emotive Therapy, according to Ellis (1962), "is based on the assumption that human beings normally become emotionally disturbed through acquiring irrational and illogical thoughts. [The therapist analyzes the client's feelings of hurt, anger, fear, and guilt, and shows] him that these emotions arise not from past events but from his present irrational attitudes or illogical fears about these events or situations." To Ellis, therefore, "Emotion itself is conceived of as *largely* being a certain kind, a biased, prejudiced kind, of thought" (p. 3).

Illogical Thoughts

Some of the major illogical ideas or philosophies that have been learned in Western culture are described by Ellis (1958) in the following excerpts. They are presented in order to aid the reader in getting a more complete picture of the kinds of values and ideas that Ellis suggests as replacements for what he regards as "irrational thinking."

1. The idea that it is a dire necessity for an adult to be loved or approved by everyone for everything he does—instead of his concentrating on his own self-respect, on winning approval for necessary purposes (such as job advancement), and on loving rather than being loved.

2. The idea that certain acts are wrong, or wicked, or villainous, and that people who perform such acts should be severely

punished—instead of the idea that certain acts are inappropriate or anti-social, and that people who perform such acts are
invariably stupid, ignorant, or emotionally disturbed.

3. The idea that it is terrible, horrible, and catastrophic when
things are not the way one would like them to be—instead of
the idea that it is too bad when things are not the way one
would like them to be, and one should certainly try to change
or control conditions so that they become more satisfactory,
but that if changing or controlling uncomfortable situations is
impossible, one had better become resigned to their existence
and stop telling oneself how awful they are.

4. The idea that much human unhappiness is externally caused
and is forced on one by outside people and events—instead of
the idea that virtually all human unhappiness is caused or sustained by the view one takes of things rather than the things
themselves.

5. The idea that if something is or may be dangerous or fearsome
one should be terribly concerned about it—instead of the idea
that if something is or may be dangerous or fearsome one
should frankly face it and try to render it non-dangerous and,
when that is impossible, think of other things and stop telling
oneself what a terrible situation one is or may be in.

6. The idea that it is easier to avoid than to face life difficulties
and self-responsibilities—instead of the idea that the so-called
easy way is invariably the much harder way in the long run and
that the only way to solve difficult problems is to face them
squarely.

7. The idea that one needs something other or stronger or greater
than oneself on which to rely—instead of the idea that it is
usually far better to stand on one's own feet and gain faith in
oneself and one's ability to meet difficult circumstances of
living.

8. The idea that one should be thoroughly competent, adequate,
intelligent, and achieving in all possible respects—instead of
the idea that one should *do* rather than always try to do *well*
and that one should accept oneself as a quite imperfect
creature, who has general human limitations and specific
fallibilities.

9. The idea that because something once strongly affected one's
life, it should indefinitely affect it—instead of the idea that one
should learn from one's past experiences but not be overly
attached to or prejudiced by them.

10. The idea that it is vitally important to our existence what other people do, and that we should make great efforts to change them in the direction we would like them to be—instead of the idea that other people's deficiencies are largely *their* problems and that putting pressure on them to change is usually least likely to help them do so.

11. The idea that human happiness can be achieved by inertia and inaction—instead of the idea that humans tend to be happiest when they are actively and vitally absorbed in creative pursuits, or when they are devoting themselves to people or projects outside themselves.

12. The idea that one has virtually no control over one's emotions and that one cannot help feeling certain things—instead of the idea that one has enormous control over one's emotions if one chooses to work at controlling them and to practice saying the right kinds of sentences to oneself. (pp. 40-41)

Ellis does not believe that it is necessary, as in psychoanalysis, to focus on historical events to show the client how he *became* disturbed or to depend on relationship variables for behavior change. Rather, he says that emphasis should be placed on *attacking* the client's irrational beliefs and on showing how he is *sustaining* his neurosis by still holding these beliefs. Ellis then stresses how the client can *reverbalize* and *rethink* these ideas in a more logical, self-helping way. Finally, he encourages the client to engage in homework *activity* that will prove the validity of his newly formed assumptions about life.

BODY TECHNIQUES

One of the most obvious ways to help people get in touch with their bodies is to help them become aware of the many expressions in common parlance that express body messages. The following phrases all increase awareness of the body and of the way it speaks to us: "You *rub* me the wrong way." "I feel *touched* by that." "You get under my *skin*." "Get off my *back*." "I can't *stomach* this." "You give me a pain in the *neck*." "I can't *stand* that." "I don't have the *guts* to do it." "You *depress* me."

Everyone has heard or used these expressions many times, and yet most people are not usually aware of the significance and accuracy of the body as it expresses itself.

A here-and-now approach to living requires continuous attention to the body and what it is expressing at every moment. This assumes that one's body can be trusted as a source of one's feelings, and therefore, places the "body" at the core of one's being. The recent body therapies hold this as a fundamental assumption. In particular, the Reichian and Bioenergetic Therapies make this important assumption. Alexander Lowen (1967) says:

> A person experiences the reality of the world only through his body. The external environment impresses him because it impinges upon his body and affects his senses. . . . If the body is relatively unalive, a person's impressions and responses are diminished. The more alive the body is, the more vividly does he perceive reality and the more actively does he respond. . . . The aliveness of the body denotes its capacity for feeling. In the absence of feeling the body goes "dead." . . . The emotionally dead person is turned inward: thoughts and fantasies replace feelings and actions. Despite this mental activity, his emotional deadness is manifested physically. We shall find that his body looks "dead" or unalive. (pp. 5-6)

Lowen (1972) further describes the therapeutic task and the relating of the body to feeling:

> Looking at the body and listening to it is a continuous process. A patient's tone of voice tells me where he is, not his words. His words can lie. The body doesn't lie. The eyes may lack feeling, i.e., be dull or vacant, but that says something. His voice may be a monotone and that, too is a sign. The lack of movement is as revealing as movement itself. But of even greater importance is the way a person holds himself, i.e., his psychological character structure. (p. 4)

To be able to feel fully requires that one get in touch with one's body. In order to do so, one must *breathe,* but most people hold their breath. Perls, in fact, equates holding one's breath with anxiety. Breathing opens up one's excitatory processes and helps one to feel. Anger, for example, is a feeling that is not the same for every person. As with other feelings, one can measure the depth of anger. Thus an energetic concept helps us to evaluate the aliveness or depth of a person's feelings. Since breathing is the key to the energy metabolism, it helps one to release one's feelings. By breathing one also gets in touch with the muscular tensions and rigidities in the body that contract to block one's excitation.

Nonbeing comes from the investment of energy in the facade of manipulations and blocks that prevent core actualizing. When the client becomes aware of his body, he gradually becomes aware of his feelings, and when he is aware of his feelings, he becomes slowly aware of the postulates of life that control his behavior.

Body awareness is learned through individual therapy, and the ability to experience and express one's feelings comes in group therapy. Individual and group therapy work coactively to energize the core being and reduce facade living.

A human being needs to be understood not only as an emotional entity but as a body. The relationship between the human being as a person and the human being as a body can be illustrated by an analogy with that elementary, one-celled creature, the amoeba. If stuck with a pin, the amoeba contracts. As soon as the pin is withdrawn, it expands again. But after several attacks, it expands anxiously and incompletely. Eventually, if it is repeatedly attacked, it becomes permanently contracted. It has defended itself from its environment by reducing its size.

Physically, human beings are constantly expanding and contracting. This is true of all the tissues of the body and is most easily observed in pulse and respiration. People themselves are always either reaching out toward the environment or withdrawing from it, in a process call contact and withdrawal. Emotions can be thought of as either expansive or contractile. Anger, for example, is expansive, as energy flows to one's muscles. Anxiety, or fear, is a contracting emotion in which one constricts himself. Sadness is also a constrictive emotion: the withdrawal seems to take place in one's arms and chest. When withdrawal is permanent, the emotions become bound up in muscle contractions and the normal expansion and contraction process is stopped. This is what happens to many people who have been hurt by the environment and by others. They tend to withdraw permanently and to contract themselves and their bodies rather than to find a homeostatic balance between contraction and expansion.

Maintaining a rhythm of contact and withdrawal requires an understanding of oneself and of one's body, of the fact that people *are* their bodies. It also requires hearing other people, touching other people, seeing other people. Such contact is not possible without an awareness of the physiological processes that make human contact possible, for contact is a bodily process as well as an emotional one.

First one must learn to breathe correctly. Breathing is the means by which a person feels excitement, an identification with his body. Most people, when they are anxious or afraid, hold their breath to some degree, whereas they should try to breathe as a baby breathes, from the diaphragm, in and around the area of the stomach. In doing the exercises that follow, one should concentrate on fully experiencing his or her breathing from the diaphragm. This can be accomplished by thinking of the diaphragm as a balloon. When breathing *out,* one should push the breath out, collapsing the balloon and, therefore, the stomach. When breathing *in,* one should enlarge the stomach as if it were the balloon.

The following are ways in which body-expression exercises help people to develop contact with the polar dimensions of anger, love, strength, and weakness.

The Anger Dimension

One of the easiest ways to start to express *anger* is simply to have a "family argument." One person is asked to say "Yes" to another, and the other is asked to respond "No," while at the same time reflecting on past experiences of being required to do something he did not want to do. The technique is to go back and forth, "Yes," "No," gradually increasing the volume and bodily participation. The exercise puts the participants in touch with their anger, their wants, and their willing. Standing up to the other person, even making a fist, increases bodily involvement. It has been suggested that the jaw is the place where repressed hostility seems to center, so people are encouraged to stick out their jaws to one another in such a "fight." This also facilitates awareness of anger in the body.

A second way to get in touch with anger or hostile feelings is for two participants to turn back to back and begin pushing each other, gently "fighting" each other with their buttocks. During such an exercise one can easily discover that he really does have feelings of anger. Although some people feel rather childish and foolish at first, these feelings, too, serve the purpose of the exercise, which is to help reactivate a more basic, childlike approach to one's feelings.

A third method for getting in touch with anger is for two people to interlock hands and push each other. If they can find a rhythm in their pushing and in allowing themselves to be pushed, they can discover the "joy" that comes from being able to communicate anger. It is joyful to feel one's capacity to relate rhythmically.

The Love Dimension

The opposite end of the anger dimension is the caring dimension, or *love dimension.* In exercises for expressing this dimension, the two participants, working together, can first begin to feel their caring for one another by both saying "Yes" instead of saying "Yes" and "No." Warmly saying "Yes" to each other can help two people discover their caring. Second, turning their backs to one another, they can rub each other's backs—this time tenderly. Each begins to feel that there is a warmth—a loving, caring feeling—that he can easily express in a physical way to, and receive from, another human being.

A third caring exercise is the "facial touch." Most people, as children, were touched often by their parents. At moments of greatest tenderness, a mother or a father would touch them on the face. One of the best ways for people to discover their ability to care for one another is to touch each other facially as a parent might touch a child. For example, one person may say to another, "I'd like you to close your eyes now and I'm going to touch your face. I'd like you to feel that I'm your father [or mother]." Then he or she may go through a touching and talking sequence something like this: "This is your hair, and it's very soft. This is your forehead, and beneath your forehead is one eyebrow, which comes down here and goes up there, and the other one goes up like this and down like this. And these are your eyes [touching the eyes very softly]. Your eyes are soft, delicate, wonderful. One eyelash comes out here and one eyelash comes out over here. And this is your nose, the bridge of your nose comes out to a very nice point and then goes out here toward your cheeks. Your cheeks are red and soft and beautiful. Below your cheeks are your lips. This is your upper lip, and it's soft and red and very lovely, and below your upper lip is your lower lip, and it's very nice and soft and beautiful. Below your lips is your chin, and your whole face comes down like this toward your chin and is very, very pretty."

Simply to say this to another person while touching him often brings tears to his eyes. This may seem a simple exercise, but if one is willing to take the risk of going through it, this physical expression of tenderness can be a very meaningful demonstration of the importance of caring in our existence.

The Strength Dimension

We have found, first, that stamping one's feet firmly into the ground gives a real sense of the feeling of one's own *strength*, for the lower half of the body is where people get their support, whereas the upper part is where they make contact. In this series of exercises, people try to get in touch with their own strength. If one *stamps his feet* firmly into the ground until he begins to feel the muscle strain in his calves and thighs, his feet will seem to become firmly planted in the ground, like the roots of a tree. This helps one feel his sense of strength and self-support.

A second exercise, helpful for developing strong resistance to manipulation in one's environment is to lie on a bed with both knees up and to pound the bed with both fists and say, "I won't give up." Both movement and voice should express conviction. Often, when intense holding and resistance is felt, the client moves to the opposite polar dimension and cries.

A third method for feeling strength is for the client to hold the weight of someone's head in his hands. The client's partner sits or lies down, and the client then lifts his or her head. In lifting or holding the partner's head, one begins to feel the strength of being trusted by another.

The Weakness Dimension

A technique for physically expressing strength also allows one to feel its opposite, *weakness.* Just as holding another person's head enables one to feel his strength, the ability to put one's head into another's hands helps one feel weakness or vulnerability. The person playing the weak role in this exercise lies on the floor and pretends that he is a child again, perhaps only six months old and still not able to get out of his crib. The other person acts as his parent, and tries to make the "infant" feel his vulnerability, his weakness, as he lies on the floor. When the "infant" is ready, he raises his hands, reaching for the "parent" and saying to him, "Will you help me?" It is important that this be a plea, not a demand. It should express great need: "I want you to help me, I need your help, will you please help me?" When this exercise is done seriously, it often brings tears to the eyes of the person playing the weak role. It also brings a feeling of strength and worth to the parent figure, who experiences having another person reach out to him. In the last part of the exercise, the "infant" reaches for the "parent" and allows himself to be lifted up. As he is lifted off the floor, he can rest in the arms of the parent figure—rest his weight on his body. In doing so, the "infant" experiences, more fully than in any other exercise, his own weakness, vulnerability, and need. Conversely, the parent figure feels great strength, capacity, and ability to cope.

A second technique for getting in touch with one's weakness is to stand in front of a couch, bent forward, with all weight on one's feet. The feet should be approximately fifteen inches apart, with toes turned in slightly. The fingers touch the floor out in front for balance. The knees are bent forward, and then slowly brought back so that a tremor in the legs begins. The vibration is accompanied by a tingling sensation in the feet and legs. Respiration now begins to deepen. When standing this way becomes painful, the client may be told to fall backward onto the couch. He is usually in tears by this time, and group members are instructed to touch and comfort him. This exercise is shown in the movie *Three Approaches to Group Therapy,* described in Chapter 9. It is illustrated in Figure 38. The point of the exercise is to experience falling and surrendering to one's weakness.

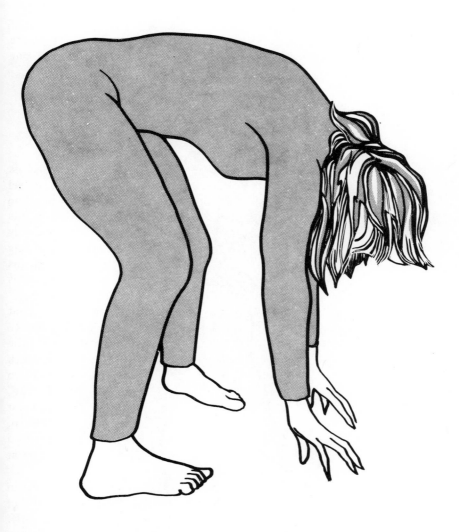

Figure 38. The Weakness Exercise (adapted from Lowen)

A third exercise to get in touch with one's vulnerability, or weakness, is shown in Figure 39. The client is asked to stand with his feet about thirty inches apart, toes inward, knees bent as much as possible, back arched, and hands on hips. The therapist then grasps the client's arms at the elbow and pushes him forward and down. As the client slowly lets himself down to the floor, he experiences deep feelings of vulnerability and surrender.

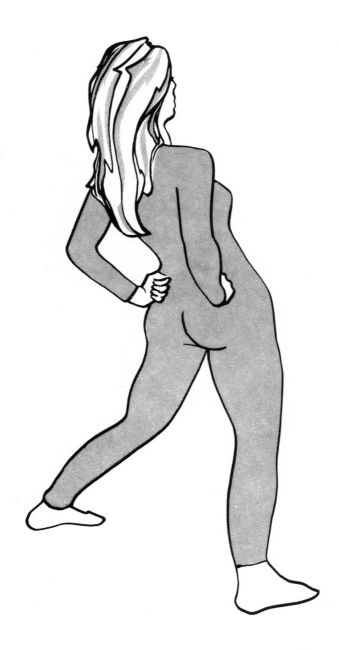

Figure 39. The Vulnerability Exercise (adapted from Lowen)

The ability to surrender to one's feelings of weakness and vulnerability is a central feat of Actualizing Therapy. Everyone is afraid to give in to his feelings, but in particular people are afraid of being weak. They feel they must be in control at all times. To surrender is to accept one's losses. The fear of falling is related to the fear of surrendering to another, especially parents and others who have manipulated one. As individuals overcome their fear of falling, they give in more readily to their bodies and their feelings.

FOCUSING: INTEGRATING THINKING, FEELING, AND BODY

Gendlin (1969) has developed a procedure whereby one can understand the relationship between the three aspects in the verbal interchange between therapist and client. He calls this "experiential focusing." His hypothesis is that words can come from a "felt sense," and this is a freshly sensed bodily version of one's problem. The following verbal exchange in therapy illustrates:

Client: I just never get close to anyone. It's because I got too much hostility from my mother. [*Intellectualizing.*]

Therapist: Let everything you know wait awhile. Feel toward closeness, and get a sense of what the whole thing feels like.

Client: [*Silence, then:*] It makes me very uncomfortable. [*Felt sense of whole problem.*]

Therapist: Stay with this "uncomfortable" sense.

Client: [*Silence, then:*] It's scary and tight.

Therapist: Stay with that "scary and tight." Just welcome it, stay next to it, ask it what is that? Don't answer, let it answer you. It takes a little while.

Client: [*Silence then:*] Whew! . . . [*Deep exhale, crying*] It's lonely, it wants to come out, but it can't. [*Felt shift and release.*]

Therapist: Now, really welcome that. For a whole minute. Then we'll try to get the whole felt sense of this "can't."

Gendlin gets his patients to work with thinking, feeling, and bodily responses in one, before these are ever split. He believes that all therapeutic interaction, when it works, is a bodily shifting of meaningful felt senses. While Actualizing Therapy would follow the above with the body techniques of the previous section, Gendlin's point is that in one bodily felt shift all three aspects of being change.

ACTUALIZING THERAPY AS MUTUAL EXPOSURE OF WEAKNESS

Sidney Jourard (1964) has suggested the following:

> Let's tune in on an imaginary interview between a client and his counselor; the client says, "I have never told this to a soul, doctor, but I can't stand my wife, my mother is a nag, my father is a bore, and my boss is an absolutely hateful and despicable tyrant. I have been carrying on an affair for the past ten years with the lady next door, and at the same time I am a deacon in the church." The counselor says, showing great understanding and empathy, "Mm-humm!"
>
> If we listened for a long enough period of time, we would find that the client talks and talks about himself to this highly sympathetic and empathic listener. At some later time, the client may eventually say, "Gosh you have helped me a lot. I see what I must do and I will go ahead and do it."
>
> Now this talking about oneself to another person is what I call self-disclosure. It would appear, without assuming anything, that self-disclosure is a factor in the process of effective counseling or psychotherapy.
>
> Would it be too arbitrary an assumption to propose that people become clients because they have not disclosed themselves in some optimum degree to the people in their life? (p. 21)

It is through self-disclosure that an individual reveals to himself and to the other party just exactly who, what, and where he is. Just as, in medicine, thermometers and sphygmomanometers disclose information about the real state of the individual, so the POI performs this same function in psychotherapy and education.

Just as the patient's expressions about himself cause change, so, too, must the therapist do the same. Kopp (1971) has stated the orientation of a self-actualizing therapist well:

> My pain hurts as yours does. Each of us has the same amount to lose—all we have. My tears are as bitter, my scars as permanent. My loneliness is an aching in my chest, much like yours. Who are you to feel that your losses mean more than mine. What arrogance! . . . I feel angry at your ignoring my feelings. I live in the same imperfect world in which you struggle, a world in which, like you, I must make do with less than I would wish for myself. . . . And too, you seem to feel that you should be able to succeed without failure, to love without loss, to reach out without risk of disappointment, never to appear vulnerable or even foolish. . . . Why? While the rest of us must sometimes fall, be hurt, feel inadequate, but rise again and go on. Why do you feel that you alone should

be spared all this? How did you become so special? In what way have you been chosen? . . . You say you've had a bad time of it, an unhappy childhood? Me too. You say that you didn't get all you needed and wanted, weren't always understood or cared for? Welcome to the club! (p. 153)

Freud established the role of counselor or therapist as that of a blank screen on which the client could express himself. The analyst sat behind the client as he free-associated on the couch, and no encounter was possible. As Jourard has said, such avoidance of being oneself with the patients can be considered a form of resistance. Hora (1960) contrasts the existential therapist as follows: "The existential therapist does not 'do' psychotherapy, he lives it. He meets his patient in the openness of an interhuman existential encounter" (pp. 498-499). Rogers (1961) states: "To be transparent to the client, to have nothing of one's experience in the relationship which is hidden . . . this is, I believe, basic to effective psychotherapy" (pp. 5-7). Buber (in Kopp, 1971), in speaking of genuine dialogue, states: "No one . . . can know in advance what it is that he has to say" (pp. 112-113).

Actualizing Therapy is a process of actualizing weaknesses or facing one's failures and illusions in life. Self-actualizing results from an analysis, and facing, of one's failures, not simply a listing of one's successes. In this light, the POI could be described as a "profile of weaknesses and strengths." It is sometimes overlooked that Maslow (1954) described his self-actualizers as "not free of guilt, anxiety, sadness, self-castigation, internal strife, and conflict" (p. 299).

Thus, the therapist-client relationship needs to be radically revised from that of a wise expert dealing with a failure to that of one human being with weaknesses plus some wisdom dealing with another human being with strengths as well as special weaknesses.

Actualizing Therapy places therapist and client in a kind of *therapeutic alliance,* rather than a strict professional-patient relationship. A kinship between two persons is established, and it is apparent that the therapist must be willing to risk vulnerability in the service of the therapeutic process. Actualizing Therapy is, in this sense, a healing partnership between client and professional.

THE IMPORTANCE OF POLARITIES

As therapists, we develop each day our technical skills, but also each day makes us aware of our humanness. Some of our Western thinking does not help us here, because of some Puritanistic and Christian teaching from which we have learned to evaluate in terms of good and bad.

Actualizing Therapy draws from Eastern thought in resolving the problem of human weakness. Instead of focusing on good and bad, some Eastern thought holds that everything in the universe shows the interplay of two interacting forces: Yang and Yin. Yang (red in design) is the positive force. It is found in everything that is warm and bright, in everything that is firm, dry, and steadfast. It is the sunlight and fire, the sunny south of the hill.

Yin (black in design) is the negative force. It is found in everything cold and dark, in everything soft, moist, mysterious, secret, and changeable. It is the shadow and water, the shade on the north side of the hill. The movement of the sun, the moon, and the stars, the predictable circling of the seasons, the growth of plants—all of nature reflects these interflowing principles.

Most importantly, in each person's life the changing balances of Yang and Yin bring now failure, now success, again success, now flowering, now decay. Both Yang and Yin are necessary to the order of the universe and to life. They are not in conflict, like good and evil, but rather they are always in harmony. This is the way, the road, the law of life, the Tao. It is perhaps the most important value a therapist can communicate to the client. To live by Yang and Yin is to accept the rhythm of life, the relationship between ups and downs, the naturalness of life. If one can live by the Tao, one can accept his weaknesses and strengths, his successes and failures, and he can flow with life rather than blame himself and others. In Chinese, the word *crisis* is defined as *danger* and also as *opportunity*. The principle of rhythmic balance gives one a principle by which humanness can be lived and enjoyed.

Choosing Priorities

When thinking, feeling, and bodily responses are expressed and integrated on each of the polarities, a feeling of "having it all together" results. When one is together, decisions are possible. In Actualizing Therapy, decision making is expressed by "priortizing" one's values, or choosing priorities.

Priorities are considered statements of one's *existence* or "isness" at any one moment, of one's *needs* at any one moment, of one's *freedom* at any one moment, and of one's *wants* at any one moment. All these dimensions of personality come together in a statement of one's priorities, in that each is important in itself as well as being important as an aspect of one's integrated total being. In a sense, expressing one's priorities is a part of having one's polarities all together.

Dealing with priorities involves a wide perspective of future goals and past learning experiences. Priorities often conflict, and there is a certain challenge and satisfaction in the creative synthesis of choosing from all available knowledge and data and applying the most useful for the present. Priority choosing is not just decision making; it requires time for assimilation and digestion. It also involves a cognizance of the intellect, which is considering outside alternatives and evaluating them, of the feelings and gut-level intuition, and of the body, which may signal a detrimental decision by its tension or a beneficial decision by its relaxation. Priority choosing is an organismic process involving an integration of all three levels of being.

A practical method of choosing priorities can be expressed in periodically rearranging one's priorities by listing, in order, the concerns that are most important in one's life. This procedure enlightens the person as to how to invest himself and as to what changes he needs to make to act on future goals and present desires. Sometimes this requires and fosters the developing of courage. For example, a young female client who was so diversely involved that she was not able to invest herself enough for personal satisfaction in any one area made a list of her personal priorities for growth and fulfillment. She found that her current boyfriend, with whom she had spent much of her time, was not even on her list. After discussing this with her therapist and group, in what we call a "priority recital," she concluded that the relationship was not conducive to her growth—that it was in fact excess baggage—and she decided to give up her boyfriend. In taking this risk, she validated her personal courage.

The actualizing person eventually develops a system in which he is constantly aware of his priorities and of their changes, with a readiness to act in terms of his committed-to values. Operating from his deep core values, he can take satisfaction and joy in the spontaneity of the expression of his life.

ARTISTIC AND SCIENTIFIC BALANCE

All of the foregoing discussion leads to an important principle of Actualizing Therapy: Therapists have two strong, balanced components—personal-artistic relationship skills and scientific-technical qualifications. In addition, the therapist must always be in a conscious process of personal growth, so that his actualizing personhood will serve him as well as his scientific methodology does. There are abundant data to validate the view that therapeutic effectiveness is maximal when the therapist can relate to clients in warm, accepting ways. Thus the therapist becomes a behavioral "model" for the client. Technical competence in interpretation, information-giving, test usage, and application of theory are also related to therapist effectiveness.

The problem in therapist or counselor selection is to find means for reliably assessing these characteristics. A study by Foulds (1969) has demonstrated that the concepts of self-actualizing as measured by the scales of the Personal Orientation Inventory do effectively discriminate between two groups of counselors with respect to the ability to communicate genuineness, warmth, understanding, and positive regard within the counseling situation. The POI Inner-Direction scale and six of the subscales significantly differentiated between a group of counselor trainees rated high on facilitative genuineness and a group rated low on this quality.

Before integrating the foregoing ideas, we wish to reemphasize some focal points of the therapist-client relationship (adapted from Brammer & Shostrom, 1968):

1. The therapist is engaged in helping others in a professional capacity, but more importantly, he is a human being with personal weaknesses and problems of his own. The therapist must take the responsibility for constant personal growth through personal therapy, group experience, and other growth experiences.

2. The professional therapist is an expert in helping others, but he has no mystical or technical solutions. Technical training can be helpful, but only continuous attempts to increase self-understanding and self-awareness make him believe in what he attempts to do with clients. Therapy is only partly technique; the rest is subtle human relationship effectiveness.

3. Each client is a unique expression of human nature; hence, the textbook never completely applies. In addition, the therapist must respect *himself* as someone who is completely unique.

4. Therapy can be viewed as a *workshop* for the *growth* of both participants. Each client can help the therapist shed new light on his own personal integration.

5. A central emphasis for any enlightened therapist must be the development of a core of valid techniques, along with flexibility for learning new ideas each day and for discarding old approaches that no longer seem to apply. Psychotherapy techniques thus develop acceptance of change for the client and, most of all, for the therapist. Actualizing Therapy must be viewed as the dynamic interplay of a unique, existential relationship between two distinctive personalities.

In addition to the study by Foulds (1969), cited above, a number of other studies have attempted to establish relationships between self-actualizing and counselor effectiveness. McClain (1970) has presented evidence that the POI is highly related to the rated self-actualizing of school counselors. Thirty counselors participating in a summer institute rated each other for self-actualizing according to criteria found in the writings of Maslow. Composite self-actualizing scores for each counselor were correlated with POI scales. The high relationship with the Inner-Direction (I) scale ($r=.69$) adds further evidence that the POI does in fact measure concepts seen by counselors as representing self-actualizing behavior.

EXAMPLES OF SYNTHESIZING THERAPEUTIC INTERACTION

The therapist's manner of response to clients can be thought of in terms of the three aspects of being. Therapists of various persuasions respond either in terms of feeling, thinking, or bodily response. Figure 40 shows how therapists of currently popular approaches might react to certain client statements. What this chart reveals is that each therapist focuses on the truth of a person's being as the therapist sees it. One approach is not "right" and another "wrong." Each is right as he sees it. *It is important to understand that the Actualizing Therapist uses both the "primary actualizing responses" and the "secondary actualizing responses" at all three levels of being. He is truly a creative synthesizer.*

Thinking Responses

As illustrated in Figure 40, Actualizing Therapists, Decision Therapists, Rational-Emotive Therapists, Behavior Therapists, Transactional Analysts, and Psychoanalysts make up the six therapeutic schools reflecting the thinking area.

Responding to the client's statements as the top of Figure 40, the Actualizing Therapist reacts to client statement number 1 with "That's growth for *you* because your responses to the POI show that anger is hard for you to express." The data-response technique is utilized to confirm the fact that the client is now expressing the opposite of the original responses to the POI. To client statement number 2 the Actualizing Therapist replies, "Your POI shows you feel angry inside but you are often afraid to *be* it," indicating that there is a difference between a feeling response on the inside and one on the outside. This is one of the important POI learning dimensions. From an actualizing point of view it is not sufficient simply to

TYPICAL MALE CLIENTS' STATEMENTS:

1. "I am really very angry at him."
2. "I don't like you either."
3. "I care a lot about my mother."

RESPONSES IN TERMS OF VARIOUS SCHOOLS OF THOUGHT:

PRIMARY ACTUALIZING RESPONSES		SECONDARY
A. THINKING		
I. Psychometric (Shostrom; POI)	II. Decision Therapy (Greenwald)	III. Rational-Emotive Therapy (Ellis)
1. That's growth for you because your responses on your POI show anger is hard for you to express. 2. Your POI shows you feel angry inside but you are often afraid to *be* it. 3. Your scores show you can admit to your anger more easily than to your caring.	1. What does that do for you? 2. So what's wrong with hating me? 3. When are you going to tell her?	1. Your assumption is that things should always happen the way you want them to or you have the right to be angry. 2. You keep trying to make everybody else love you — it's O.K. to disagree with me. 3. Do you assume you should feel guilty about that?
B. FEELING		
VII. Sharing Experiences (Shostrom)	VIII. Gestalt Therapy (Perls)	IX. Client Centered Therapy (Rogers)
1. You make me angry when you don't admit your hurt. 2. I feel warmly toward you when you admit to both your anger and your caring. 3. I know about that — but I often feel hatred toward those I love most.	1. You say that you are angry but your eyes say to me you are hurting inside. 2. Be your anger at me. 3. Put her in the empty chair and tell her about it.	1. You are very resentful toward him. 2. You want me to know how much you dislike me also. 3. You deeply love her?
C. BODILY EXPRESSION		
X. Polarity Bodily Expression (Shostrom)	XI. Bioenergetic Therapy (Lowen)	
1. Your muscles in your neck and shoulders show you are holding in a lot of anger. Can you hit the couch and let it out? 2. I accept that, but can you express your anger with your body too? Let me massage your neck and shoulders and see if you can express the anger lodged there. 3. If you can let your chest collapse and surrender to the ground, then you can really love.	1. When did you first feel such anger in your body? 2. Do the feelings in your body remind you of feelings you had toward your father? Why don't you lie down and kick and hit to express these feelings? 3. Notice that your body tightens up when you talk about your mother.	

Figure 40. Three Levels of Therapeutic Responses in Terms of Various Schools of Thought

---

ACTUALIZING RESPONSES

IV. **Behavior Therapy**

1. What are you doing to show that?
2. It's O.K. not to like me, I don't like everybody either.
3. I'm sure your mother would appreciate that.

V. **Transactional Analysis**

1. Is that your child speaking?
2. I have the feeling you're making a parent of me.
3. Do you feel you have to love her?

VI. **Psychoanalysis**

1. Who does he remind you of?
2. I think that's very significant.
3. Aha! Tell me more about that.

Figure 40. Three Levels of Therapeutic Responses in Terms of Various Schools of Thought

experience something on the inside; it is necessary to express that feeling verbally to other people. To client statement number 3 it is asserted, "Your scores show you can admit to your anger more easily than to your caring." Here, again, through the medium of the POI, the suggestion is made that caring and anger are synergistic concepts and that the client is, to some extent, able to express one but not the other.

Decision Therapy attempts to align itself with the client's resistance. Instead of fighting the client's assumptions, the Decision Therapist goes along with them and urges the client to carry them to their often illogical conclusions. To client statement number 1 the Decision Therapist might suggest, "What does that do for you?" Concern is with the payoff or advantage that one gets from a particular form of behavior. To client statement number 2 the reply is, "So what's wrong with hating me?" This is a joining-the-resistance type of therapeutic response, in which the therapist aligns himself with the client's statement. The response to statement number 3, "When are you going to tell her?" is a decision-type response, in which the therapist attempts to tell the client that a decision response is the ultimate goal.

In the Rational-Emotive approach, the therapist might respond to client statement number 1 with, "Your assumption is that things should always happen the way you want them to or you have the right to be angry." Here, this therapeutic technique is used to demonstrate that the basic approach is to help the client, by rational means, to reevaluate his assumptions about life—in this case, the belief that if things don't happen the way the client wants them to happen, he or she has a right to be unhappy. According to the Rational-Emotive frame of reference, this is an unnecessary assumption. To client statement number 2 the therapist responds, "You keep trying to make everybody else love you—it's O.K. to disagree with me." Here, the suggestion is made that it is O.K. to disagree with therapists; therapists are not God, and it is perfectly acceptable to be annoyed with them. To statement number 3, the Rational-Emotive Therapist asks, "Do you assume you should feel guilty about that?" In asking the question, the therapist is attacking the assumption that one should always feel guilty about being overly loving toward one's mother. Here Ellis is attacking the psychoanalytic concept of the Oedipus Complex.

In the Behavior Therapy approach, the therapist might respond to client statement number 1 with "What are you doing to show that?" Here the therapeutic emphasis is on doing, or behavior, rather than just verbal response. To client statement number 2 the Behavior Therapist responds, "It's O.K. not to like me. I don't like everybody either." Here the attempt is to teach a principle or idea to the client. To client statement number 3 the Behavior Therapist responds with "I'm sure your mother would appreciate that." Again the Behavior Therapist is attempting to suggest that the client *act* on this feeling of caring about the mother and not simply talk about it.

Transactional Analysts are principally concerned with the tripartite system of therapy, in which the client is broken down into the child, parent, and adult parts. The first two therapist responses reflect the first two ego states (child and parent), while the last, "Do you feel you have to love her?" means that the life "script" of the client can change from loving everybody to not having to love everybody. This is considered to be an "adult" choice.

In the psychoanalytic responses, "Who does he remind you of?" is a historical referent, usually to a parent. When the analyst says, "I think that's very significant," he is responding to the transference dimensions of the therapeutic relationship. And when he says, "Aha! Tell me more about that," he is interested in the Oedipal situation that exists within the client.

Feeling Responses

In the feeling area, the Actualizing Therapist shifts to sharing experience. The reply to client statement number 1 is, "You make me angry when you don't admit your hurt." In effect a personal response is given to the client's verbalizations. The Actualizing Therapist responds to client statement number 2 with, "I feel warmly toward you when you admit to both your anger and your caring." Here, in terms of the theory of polarities, response is in terms of the therapist's own warmth to the client's admission of the anger dimension. In response to client statement number 3 the Actualizing Therapist, drawing on his own experience, says, "I know about that—but I often feel hatred toward those I love most." By saying this he is teaching the client something about the universality of feeling in the area of parental relationships.

The Gestalt Therapist's response to client statement number 1 might be, "You say that you are angry but your eyes say to me you are hurting inside." Thus, Perls goes beyond Client-Centered Therapy to describe what the body is saying, rather than responding only to verbal expressions. To client statement number 2 the Gestalt Therapist responds, "Be your anger at me," stressing being rather than talking. The reply to client statement number 3, "Put her in the empty chair and tell her about it," is an instance of the empty-chair role-playing technique.

Reflection of feeling is manifest in the Client-Centered Therapist's reaction to the first client statement. The Client-Centered Therapist would respond, "You are very resentful toward him." To statement number 2 he replies, "You want me to know how much you dislike me also." And to statement number 3 he responds, "You deeply love her?"

Bodily Responses

The Actualizing Therapist's polarity response to statement number 1 is, "Your muscles in your neck and shoulders show you are holding in a lot of anger. Can you hit the couch and let it out?" Here, a bodily expression technique is used to help the client release pent-up anger. To client statement number 2, the polarity response is, "I accept that, but can you express your anger with your body, too? Let me massage your neck and shoulders and see if you can express the anger lodged there." Again, the client's verbalizations are put in terms of the body. To client statement number 3, the Actualizing Therapist replies, "If you can let your chest collapse and surrender to the ground, then you can really love." Rather than simply using words, the therapist begins to work on that part of the body that relates to surrender and love.

Emphasizing the relationship between the body and past experiences, the Bioenergetic Therapist responds to statement number 1 with, "When did you first feel such anger in your body?" and directly relates the client's verbalization to bodily response. To statement number 2 he replies, "Do the feelings in your body remind you of feelings you had toward your father? Why don't you lie down and kick and hit to express these feelings?" Again, he refuses to accept more verbalization, but rather he relates the client's words to inner body response, linking the client's feelings for the therapist with those for his father. To client statement number 3, the Bioenergetic Therapist draws a direct physical parallel. The client is told, "Notice that your body tightens up when you talk about your mother," making him immediately aware of his overt bodily expression.

In summary, therapists of different persuasions respond to therapeutic situations in terms of their own biases. This does not mean that one system is better than another. Figure 40 illustrates this book's thesis: In the process of becoming an Actualizing Therapist, the therapist can relate to a client in terms of his thinking, his feeling, or his bodily responses. The creative synthesis approach is an attempt to help people realize that there are not right or wrong answers in therapy, but rather that there are *different* responses, based on one's ability to understand various persuasions and to use them in a flexible manner. The Actualizing Therapist must be aware of all the choices of response available to him, and then let the situation determine his response.

THE LEVELS OF PERSONAL ACTUALIZING

Personal actualizing may be seen as the client going through a *personal development process* (in seeking the answers to life's questions) parallel to the therapist's professional development (see Chapter 1). This continuous personal process, which we call self-actualizing, proceeds as follows:

1. *General level.* The individual is heavily *influenced* by the parameters of his parents, teachers, and friends.

2. *Personalized level.* The individual *adapts* his original ideas to his own *experience,* evolving a more personal philosophy of life.

3. *Stylized level.* Through therapy and experience, the individual *commits* himself to selected theories that "fit" with his developing personal philosophy, which becomes a unique gestalt that he defines as his "self."

Thus, a growing person can be thought of as a "creative synthesizer" in that his commitment to his own theoretical view of life is a composite of everything he has heard or seen. Actualizing is seen as a process of constantly expanding one's approach to understanding life. One's personal growth requires that he continually evolve and emerge personally. Not to grow emotionally, intellectually, or bodily is to slowly die. Thus, the whole point of actualizing is to become one's true self—to realize all of one's potentialities and to become actualizing as a responsible human being.

Epstein (1973) has defined the "self" as a person's developing theory about life. We believe that the Actualizing Assessment Battery provides the individual with universal dimensions to consider as he develops a personally meaningful understanding of his own intrapersonal and interpersonal theories of life that work for him. Thus, Epstein defines the self-concept as a *theory*—a theory the individual continually constructs about himself as an experiencing, functioning human being. Each person is either consciously or unconsciously developing postulates about the *nature of life* and *himself* and *his work.* He is continuously organizing the data of his experience so that he can more effectively cope with life.

Like the therapist, then, each person is continually ordering and testing hypotheses for living. He organizes his data in a network of postulates called theories. Without such a system he would be overwhelmed by innumerable isolated details. The system maintains its self-actualizing qualities, however, only as it remains both firm and flexible. Changes in each individual, as well as changes in circumstances, may cause a person to alter, amend, or modify his postulates in terms of his own growth. Self-actualizing is a *process,* not a fixed state.

Therapists, therefore, are *guides* for the individual; they aid him in his search for suitable theories of life for himself. The parameters suggested in Chapter 1 cover the three basic functions of any actualizing therapist:

1. The therapist serves as a *model* by *caring* for the client, by *encountering* the client, and by *ego-strengthening* himself and the client in the developing of thinking, feeling, and bodily expression.

2. The therapist serves as a *teacher* by *pattern analysis* of the client's workable and unworkable theories of life, by encouraging the client to stand behind his theories and test them under fire in group therapy, by *analyzing* the client's interpersonal theories as they function in group therapy, and by disclosing the therapist's own adaptive or maladaptive theories, thereby encouraging the client to do the same thing.

3. The therapist serves as a *change agent* by encouraging the continuous *value reorientation* of the client's theories and valuing the continuous emergence of change in the client, by encouraging *reexperiencing* of the past influential learnings and desensitizing the effects of maladaptive learnings on present functioning, and by *reinforcing* behavior felt to be growth-enhancing.

The Actualizing Therapist believes that he must be broadly committed to an understanding of all extant theories of life. As the Actualizing Therapist is truly a scientist-philosopher, so each person who is committed to growing is a scientist-philosopher in the search for personal truth.

CHAPTER 8. GROUP THERAPY AND ENCOUNTER GROUPS

The increasing popularity and widespread use of the group experience as a force for personality change is attested to by Carl Rogers (1968):

> . . . the intensive group experience is one of the most rapidly growing phenomena in the United States . . . because people . . . have discovered that this group experience alleviates their loneliness and permits them to grow, to risk change. The encounter group brings persons into real relationships with persons. . . . It has been estimated that at least 5 million persons have now had an encounter group experience in the United States. (p. 29)

Maslow (1970) has said, "If ordinary [individual] therapy may be conceived of as a miniature ideal society of two, then group therapy may be seen as a miniature ideal society of ten . . . in addition we now have empirical data that indicate that group therapy . . . can do some things that individual psychotherapy cannot" (p. 263).

While Rogers' and Maslow's comments have demonstrated the need that group therapeutic procedures serve, we believe that the work of Kagan and Yalom points to the importance of Actualizing Therapy theory as a grounding for group therapy procedures.

Kagan (1970) has asserted that clients in groups have vague irrational (or interpersonal) fears that seem to be nearly universal. These are:

1. The counselor might hurt or reject them. [Fear of exposing weakness.]

2. The counselor might make an affectionate, intimate, or dependent demand on them. [Fear of love.]

3. The client's own hostile impulses might be expressed toward the counselor. [Fear of anger.]

4. The client's own affectionate, intimate, or dependent needs might be
acted-out toward the counselor. [Fear of loving.] (p. 47)

To these four we add a fifth: The client might have to assert his own
strengths or competencies. [Fear of strength.]

As suggested by our bracketed interpretations after the above comments,
it is apparent that Kagan is referring to the fundamental polarities of
Actualizing Therapy. Kagan asks, "Would it be possible to confront people
with these general concerns? Would such confrontation serve as a stimulant
or facilitative device to encourage clients to become aware of their own
specific interpersonal concerns?" (p. 47). We believe that our interpersonal
system does exactly this.

Yalom (1970) has stated, "New procedures which focus primarily on
interpersonal behavior must be developed [for group therapy]" (pp. 183-
184). Enlarging on Maslow's idea of group therapy as a miniature society of
six to ten, we have constructed such a miniature society to show its potential
for multiple means of relating, as depicted in Figure 41. In this figure, the
familiar polarities of Actualizing Therapy are shown as existing not simply
between opposites, but also among all members of the group.

Yalom has stated that Leary's (1957) system is too complex and cumbersome in its present form, but we believe our modification of Leary illustrates
a complex system rather simply. For example, within the person there is a
rhythm between his own primary polarities, as shown in the eight circles
representing individuals in Figure 41, but as he broadens his perspective,
he interacts rhythmically with the polarities of the other members of the
group. At any one moment, in a simple group of eight, there are 1,367
possibilities of interactive combinations! Figure 41 may also be seen as a
symbolic representation of the group as a second family with various sibling
and parental roles.

Another model that illustrates the importance of the group as a universal
therapeutic modality comes from literature. All good literature expresses
various levels of conflict or interaction: first, that within the individual
himself; second, that between the individual and others; and third, that
between subgroups.

In individual Actualizing Therapy, the emphasis is on the *bodily* dimension and the *intellectual* dimension in considering the individual values for
a person's life. Group therapy is a miniature society in which interpersonal
expression of *emotion* becomes a primary focus. Individual therapy is
analogous to a lecture session in college, whereas group therapy is the
laboratory session—each is necessary for total learning. In the laboratory of

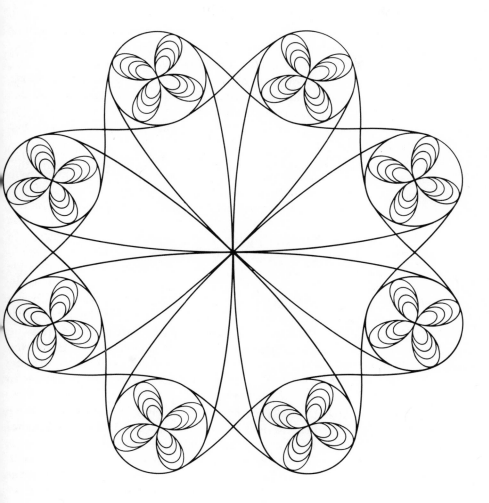

Figure 41. The Rhythmic Expression of the Polarities in a Group Setting

the group, the client is afforded the opportunity to try out a new "stance" in life and to experience and express the values to which he is committing himself. If the number of people going to group therapy is added to the number of those who have sought encounter group experiences, Rogers' estimate of 5 million (originally made in 1968) should perhaps be increased to 10 million. Those seeking encounter group experiences as well as those seeking group therapy are well people who want to be weller and who want to give new meaning to the word courage. The fact of their numbers seems to have taken away the stigma of attending a group experience and has measurably reduced even the stigma of going to therapy in general. Psychotherapy is now a privilege of the middle class.

Those who choose *therapy* are more often people who are *hurting* inside and are choosing individual and group therapy even though they are not "sick" in the old-fashioned psychiatric sense. Those persons choosing the *encounter* experience are often actualizing persons who wish to enhance their own functioning.

Research with the POI has suggested that, generally, it is the comparatively more actualizing person who seeks out the encounter group experience. Using a college sample of introductory psychology students, Gilligan (1973) administered a questionnaire designed to determine interest in participating in a weekend sensitivity experience. The POI was administered to samples of fifty-three selectors and fifty-five nonselectors of the offered experience. Those indicating above average interest in participation were significantly higher on the major POI Inner-Directedness (I) scale as well on subscales of Existentiality (Ex), Spontaneity (S), and Capacity for Intimate Contact (C). Gilligan concluded that these results support the notion that T-groups are composed of well-functioning individuals and that the results challenge the hypothesis that many who seek sensitivity training are really in need of counseling or psychotherapy. Similarly, a study by Noll and Watkins (1974) reported higher POI scores for females seeking encounter group experiences than for those declining to participate in such groups.

As we have stated, group methods are growing in popularity, not so much as clinical methods to help the seriously disturbed, but as media for assisting the already functional person to become more actualizing. In the preceding chapter we expanded on the concept that intellectual, emotional, and body awareness is learned through intrapersonal therapy. Through the group process persons develop the ability to experience these three dimensions in an interpersonal setting. Thus this awareness in turn can lead to increased effectiveness, greater humanness, and further actualizing of potential.

We have already made one distinction between "group psychotherapy" and the "encounter groups." "Group psychotherapy," a standard term for many years, refers to a problem-centered, crises-oriented method for clinical and private practice settings. The "encounter group" technique has a wider use among educational, business, and religious settings. The most significant differences between the two terms are intensity of emotional involvement and agency setting. The encounter experience deals more with present attitudes and behaviors and less with past difficulties. Depth of feeling is usually more controlled during the encounter experience than it is in group psychotherapy, which not only permits but encourages members to express intensive core feelings. For example, during group therapy a member might elaborate on such feelings as his intense hatred of women in his past and present life, or his deep anxieties about loneliness. This intensive therapeutic approach is more applicable to clinics and private practice settings, whereas in a "weekend workshop," conducted in a growth center or educational institution, the emphasis might be more on here-and-now feelings only.

A number of additional terms are commonly used in group literature: "Group dynamics" refers to the general principles of group interaction and communication, while specific groups are described variously as "sensitivity training groups" (largely from industry), "T-groups" (training in group dynamics), "confrontation" or "encounter" groups (in growth centers conducted by paraprofessionals), and "conjoint family groups." Applications of group principles, stressing openness with feelings, leading to self-awareness and improved human relations, have been made in industrial, educational, governmental, clinical, religious, and family settings. These general approaches emphasize actualizing for people already functioning well, rather than solving intense personal problems.

A new approach to group work is the self-actualizing workshop, an intensive group experience conducted for as long as twelve weeks or as short as a three-day weekend. The emphasis is both didactic (lectures, films, demonstrations) and experiential (actualizing or encounter groups). These workshops emphasize the three aspects of being: intellectual, feeling, and bodily approaches.

Self-actualizing workshops can be conducted as courses for credit, but such programs are not conducted in the usual academic manner. They are held in settings that maximize small group relaxation and involvement, and they are coordinated with lectures that provide structure and theory.

ACTUALIZING GROUP THERAPY

In Actualizing Therapy, the group is a training ground for inner-directedness. As we have seen, the manipulative person and the person at the character styles level are both other-directed, in that both try to please others or try to give them what they want—or they give others what they themselves want. The group functions as a laboratory in determining what deepest needs are at the core level and in trying to satisfy those needs (see Figure 42). Most people have their physiological and safety needs met, but it is at level 3, love needs, that they break down. Instead of really feeling

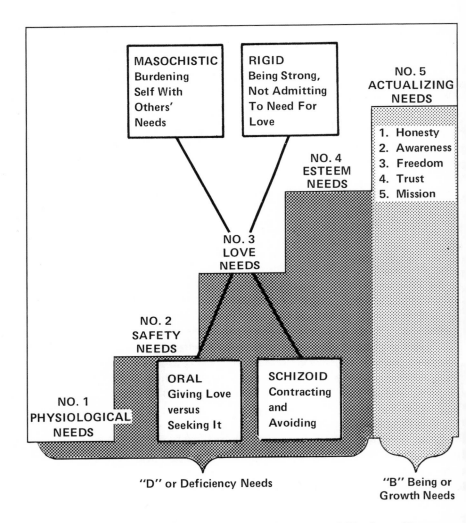

Figure 42. The Relationship of Maslow's Hierarchy of Needs to Character
Styles in Actualizing Therapy

their biological-child-wanting-love-contact aggressively, as suggested in the
discussion in Chapter 4 on character styles, they become schizoid and
contracting and avoiding; they become oral and give love rather than seek
it; they become masochistic and burden themselves with others' needs; or
they become rigid, being strong for others but not admitting their own need
to love.

Group therapy helps people to be their need for love, squarely and straightly rather than crookedly, as the character structures express their loves. This means they can then move on to esteem needs and feel their self-actualizing needs from within.

As suggested in Figure 41, a fundamental theory of Actualizing Group Therapy is that the "group is the individual turned inside out." Also, each person, paradoxically, is such a group, with all these manipulative potentials. The reply of the so-called Gadarene demoniac (Mark 5:9), "My name is legion: for we are many," applies to the healthy personality as well. The complexity of intrapersonal relationships is as formidable in its dimensions as the maze of variables involved in interpersonal relationships.

The basic theory of actualizing group change is to modify the manipulative patterns shown in Figure 33 (page 139). Thus, Figure 35 (page 142) shows how each person, with various self-defeating manipulative techniques, can be modified into an actualizing person. The processes by which these changes take place have been discussed in Chapter 6. In Chapter 9 we present an actual transcript of an Actualizing Therapy group in action.

THE CURATIVE DIMENSIONS OF GROUP THERAPY

How does group therapy help patients? To date, perhaps the single most important answer to this question is found in Yalom's (1970) research. His data from group therapists, group therapy patients, and systematic research suggest that there are ten curative factors that assume differential importance in measurement of effectiveness in group process. The data further suggest that these dimensions operate in all therapy groups but that they assume a differential importance depending on the goals and leadership of the group.

Based on Yalom's work, Magden and Shostrom have constructed a rating sheet of eight dimensions of effectiveness in groups that can be used by trained observers watching groups or films of groups in process.

The following are the dimensions used in this rating form:*

1. *Catharsis.* Group members often ventilate feelings and/or experiences.

2. *Group as a second family.* Group members identify the therapist and/or other members in family roles.

---

*The complete rating forms are available from EdITS, Box 7234, San Diego, California 92107.

3. *Awareness.* Group members become more aware of their thoughts, feelings, and/or bodily responses.

4. *Group cohesiveness.* Group members appear involved in the group.

5. *Receiving information.* Group members appear open to instructions, advice, and suggestions from the therapist.

6. *Imitative behavior.* Group members model their behavior after that of the therapist.

7. *Faith in the process.* Group members' behavior suggests that the group process will work for them.

8. *Giving and receiving help.* Group members appear to help one another through support and reassurance.

The two additional dimensions listed by Yalom, but not utilized on the rating sheet, are:

9. *Universality.* Group members appear to get insight into the "universal commonness" of their ideas, feelings, and behavior.

10. *Altruism.* Group members appear to feel a sense of caring or love for one another, which facilitates each other's expression.

The rating form was used in research conducted at the meetings of the American Psychological Association in New Orleans in September 1974. The film series *Three Approaches to Group Psychotherapy* was rated by over 200 psychologists attending this meeting. The three group sessions in the film series were conducted by Everett L. Shostrom (Actualizing Therapy), Albert Ellis (Rational-Emotive Therapy), and Harold Greenwald (Direct Decision Therapy). The psychologists rating the films were asked to specify their therapy orientation in terms of these three leaders. Approximately three quarters of the psychologists in the sample were divided equally in terms of their professed orientation, while one quarter expressed no preference. The purpose of the study, reported by Magden (1975), was to relate the eight dimensions measured by the rating form to the three approaches to group therapy presented in the films. Analysis of the data indicated that, in an overall comparison of the therapy group leaders, Shostrom averaged highest on all dimensions of effectiveness. Ratings were significantly different on all dimensions except dimension five, and the rankings were consistent for all rating groups, regardless of their orientation. Results of this study are shown in Figure 43.

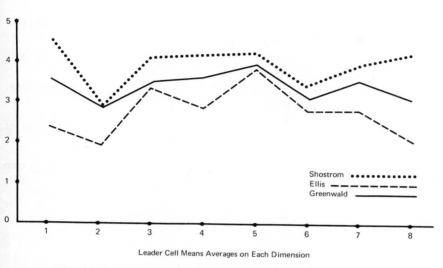

Leader Cell Means Averages on Each Dimension

Figure 43. Comparison of Three Group Leaders in Terms of Ratings on Eight Dimensions of Effectiveness

Preliminary analyses of the results show that this rating form easily lends itself to an evaluation of the effectiveness of a group session within a two-minute period.

The Concept of Orchestration

Foulkes (1949) has suggested that the term "conductor" be used to designate the role of group therapists. Because we see many parallels between conducting a symphony orchestra and leading a group, we would like to pursue such an analogy.

An orchestra has four basic families of instruments: string, woodwind, brass, and percussion. The strings and woodwinds are softer—parallel to *passive* expression—while the brass and percussion instruments are parallel to *active* expression.

The term "orchestrate" means "to arrange or combine so as to achieve maximum effect," which is what we believe the actualizing "conductor" of a group does. His primary method for achieving maximum effect is encouraging passive people to be more actively expressive and encouraging active people to be more passively expressive. As a conductor, the therapist brings out the fine expression of each person's core being in the group, just as a conductor brings out the appropriate instrumental voicings in an orchestra. Each person in a group is like a unique musical instrument—he has his own unique quality of being that he needs to actualize, and when he is actualizing he can be said to be "in tune." To realize full expression of musical quality, the conductor must evoke the complete dynamic range from the orchestra—from pianissimo (very soft) to fortissimo (very loud). Similarly, in group, the therapist's primary task is to evoke the fullest possible range of modulation of affect from the group members.

A useful extension of this analogy is that an actualizing person has the ability to "play" all four basic instruments; that is, he can move freely among the four basic polar dimensions: strength, weakness, anger, and love. A nonactualizing person, on the other hand, is limited in his personal repertoire of emotional "musical" expression.

PRECAUTIONS FOR JOINING GROUPS

A number of precautionary issues should be raised regarding joining a group. These precautions (Shostrom, 1969) have been widely recommended by psychologists to prepare people for selecting a group experience:

1. Never respond to a newspaper ad. Groups run by trained professionals, or honestly supervised by them, are forbidden by ethical considerations to advertise directly. Modest and tasteful informational brochures are circulated among professionals in relevant disciplines, and referral by a reputable and well-informed counselor is one of the surest safeguards. Cheap mimeographed flyers promising marvels, especially erotic ones, are danger signals, as are donations or fees of less than $5.00. A good group is backed by a lot of labor and experience, which are today in very short supply.

2. Never participate in a group of fewer than a half-dozen members. The necessary and valuable candor generated by an effective group cannot be dissipated, shared, and examined by too small a group, and scapegoating or purely vicious ganging-up can develop. Conversely, a group with more than sixteen members generally cannot effectively be monitored by anyone, however well trained or well assisted.

3. Never join an encounter group on impulse—as a fling, binge, or surrender to the unplanned. Any important crisis in your life has been a long time in preparation and deserves reflection. If you are sanely suspicious of your grasp on reality, be doubly cautious. The intense, sometimes apocalyptic experience of the group can be most unsettling, particularly for persons who feel that they are

close to what one layman calls "controlled schizophrenia." A trained person responsible for a meaningful session would not throw precariously balanced persons into a good encounter group. Nor would he allow persons who are diabolically experienced in the ways of group dynamics to form a group. If you find yourself in a group in which everybody talks jargon, simply walk out.

4. Never participate in a group encounter with close associates, persons with whom you have professional or competitive social relations. Be worldly wise, or healthily paranoid, about this. As a corollary, never join a group that fails to make clear and insistent distinctions between the special environment of the group and the equally special environment of society. You should be told crisply that everything occurring within the group must be considered vitally privileged communication. You should always feel that the warm, vigorous disalienation that flowers in a good group is to a certain extent designed to suggest the richness of possibilities—in terms of self-knowing and other-knowing—and does not by any means imply a rigid code of behavior. In these matters, consult your common sense—it may be one of the worst enemies you have, but it still is an entirely internalized enemy, hence deserving of notice.

5. Never be overly impressed by beautiful or otherwise class-signaled surroundings or participants. Good group sessions can be held in ghetto classrooms, and all good sessions will include persons and life styles with which you do not identify intimately or on a day-to-day basis. Social or intellectual homogeneity in a group usually suggests an unimaginative, exploitative hostess mentality. A good group session should, I think, eventually unfold itself to every member as a kind of externalization or dramatization of himself—himself as fawner and snob, weakling and bully, villain and victim, poet and bureaucrat, critic and nice guy—himself as a small but complex galaxy of contraries. If you have a strong feeling that, as Huck Finn said, you've "been there before," you most probably have.

6. Never stay with a group that has a behavioral ax to grind—a group that seems to insist that everybody be a Renaissance *mensch,* or a devotee of *cinéma vérité*—or a rightist or leftist, or a cultural, intellectual, or sexual specialist. This is narrow, destructive missionary zeal, or avocational education, and it has nothing to do with your self, your sweetest goals, or your fullest life as a self-knowing, self-integrating human being.

7. Never participate in a group that lacks formal connection with a professional on whom you can check. Any reputable professional has a vital stake in any group he runs or in any group whose leader he has trained and continues to advise and consult. Such a professional may be a psychiatrist (M.D.), a psychologist (M.A. or Ph.D. in psychology), a social worker (M.S.W.), or a marriage counselor (Ph.D.). One of the most significant questions to ask is, *Are you, or is your professional consultant, licensed to practice in this state?* If he has a Ph.D. and is not licensed, find out why not. Most reputable professionals are members of local, usually county, professional organizations; such organizations in many instances determine who may be listed where and how in your local Yellow Pages. If you can't find your group leader or the group's adviser in the Yellow Pages, check with the professional organization to find out why. It must be said at this point that all the training and accreditation in the world will not guarantee that every man in every place will be a good, efficient, worthy, or honest practitioner. . . .

Any encounter group that uses the words *psychologist, psychiatrist, psychotherapy, psychotherapist, psychology, or therapy* in describing itself is usually subject to regulation by state laws and by the American Psychological Association, the American Psychiatric Association, [the American Association of Marriage Counselors, the American Association of Pastoral Psychology], or the National Association of Social Workers. In the past decade or so, however, humanistic psychology has explicitly and implicitly de-emphasized therapy, in the sense of curing or treating people who are, on the analogy with physical medicine, mentally sick. Humanistic psychology, from whose passionate forehead the encounter group has sprung, tends to talk about *emotional growth, fulfillment of one's potential, feeling, contact* and the participative *experiencing* of one's self and others with *honesty, awareness, freedom,* and *trust.* It has dealt usually with persons who are performing within socially acceptable parameters of legality, productivity and success. It speaks usually to those who are not sick but rather normal—normally depressed, normally dissatisfied with the quality of their lives, normally tormented by irrelevance, meaninglessness, waste, loneliness, fear, and barrenness. Anyone can appropriate this humanistic vocabulary, set up shop as a lay encounter leader, and evade all professional legal regulation by omitting psychological, psychiatric, and therapeutic terms from his descriptive catalogue or notice.

There are dangers in all group encounters—groups are crucibles of intense emotional and intellectual reaction, and one can never say exactly what will happen. It can be said generally, however, that well-trained people are equipped to recognize and deal with problems (and successes) before, while, and after they happen, and that ill-trained or untrained people often are not. Yet training—in the sense of specialized, formally accredited education—will not guarantee that a man or woman will be a helpful or successful group leader. Indeed, such researchers as Margaret Rioch have shown that natural group leaders with [basic M.A. level] training can facilitate precisely the kind of ideal, joyful, alive, tender, and altogether marvelous self-learning that the most highly trained leaders strive for. Since there are not enough trained professionals to go around, the problem is to get good group leaders—to develop a set of standards that will allow us to enroll good people, teach them the necessary skills, and send them out with some formal approval that will give the public a fair chance to stay out of trouble.

Such well-selected, well-trained leaders should have a title and a certificate of some sort indicating that they have met certain nationally accepted standards. They would stand in some fairly well-defined relationship to professionals and to other licensed counselors. The analogy that most quickly, and perhaps most unhappily, comes to mind is the relationship of registered nurses to physicians. . . . I'd like to propose that persons with such training call themselves facilitators and refer to their work in such a way that they distinguish themselves from certified counselors who work in institutional settings, and from licensed psychotherapists in professional practice. . . . the public is entitled to some ready means for distinguishing a rigorously selected and coached facilitator from, for instance, [an untrained and unskilled layman]. (pp. 36-40)

Research is badly needed to evaluate and measure competence and to codify standards. State licensing laws need to be updated, to include specific mention of groups, group therapy, encounter groups, and growth groups. Presently there is an impression, in some quarters, that anyone can lead a group. But the responsibility involved in group experience is no less significant than that in individual treatment. One possible compromise would be a legal requirement that all group leaders be under the direct supervision of a licensed clinical psychologist, board certified psychiatrist, licensed clinical social worker, or licensed marriage counselor.

Encounter groups in all their forms are far too valuable—and the demand for such groups is far too clamorous and desperate— for us to let ignorance, psychosocial greed, or false prophecy tarnish them. (p. 40)

GUIDELINES FOR PSYCHOLOGISTS
CONDUCTING GROWTH GROUPS

In addition to the above suggestions for potential group members, the American Psychological Association (1973) has prepared some guidelines* to assist psychologists in group methods:

> The following guidelines are presented for the information and guidance of psychologists who conduct growth or encounter groups. They are not intended to substitute for or to supplant ethical practices for psychologists specified elsewhere.
>
> The development of these guidelines was prompted by the concern of several units within the American Psychological Association that there be a set of operating principles for the use of psychologists active in such groups. The guidelines do not presume to specify or endorse any professional procedure or technique used in a group, but only to aid psychologists who offer groups to present themselves in a manner that is ethically sound and protective of the participant.
>
> The present statement attempts to accommodate those suggestions from various psychologists in response to the draft statement published by the Board of Professional Affairs in the *APA Monitor* of December 1971 (Vol. 2, No. 12, p. 3). It is to be expected that these guidelines will be subject to modification as they are put to use, and also in the light of the evolution of new knowledge and practices in the utilization of growth groups.
>
> 1. Entering into a growth group experience should be on a voluntary basis; any form of coercion to participate is to be avoided.
>
> 2. The following information should be made available in writing to all prospective participants:
>   (a) An explicit statement of the purpose of the group;
>   (b) Types of techniques that may be employed;
>   (c) The education, training, and experience of the leader or leaders;
>   (d) The fee and any additional expense that may be incurred;
>   (e) A statement as to whether or not a follow-up service is included in the fee;
>   (f) Goals of the group experience and techniques to be used;

---

*Approved for publication by the Board of Directors of the American Psychological Association on February 15, 1973. An ad hoc committee consisting of Donald H. Clark, Wilbert Edgerton, and John J. McMillan (Chair), the Board of Professional Affairs, and the Board of Directors were successively responsible for development of the statement in its final form. Reproduced with permission.

(g) Amounts and kinds of responsibility to be assumed by the leader and by the participants. For example, (i) the degree to which a participant is free not to follow suggestions and prescriptions of the group leader and other group members; (ii) any restrictions on a participant's freedom to leave the group at any time; and,

(h) Issues of confidentiality.

3. A *screening interview* should be conducted by the group leader prior to the acceptance of any participant. It is the responsibility of the leader to screen out those individuals for whom he or she judges the group experience to be inappropriate. Should an interview not be possible, then other measures should be used to achieve the same results.

At the time of the screening interview, or at some other time prior to the beginning of the group, opportunity should be provided for leader-participant exploration of the terms of the contract as described in the information statement. This is to assure mutual understanding of the contract.

4. It is recognized that growth groups may be used for both educational and psychotherapeutic purposes. If the purpose is primarily educational, the leader assumes the usual professional and ethical obligations of an educator. If the purpose is therapeutic, the leader assumes the same professional and ethical responsibilities he or she would assume in individual or group psychotherapy, including before and after consultation with any other therapist who may be professionally involved with the participant. In both cases, the leader's own education, training, and experience should be commensurate with these responsibilities.

5. It is recognized that growth groups may be used for responsible research or exploration of human potential and may therefore involve the use of innovative and unusual techniques. While such professional exploration must be protected and encouraged, the welfare of the participant is of paramount importance. Therefore, when an experience is clearly identified as "experimental," the leader should (a) make full disclosure of techniques to be used, (b) delineate the respective responsibilities of the leader and participant during the contract discussion phase prior to the official beginning of the group experience, and (c) evaluate and make public his or her findings. (p. 933)

PROFESSIONAL ISSUES IN GROUP THERAPY

Other considerations are also important in the structuring of groups, from a professional viewpoint. The balance of this chapter will consider some of these critical issues.

Selection of Group Members

When a client comes for therapy, he is first seen by the psychotherapist, so that the therapist gets to know the client well before placing him in a group. A group is selected that seems to meet the needs of the client, as well as the client's meeting the needs of the group. The client may then continue to meet his therapist individually once a week in addition to working in his group once a week, or he may reduce the number of individual visits, depending on the setting and the problem.

Bach (1954) has introduced a theory of grouping that he calls the "nuclear expansion theory." In this model, the group is started with two or three members and the expansion is made according to the identification and similarity needs of these particular individuals. We generally tend to subscribe to Bach's point of view on selection of members.

In Actualizing Therapy, all new group members are provided with a preparation sheet on which critical dimensions are included (see Figure 44A for an example). In addition, a copy of "Ground Rules for Groups" (Figure 44B) is given to new group members to help them function more effectively in the group.

Placement

The concept of "role vacancies" is fundamental to the decision of placement in a group. Actualizing Group Therapists feel that groups should have a balance of personalities representative of the *polarities*. These various personality types give the group material with which to provoke discussion of common human problems and transference relationships. An Actualizing Group Therapist's first consideration is the selection of appropriate group membership. He or she is constantly aware of the need for a balance of personalities representing the four polar dimensions of anger, love, strength, and weakness. Only when there is a personality in the group to represent each polar dimension does the group have sufficient balance to potentiate growth in each member. This idea is shown in Figure 45.

PREPARATION SHEET FOR NEW GROUP MEMBERS

1. *Size of group.* The group's size is limited to a minimum number of six and a maximum number of ten patients.

2. *Admission of new members.* When an old member leaves the group, his or her place in the group will be filled by a new member. The selection is made on two bases: which group is best for the prospective member, and which prospective member is best for the group.

3. *Post sessions.* The regular office meetings of the group with the therapist, while of central therapeutic importance, are only part of the total program. Experiences during the post session between members of the group provide important material for self-observation and analysis.

4. *Extra office meetings.* No extra office meetings, other than post-session meetings are allowed. Your own reputation, as well as the reputation of the Institute, is at stake in this matter and it is important to consider seriously.

5. *Sharing of mutual experiences.* Group members usually adhere to the principle that everything anybody says, thinks, or does that involves another member of the group, is subject to open discussion in the group. In other words, the emotionally important experiences of any members are shared by all members. There are no secrets *inside* the group.

Figure 44A. Preparation Sheet for New Group Members (continued)

6. *Ethical confidence.* In contrast to Principle Number 5, everything that goes on within the group—*everything*—must remain in absolute secret as far as any outsider (nonmember) is concerned. This especially includes spouses. Anyone participating in group therapy automatically assumes the same professional ethics of absolute discretion that bind professional therapists.

7. *The group's goal.* The group's goal is free communication on a nondefensive, personal, and emotional level. This goal can be reached only by the group effort. Experience shows that the official therapists cannot "push" the group; the group has to progress by its own efforts.

Each member will get out of the group what he puts into it. As every member communicates to the group his feelings, perceptions, and associations of the moment as openly as he can and as often as he can, the group will become a therapeutically effective medium. The goal of free communication is freedom to be oneself most fully and comfortably.

I have read the above and agree to cooperate fully.

Signed _____

Figure 44A. Preparation Sheet for New Group Members

GROUND RULES FOR GROUPS

1. To stay together in the same place and not leave until the group breaks or ends at its prearranged time. Everyone attends to and reacts to how each individual acts in the group situation. This means that there must be no subgrouping, such as is common at ordinary social gatherings and parties.

2. All forms of physical assault or threats of physical violence are outlawed. Attacks must be confined to verbal critiques. However, there are no limits as to the straightforward use of Anglo-Saxon words or slang.

3. The encountering experience is a four-phase process: Individual expressions are a) reacted to; and b) these reactions are shared in a "feedback"; c) the "feedback" in turn generates counter-reactions from the original expressors as well as d) from the rest of the group. Members are expected to facilitate each of these phases by active participation in the following manner:

   a. Sharing true feelings as clearly and transparently as possible. The expressor is himself responsible for drawing, and keeping, the full attention of the group on himself. No one should wait to be "brought out." Every participant is expected to voluntarily put himself into the focus of the group's attention, to seek out the group and to turn attention to himself, preferably a number of times.

   By being an attentive audience, the group rewards the expressor. The expressor will remain in focal-position (or the "hot seat") until his feeling-productivity wanes and/or until the expressor himself has had "enough" of the "hot seat," or until group interest and group pressure are dissipated.

Figure 44B. Ground Rules for Groups (continued)

b. In the "feedback" reactions to the expressor, no holds are barred! Candid *"leveling"* is expected from everyone; which means participants explicitly share, and do *not* hide or mask, their here-and-now, on-the-spot reactions to one another! Tact is "out" and frankness is "in." Any phony, defensive, or evasive behavior (such as playing psychiatric games or reciting old "numbers") is fair game for the group's critique and verbal attack. "Oughtmanship" (advising others how to solve their problems) can deteriorate into a time-consuming, dulling routine that suppresses spontaneous encounter. Excessive advice-giving is, therefore, undesirable.

c. Trying to make people "feel better" is *not* the purpose of the group. Self-appointed tactful diplomats, amateur "protectors" and "Red Cross nurses" distract and dilute the leveling experience. Any kind of protective "cushioning" spoils (for the central "hot-seat" person) the experience of standing up alone to the group, as he must to the world.

4. *"Show me now . . . do not tell me when"* is *the* group leitmotif. Owning up to feelings, *here and now,* and sharing them, is *the* mode of participation. Telling the group about how one behaves outside the group and telling how "he" then and there reacted—in bygone times and other places (back home or back at the office)—is only warm-up material. The thing to do is to let yourself feel your presence in the group and let the currently active impact of the others get to you!

5. *"As you are in the group, so you are in the world."* As you learn to exchange feelings in the group, a pattern of participation automatically emerges that the group will mirror back to you. In the long hours of a group you cannot help being seen for

Figure 44B. Ground Rules for Groups

what you really are and seeing what you can become. The group simulates the world of emotionally significant others, and the ways in which you relate to this world reflect the core pattern of your being. The group members' reactions will give you cues as to the effect your behavior patterns have on the world. You have the option to try out new, improved ways of being.

6. Giving affectionate recognition to growth and new learning is as much in order as defensive behavior is out of order. Reinforcement of new learning is the loving side of critical leveling.

7. *"Rule of discretion."* While nothing is sacred within the group, the information gained during a group is confidential—in the nature of professionally privileged communication. Nothing is revealed to anyone outside. Objective research reporting in anonymous format is the only exception.

Figure 44B. Ground Rules for Groups

Potentiation and Synergy as Applied to Groups

The above concept of placement is based on the theory of *potentiation* of polarities, or the idea that a representative of each polar dimension in the group tends to encourage the expression of that dimension in other members of the group. When there is a primary person representing each of the polar dimensions in the group, then the group has potential for total expression.

In the group context, potentiation is based on the idea that because the individual belongs to the group, he has at his disposal the power of the entire group. *Synergy* is the "tertium quid," the power beyond, which exceeds the summated power of each of the individual members of a group. The primary means for achieving the goals of potentiation and synergy is to expose an individual member who is weak on a particular polar dimension to another member who is strong on that same dimension. For example, a client who is able to express loving but not anger needs another person in the group who can stimulate him to express his power to be angry. Furthermore, exposing such a person to an even weaker person provides him with the disgust of seeing himself mirrored by this person. Thus "modeling," in a positive or negative sense, is an important principle that is utilized in Actualizing Therapy. In addition to modeling, members can stimulate an individual's growth on a particular polarity by various forms of group pressure, such as encouragement, disappointment, and caring.

A group is a synergistic assembly of persons that has a power greater than the individual members alone. It has a power greater than individual therapy in that the power of co-members, acting in a therapeutic manner toward a particular member, provides dimensions of growth that even a trained therapist would not have, since therapists themselves never totally have "all their polarities together." Furthermore, the therapist is simply one individual, in comparison to six or seven other facilitators—the group members—who augment and amplify *energy for change.*

The twin principles of potentiation and synergy thus enable the group to be a field of energy that vitalizes the potential for growth on each polarity for each individual. Thus it can be seen that placement in a group requires an understanding of polarity theory and a comprehension of the growth possible through synergy and potentiation.

Figure 41 suggests the rhythm expressive of the polarities in a group setting. As each member learns to "rev up" the power of his own polarities, the accumulated polarities of the group create power in a manner like the movement of cylinders in the dynamic motion of a motor engine.

Manipulation Analysis in Groups

Another dimension of Actualizing Group Therapy has to do with the ability of a group to encourage expression of common manipulative or controlling patterns in one another. Since each person manipulates to some degree, simply staying in the moment and being oneself will eventually facilitate expression of one's own manipulations. The therapist's skill in recognizing manipulations, as well as the ability of more experienced members to do the same, creates an arena for the awareness of manipulations that, again, goes beyond individual therapy.

Theoretically, we say that the group is the individual turned inside out. So clients can not only see their own *potentials* in others, but they can see their own *manipulations* in others as well. While individual therapy often focuses more on body work and intellectual awareness, the group is unsurpassed as a means for facilitating change in feeling awareness.

Some of the many possible role needs for a mixed group are suggested by our research on the Pair Attraction Inventory (PAI). Figure 45 illustrates the six basic pairings, which cover most of the problem pairs seen in pairing and marital therapy. Selection of similar "opposites" can almost guarantee good group interaction.

Criteria for Exclusion of Members from Groups

When selecting certain members for groups, Hobbs (1951) has found that there are several types of persons who tend to disrupt or hinder group progress. They are: psychologically sophisticated persons who use knowledge of psychodynamics cruelly on others; extremely aggressive or hostile people who destroy the atmosphere of acceptance and freedom essential to the success of the group; and people who are continuously in close contact with each other outside of the group.

Bach (1954, pp. 18-22) uses four personality criteria for exclusion of members from groups: insufficient reality contact; extremes of illegal or culturally tabooed behavior; the dominant character who would be a chronic monopolizer of discussion; and those with psychopathic defenses and impulsiveness.

Size of Groups

In organizing a therapeutic group for counseling or psychotherapy, the question usually arises as to how many persons should be included. Size is important because it can be a barrier to effectiveness of communication. A suggested minimum number for an effective social unit is five or six. Ten to

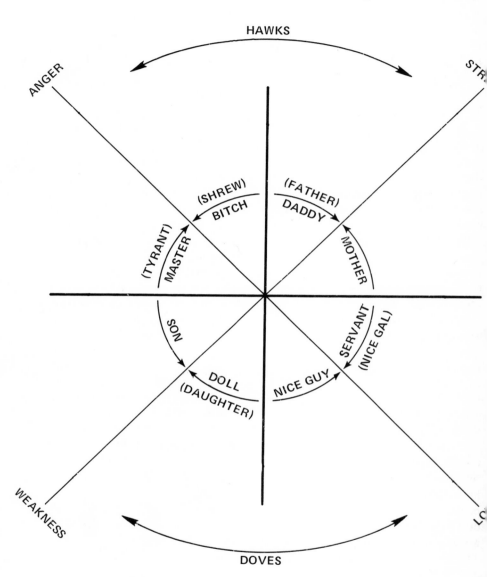

Figure 45. Pairings that Facilitate Group Expression

NOTE: In *Between Man and Woman* (1971), we tried to find commonly understood words that have male-female parallel meanings. We were unable at that time to do so completely, because the literature reflected a male characteristic bias. We have now added, in parentheses above, alternative terms that are parallel to the interpersonal roles reflecting each of the polarities. We believe these terms now reflect a more equalitarian view.

twelve would be the maximum. Group therapists generally agree, however, that eight is an optimum number.

In sensitivity or encounter groups, the number of participants often reaches fifteen or sixteen members. This keeps limits on the intimacy that develops in groups with fewer members.

Closed versus Open Groups

There are two kinds of groups: closed and open. A closed group maintains the same membership throughout its existence (often the case in educational settings, for example, where groups run the length of the academic semester) while in an open, or continuous, group, replacements are made when a member leaves.

There is some degree of speculation among therapists as to whether closed groups offer more advantages than continuous groups. Some think that the closed group has more advantages because data can be more readily accumulated when the group composition is kept constant. In many cases where a closed group has a time limit, members may get down to the "nitty-gritty" much faster. Such a group may begin in September, for example, and end in May. Some group leaders and members have noted that, if there is a definite time limit, a psychological feeling of urgency prevails, since the group members and the facilitator know that they must accomplish whatever goals they wish to attain in a certain period allotted to them. This same phenomenon has been noted during individual sessions, wherein clients sometimes work more intensely toward the end of the therapeutic hour, when they know that their time is drawing to a close.

If members do drop out of a closed group, however, it may become unduly small. An advantage of an open group is that a new member sometimes fosters a reworking of rivalries and competition in the group and may help therapeutic movement through a consolidation of group feeling. Also, because new members often reduce their defensiveness by identifying with other members who have already overcome theirs, their presence in the group appears to have some ego-strengthening effects on the older members. The old members gain therapeutically through the experience of sharing and helping new clients adjust to the group.

Actualizing Communication Skills

Alan Levy has developed a catalog of twelve communicative fouls that assists the individual in group therapy to be more authentic in his communication. Figure 46 is a copy of this form, which we have found very useful in helping group members learn communication skills.

AUTHENTICS

Authentics is a direct approach to learning the verbal language of loving. It involves identifying and understanding the most common obstacles to direct communication and replacing them with more authentic forms to promote closeness between persons.

The following is a catalog of twelve *communicative fouls.* Each will be labeled, defined, and described in terms of the avoidance mechanism involved. Then, examples of each foul and possible alternatives are offered.

It is easy, if you're so inclined, to interpret this approach to authentic communicating in an authoritarian way, and thus discount its value. What follows is not a set of "dos and don'ts," or "rights and wrongs." It is a method to increase your awareness of what kinds of verbal responses tend to bring you closer to people and what kinds tend to keep you distant from the vulnerability of intimate contact.

Level I

1. *Questioning:* Asking a question is a common way to make contact with others dependently and at a safe distance. Questions are sometimes used to disguise opinions or accusation. Questioning avoids responsibility for self-assertion. Example of foul: "Why do you look at me like that?"

   Alternative: "I feel uncomfortable with you looking at me like that. I want to know what you're feeling about me."

2. *Gossiping:* Talking *about* someone rather than *to* them. It's almost as if the object of the response were not present. Gossiping avoids direct contact with another person. Example of foul: (To Cynthia or the air) "I like Mary. She gives a great deal of herself."

   Alternative: (To Mary) "I like you. You give a great deal of yourself."

Figure 46. Authentics (continued)

3. *Shoulding:* Using tyrannical words like "should," "ought to," "have to," and so on. Making prescriptions or proscriptions for self and/or others. Shoulding is an attempt to manufacture a sense of security out of thin air, a way of avoiding the deeper issue of what one really *wants* to express.

Example of foul: "I should participate more, I know. But I have to wait until there's something the group should hear before I talk. I guess I ought to be more spontaneous."

Alternative: "I want to participate more. But I choose to wait until I believe the group wants to hear what I want to say. I have mixed feelings about being spontaneous. I want to and I want to be careful too."

4. *Blind Interrupting:* Not allowing another person to finish a sentence or expression and doing it without being aware of interrupting. No example can be cited adequately here, but it is usually obvious when brought to attention. Less obvious, but equally important, is the interrupting of someone's flow of feeling with irrelevant talk or action. An interruption that is made deliberately and with a measure of consent is not a barrier to intimacy.

5. *Sarcasm:* Saying the exact opposite of what you mean. Sarcasm is 180 degrees off center. The emotional message and the content message of a response are in conflict. Sarcasm, a classic double-bind communication, avoids direct expression of negative feeling.

Example of foul: (derisively) "I love the way you lecture people."

Alternative: "You lecture people and I don't like it."

6. *Group Spokesman:* This is a role in which the person acts as if he were the group's mouthpiece and is expressing accurately a consensus of attitude or feeling—a sheer impossibility in a

Figure 46. Authentics (continued)

spontaneous gathering. Pretending such "togetherness" is an avoidance of taking the risk to be an individual, possibly at variance with others. This occurs commonly when someone is experiencing a strong negativity while trying to prevent standing alone with it.

Example of foul: "We're not accomplishing anything with this chitchat. We didn't come here to make friends; we're here to learn how to be more effective with people."

Alternative: "I'm not accomplishing what I expected to in this situation. I don't want to chitchat or make friends here; I want to become more effective with people."

Level II

7. *Intellectualizing:* Generalizing about subject matter or issues that are distant from the here-and-now interaction. Contacting other people very indirectly through abstract discussion or argument instead of meeting the more emotionally vital present situation with personal talk. Intellectualizing usually involves an avoidance of the word "I," although a typical intellectualizing statement can be made from "I feel that . . ." This foul is used to avoid the experience of any feelings.

Example of foul: "People usually don't warm up quickly to one another in a new group. They're not likely to talk about themselves until you've established an atmosphere of trust."

Alternative: "I feel cold and distant toward you until I know you better. I don't trust you yet."

8. *Mind-Raping:* Pretending to read the mind or needs or underlying motivation of another person; acting as if you know him better than he does. Sometimes called the "Psycho-

Figure 46. Authentics (continued)

analysis Game." A favorite husband-wife ploy, mind-raping avoids examination of your own assumptions and projections and gives a false sense of security by staying "on top."

Example of foul: "You're just saying you like me. I don't believe you really mean that. You're just patronizing me."

Alternative: "I have trouble believing you like me. I don't feel it."

9. *Justifying:* Overly long explanations that serve to defend the speaker from feeling guilty. Others listening often begin to feel that the person is acting like a defendant on trial, doing his best to prove his innocence. Listeners' boredom and irritation sometimes provide a clue to this foul. Justifying avoids acknowledgment of the pain of being misunderstood and perhaps misjudged at times.

Example of foul: "Let me explain. I didn't mean anything critical by what I said. I mean, I was only going along with what the rules are here and expressing my opinions like we're supposed to, and of course, it's the way I was brought up, you know, to be honest and say what I think. That's the only way we learn, right?"

Alternative: "Well, that's the way I feel."

10. *Rescuing:* Protecting or attempting to protect another person from the criticism or confrontation of others. It may also be labeled "meddling" or "interrupting" because it sometimes serves the purpose of interfering with the honest flow of feelings. Reassuring is a mild variation of rescuing. There is a subtle difference between offering needed assistance and/or reassurance and rescuing, but the receiver usually feels it. Rescuing helps the rescuer avoid feeling helpless and vulnerable to what the rescued one is experiencing.

Figure 46. Authentics (continued)

Example of foul: "I think you're all being too harsh with Myrna. After all, she's been rejected by her husband too. Don't worry, Myrna, it'll work out all right."

Alternative: "I'm aware that I feel very protective toward you, Myrna; I know how painful it's been for me to be rejected."

11. *Blaming/Negative Predicting/Threatening:* These three are variations of one common theme: They all convey an avoidance of a present reality and a holding on to negativity about the past or future.

Blaming is an indirect expression of hostility over the past. Negative predicting is an expectation of future hurts, usually a projection of the blamer's hostility. Threatening is a hostile promise to inflict punishment; the act of threatening is usually more painful to the victim than is the threatened punishment itself.

Example of blaming: "You hurt me back then."

Example of negative predicting: "You'll hurt me again."

Example of threatening: "I'll hurt you."

Alternatives are difficult to spell out for this set of personal fouls. To chronic users of this threesome (and they often go together), professional help is often indicated to unravel the underlying confusion of rage, dependency, and panic. All of us, to the extent to which we are emotionally dependent, under stress, and desperate about our self-esteem, use this kind of avoidance at times.

Some possible alternatives:
To blaming: "I feel hurt and misunderstood about the past. I realize you're not to blame, but I am still hurt and

Figure 46. Authentics (continued)

	angry. I wonder why I am unable to let go of my resentment."
To negative predicting:	"I still feel resentful about the past and I'm afraid that unless I let go of it, I'll have trouble really liking you or anyone."
To threatening:	"When you say that, I feel helpless and afraid about the future. I just don't know what will happen to me."

12. *Praising/Positive Predicting/Promising:* These are sugar-coated relatives of the above negative threesome (blaming/negative predicting/threatening). Because they are basically positive expressions, and only toxic in a subtle sense, they are often acceptable and even sought after in relationships. The unconscious (and sometimes conscious) attempt to control with the "positive reinforcement" that underlies their use is therefore hidden and often overlooked. However, they can become effective blocks to authentic relating, particularly of unsureness and mistrust. The popular "win-friends-and-influence-people" attitude, "If you can't say something nice, don't say anything," discounts the ability of others to accept honest negativity. In other words, it hides a deep lack of faith in one's acceptability and in the world's readiness to "be there."

| Example of praising: | "Group was great tonight; everyone participated like the self-actualized people we are, and you're the greatest leader, Dr. Authentic." |

Figure 46. Authentics (continued)

Alternative: "I enjoyed being in group
                                    tonight, the way everyone
                                    participated. I feel as
                                    though something impor-
                                    tant has happened."

Example of positive predicting: "I just know that we're
                                    going to be a close-knit,
                                    loving group."

Alternative: "I hope that I grow closer
                                    to others in the group."

Example of promising: "From now on, I'm going
                                    to be more assertive and
                                    self-expressive."

Alternative: "I want to be more assertive
                                    and self-expressive from
                                    now on."

Figure 46. Authentics

RESEARCH ON EFFECTIVENESS OF GROUPS

The question as to whether group techniques do, in fact, yield enduring positive personality change (Gibb, 1971) or actually result in psychological damage in some cases (Yalom & Lieberman, 1971) has only recently been subjected to objectively quantified assessment.

Gibb (in Rogers, 1970), after analyzing 106 studies, as well as examining 123 additional studies and 24 recent doctoral dissertations, stated, "The evidence is strong that intensive group training experiences have therapeutic effects. . . . Changes do occur in sensitivity, ability to manage feelings, directionality of motivation, attitudes toward the self, attitudes toward others, and interdependence" (p. 117).

The term "interdependence" refers to interpersonal competence, teamwork in problem solving, and being a good group member. Because interdependence is also one of the chief goals of Actualizing Therapy, we believe this research summary is significant.

Encounter Groups: First Facts (1973), based on an exhaustive study at Stanford University by Morton A. Lieberman, Irvin D. Yalom, and Matthew M. Miles, is billed as the first scientific report of any magnitude to deal with *encounter groups*. In the academic year 1968-1969, 210 Stanford undergraduates were recruited and divided randomly into seventeen different encounter groups. Two of the groups were led only by tape-recorded instructions, and the others were led by professionals whose philosophical approaches included Gestalt, Transactional Analysis, Synanon games, "Esalen eclectic," and others.

In contrast to Gibb, the Stanford researchers found the rate of casualties to be an "alarming and unacceptable" 10 percent. Chances of "clear, positive benefit" proved to be about one in three. *Psychotherapy* seemed a surer route to "positive change." Only 16 percent of the participants had "peak experiences" during the course of the groups. Gimmicks and structured exercises did not prove especially valuable. In conclusion, Lieberman, Yalom, and Miles have asked the deepest possible respect for the self-preservatory functions of defense mechanisms and have emphasized that to attack a person in an effort to dislodge him from familiar defenses is crude and often counterproductive. Lieberman et al. (1973, pp. 422-424) also confirm certain tenets of Actualizing Therapy, concluding from their research that expressing anger is good but that sustained levels of anger are unproductive and need to be balanced by love and support. Furthermore, they conclude that both feeling *and* thinking need to be expressed in group, in contrast to the Rogerian myth that only feeling is important, and the layman's myth that one should use only his head and deny his feelings and his body.

We believe the contrast between Gibb's and Yalom and Lieberman's conclusions leaves the question of encounter group effectiveness in the air (although Maliver's *The Encounter Game,* 1972, suggests that trained clinical psychologists and psychiatrists conducting groups in professional settings have much greater success than untrained leaders of encounter groups).

POI Research on the Effectiveness of Encounter Groups

The major instrument used in recent studies has been the Personal Orientation Inventory. In a recently published review of instruments in human relations training, Pfeiffer and Heslin (1973) have noted:

> The POI, perhaps more than any other instrument described in this book, measures the things talked about by people in human relations training. For this reason it is an excellent training device. It awakens people to important dimensions of life and ways of viewing the world and themselves that they may well not have considered previously. (p. 100)

Many of the early studies considered here contained a number of methodological shortcomings, but due to the importance of objective data in this area a review and integration of findings to date seems appropriate.

The POI has been particularly successful in measuring the effectiveness of group work in a variety of settings. For example, of fifteen studies received by Knapp (1973), seven dealt with adult samples, seven with college student samples, and one with high-school student samples. Eight of these fifteen studies incorporated a control group. Sample sizes, an important factor in statistical interpretation, ranged from 14 to 135, with results of four of these studies being based on responses from fewer than 30 subjects.

Perhaps of greatest importance in the review of these studies, however, are the effects of such variables as length of time over which the changes are evaluated and comparisons of the effects of different encounter techniques. Before undertaking studies evaluating effects of such variables upon outcome of the encounter group experience, adequate measurement techniques were required. As mentioned, the availability of the POI has accelerated research in this area.

Studies of Change Following Encounter

A number of studies have demonstrated changes in self-actualizing following encounter group experience. A summary of the results of the major of these studies is presented in Figure 47.

In an extensive study of the effects of nonprofessionally led encounter groups with university and community volunteers, Bebout and Gordon (1972) reported the results of pre- and post-encounter group experience. The sample for which POI analyses were reported involved seventy males and sixty-five females. Pre- to post-test changes were analyzed separately for the sexes, and significant increases were obtained for the POI scales of Inner-Direction (I), Existentiality (Ex) (males only), Feeling Reactivity (Fr), Spontaneity (S), Acceptance of Aggression (A), and Capacity for Intimate Contact (C). Although the analysis suffers from the lack of a control sample, the increases are in line with those of several other studies employing smaller samples but also incorporating control samples in the design.

To examine the effects of a program of Transcendental Meditation on self-actualizing, Seeman, Nidich, and Banta (1972) administered the POI to an experimental group of twenty college students, and to a control group of twenty, prior to the initiation of the program and two months following completion of the program. The mean difference for the experimental group on the Other/Inner support dimension was significantly higher than that for the control group. Significant mean changes in the positive direction were obtained for the experimental group on scales of Inner-Direction (I), Self-Actualizing Value (SAV), Spontaneity (S), Acceptance of Aggression (A), and Capacity for Intimate Contact (C). No pre- to post-test changes were significant for the control group.

Guinan and Foulds (1970) report changes on POI scale scores following a marathon group experience. The study was designed to investigate such changes that might occur among a group of relatively "normal" college students following a voluntary, thirty-hour weekend marathon experience. Results were compared with those obtained from a selected control sample volunteering to be in "an experiment." Analysis of the data disclosed that mean POI scores for the experimental group changed in a positive direction and that, for seven of the twelve scales (Inner-Direction, Existentiality, Feeling Reactivity, Spontaneity, Self-Acceptance, Acceptance of Aggression, and Capacity for Intimate Contact), changes reached significance at or beyond the .05 confidence level. No changes for the control group reached significance.

Findings of this study were challenged by Marks, Conry, and Foster (1973) on the basis of shortcomings in the design of the study. In a sub-

POI Scales		Studies With Control Group									Without Control				
	Study	Alperson, Alperson & Levine (1971)	Byrd (1967)	Foulds & Hannigan (in press)	Guinan & Foulds (1970)	Kimball & Gelso (1974)	Seeman, Nidick & Banta (1972)	Treppa & Fricke (1972)	Walton (1973)	Young & Jacobson (1970)	Banmen & Capelle (1972)	Bebout & Gordon (1972)	Culbert, Clark & Bobele (1968)	Knapp & Fitzgerald (1973)	Reddy (1973)
Experimental Group															
Time Competence	(Tc)	**		**				*							**
Inner Directed	(I)	**	*	**	**	**	**	*	**		**	**	**	**	**
Self-Actualizing Value	(SAV)	*	*	**			*			**					*
Existentiality	(Ex)	**		**	**			**	*		**	**			**
Feeling Reactivity	(Fr)	*		**	**						**	*		**	**
Spontaneity	(S)	*	**	**	**	**	**	*	**			**	*	**	**
Self Regard	(Sr)	**		**		**	**	*						**	
Self-Acceptance	(Sa)	**		**	**	*		**	*		**				**
Nature of Man (Constructive)	(Nc)		*												
Synergy	(Sy)	*				*							*		*
Acceptance of Aggression	(A)	*	**	**	*		**	*			**	**		**	
Capacity for Intimate Contact	(C)	*		**	**		*				**	**	*		**
Control Group															
Time Competence	(Tc)														
Inner Directed	(I)							*							
Self-Actualizing Value	(SAV)														
Existentiality	(Ex)														
Feeling Reactivity	(Fr)	*													
Spontaneity	(S)														
Self Regard	(Sr)														
Self-Acceptance	(Sa)														
Nature of Man (Constructive)	(Nc)							**		**					
Synergy	(Sy)														
Acceptance of Aggression	(A)														
Capacity for Intimate Contact	(C)														

*Significant at the .05 confidence level.
**Significant at the .01 confidence level.

Figure 47. Significant Pre to Post Increases for POI Scales in Major Encounter Group Studies

sequent study, very carefully designed to meet these criticisms, Foulds, Guinan, and Hannigan (in press) obtained much the same results as those reached in their earlier study. Significantly greater increases in measures of self-actualizing were obtained for those in the encounter experience, as contrasted with a control group, in terms of the major POI Inner-Direction scale and eight of ten POI subscales. Only the Nature of Man (Nc) and Synergy (Sy) scales failed to reach significance.

In a similarly designed study by Treppa and Fricke (1972), further evidence, bearing especially on the issue of the comparative effects of control versus marathon group experience on POI test scores, has been presented. The POI, along with other personality inventories, was administered prior to, and immediately following, a weekend marathon group experience and again, six weeks later as a follow-up. Both experimental and control groups, with sample sizes of eleven each, showed significant positive changes on post-test and follow-up scores. Although changes from pre-test to post-test reached significance (beyond the .05 confidence level) for seven of the twelve POI scales in the experimental group, as compared with only two scales in the control group, the *interaction effect* between groups and test condition reached significance for only one POI scale, Spontaneity. Changes from pre-test to post-test were all in the positive direction in the experimental group while in the control group four of the twelve changes were in the negative direction. The authors concluded that the data from their study failed to adequately demonstrate the positive effects of the marathon group experience. In contrasting the results of this study with four others in which positive results were obtained, Kimball and Gelso (1974) noted that only one group facilitator, a graduate student, was used and that the number of hours of group time was not specified. Of these four studies, three used two group facilitators and the other a single highly experienced and noted facilitator. Furthermore, in the positive studies a minimum of fifteen hours of group time was involved. Thus, the authors hypothesized that, based on present research, in order to have the desired impact, growth groups should either employ more than a single leader, or should employ a highly experienced facilitator, and should continue for a minimum of fifteen hours.

Long-Term Effects of Encounter

A question frequently asked of those who espouse the intense encounter group experience is whether the effects are merely transitory or are of a more permanent nature. Several studies have evaluated the level of self-actualizing over periods ranging from six weeks to as long as one year following the encounter group experience.

Alperson, Alperson, and Levine (1971) examined the effect of a marathon encounter group experience on POI scores among high-school students. Thirty-two volunteer students were unsystematically assigned to a control (no marathon treatment) or experimental (marathon treatment) group, and completed the POI as a pre-treatment and post-treatment measure. Increases in POI scores for the experimental group reached significance for six of the POI scales including the major scales of Time Competence and Inner-Direction and the subscales of Existentiality, Self-Regard, Self-Acceptance, and Acceptance of Aggression. The Inner-Direction scale was not significantly different for the control group, and only one scale, Feeling Reactivity, showed a significant increase at the .05 level. Alperson, Alperson, and Levine concluded that marathon encounters can contribute to growth in terms of these POI scales.

In examining the effectiveness of a human relations training program among high-school teachers, Banmen and Capelle (1971) used the POI to measure pre- to post-test changes in a sample of thirty-two educators volunteering for a three-and-a-half-day program. Gains following the program (four days after) were significant for six of the POI scales: Inner-Direction, Existentiality, Feeling Reactivity, Self-Acceptance, Acceptance of Aggression, and Capacity for Intimate Contact. As a part of the design of this study, the POI was readministered to the participants three months following the training program. The follow-up scores reaffirmed the original gains made, and, in addition, the Spontaneity scale reached significance at the .05 level. None of the differences between post-test and follow-up measures reached significance. Thus, changes immediately following the program were consistent with the other studies available and were also maintained over a three-month period.

Investigating the long-term effects of a ten-day sensitivity training laboratory, Reddy (in press) administered the POI prior to the first group meeting, and again one year after the close of the laboratory. Interaction effects over time were significant for the major POI scales of Time Competence and Inner-Direction, as well as for seven of the ten subscales. The results were interpreted as demonstrating that sensitivity training group participants exhibited changes in measures of self-actualization and that these changes were maintained or continued over time. The results further suggested that participants exhibited change at different rates and at different times. Whereas some participants showed substantial gains in self-actualizing at the close of the laboratory, others exhibited major gains after returning to their usual environment. Further analysis showed that this differential rate was related to the level of anxiety of the participants as measured by the Multiple Affect Adjective Check List (Zuckerman & Lubin, 1965).

Correlations between POI changes and the measure of anxiety suggested that participants who experienced higher levels of anxiety during the laboratory did not exhibit changes on the POI at the close of the laboratory.

A number of military sponsored drug rehabilitation programs have incorporated the POI to assess the effects of encounter experience among drug users. Knapp and Fitzgerald (1973) reported on the use of the POI in assessing change among participants in a seventy-two-hour transgenerational workshop designed to establish community feeling among Navy personnel, many of whom had experienced drug abuse problems. Because evaluation of the workshop technique was concerned with personality changes of comparatively greater permanence, participants were retested one to eight months following the experience. Significant POI subscale increases were obtained for the major Inner-Direction scale as well as for Feeling Reactivity, Spontaneity, Self-Regard, and Acceptance of Aggression. Interpreting from scale descriptions, results of the workshop experience might suggest increased sensitivity to internal needs and feelings (Fr), increased freedom to express feelings spontaneously (S), increased affirmation of self strengths (Sr), and increased acceptance and understanding of natural aggressiveness (A) as opposed to defensivenesss and repression of these tendencies.

Thinking-Level versus Feeling-Level Expression

Ample evidence has accumulated to demonstrate the effects of the encounter group experience in producing significant self-reported changes toward self-actualizing. In terms of the three aspects of being, such changes reflect growth at the thinking level. It might be asked to what extent these may be reflected in changes in the feeling and bodily expression levels of this continuum. Although very little evidence has been presented to date on this topic, one study, at least, is pertinent. In their study of the effects of sensitivity training among university students, Culbert, Clark, and Bobele (1968) administered the POI before and after a series of two-hour sensitivity training meetings. When divided into initially "actualizing" and "normal" groups, those students with initially high POI scores showed significant increases on the major Inner-Direction scale and on the subscales of Spontaneity, Synergy, and Capacity for Intimate Contact. Of particular interest are correlations between the POI and a measure of self-aware verbal behavior. While the POI is a measure of self-percepts at the thinking level, self-aware verbal behavior was assumed to be a measure of self-actualizing behavior itself. In this part of their study, Culbert, Clark, and Bobele obtained no significant relationships. Thus, in this study, although POI changes for an initially low actualizing sample showed significant POI score changes (thinking level), these changes were not reflected in increased self-aware verbal behavior (bodily expression level).

In a related study, Walton (1973) administered the POI to groups of college students enrolled in a seminar in humanistic psychology. Those students in the two experimental groups received didactic content instruction as well as ten to fourteen one-hour personal growth group sessions. Students in a control group received instruction concerning counseling concepts, including the concepts and counseling procedures for furthering self-actualization. However, no systematic training experience was provided. Comparisons of pre-test to post-test changes on the POI showed that students in both groups receiving the training experience increased on the major Inner-Direction scale. Changes on this scale for the control group, receiving instruction only, did not reach significance. The subscales that changed significantly for the experimental groups were Existentiality, Spontaneity, Self-Acceptance, and Capacity for Intimate Contact. For the control group, taught by didactic procedures, only the Nature of Man scale showed significant increase. Findings were interpreted as supporting the hypothesis that personal growth groups are productive of psychological growth as defined by the POI.

Studies of attempts to "fake" POI results are of some relevance here. As pointed out in Chapter 2, instructions to fake, or make a good impression, on the POI generally result in profiles characteristic of *less* self-actualized individuals. However, Braun and LaFaro (1969), in a study of the faking of POI responses, included two experimental groups that listened to discussions of the concept of self-actualization between the standard and the "fake" administrations. Mean scores for the major Inner-Direction scale significantly increased in one group but not in the other. Results of this study suggest that the POI shows an unexpected resistance to faking but that with specific knowledge about the inventory and the concepts measured, persons *can* improve their POI scores under certain circumstances.

In a series of studies in which college students were presented with either information about the concept of self-actualizing, information about more conventional social adjustment, or no information at all, Warehime, Routh, and Foulds (1974) found that those receiving information concerning self-actualizing were able to increase their scores on the POI when asked to use this information. However, when asked to respond honestly, their scores were unaffected by knowledge about the self-actualizing person. The authors concluded that the Inner-Direction scale is more resistant to faking than many other self-report inventories and that the POI is remarkably unsusceptible to dissimulation.

Comparison of Encounter Training Techniques

An area of broad implication, but one that has barely been explored, involves comparisons between different encounter experience techniques. Using samples of thirty-three church professionals in an experimental "creative risk taking" training group and an additional thirty-eight church professionals in a standard sensitivity training control group, Byrd (1967) compared the relative effectiveness of sensitivity training procedure with other procedures collectively designated as "creative risk taking." Significantly greater increases were obtained for the experimental group on five POI scales (Inner-Direction, Self-Actualizing Values, Spontaneity, Nature of Man, and Acceptance of Aggression), thus suggesting the possible superiority, in certain circumstances, of the experimental encounter-group techniques.

Summary of Research

The collection of studies available to date suggests that encounter group experience contributes to increased self-actualizing as measured by the POI and that these effects may be comparatively long-lasting, with growth being maintained, or increasing, for periods of up to one year. The POI appears to be sensitive to the effects of different group techniques and approaches, and use of the POI, and the more recently developed POD, for evaluation of the effects of the growth group experience may be expected to yield rich insights into the dynamics and effects of such groups.

The compendium of studies measuring significant changes resulting from encounter group experiences, summarized in Figure 47, leads to the conclusion that the POI, perhaps more than any other instrument, measures the relevant dimensions of life that are shared and experienced in encounter and group therapy.

CHAPTER 9. AN EXAMPLE OF ACTUALIZING GROUP PSYCHOTHERAPY

This chapter presents a transcription of the first part of a film series titled *Three Approaches to Group Psychotherapy,* featuring Everett L. Shostrom, Albert Ellis, and Harold Greenwald, and produced in 1974 by Psychological Films (205 West 20th Street, Santa Ana, California 92706). The film was made in one day, with each of the therapists (each a Diplomate in Clinical Psychology of the American Board of Professional Psychology) conducting a group for one and one-half hours. The films were then edited to about half that length for classroom use. The series is the sequel to the famous "Gloria" film, *Three Approaches to Psychotherapy,* a portion of which was presented in Chapter 1. Only Shostrom's part, "Actualizing Therapy," is transcribed here. Comments on the significance of Shostrom's responses have been added for this volume.

FILM'S INTRODUCTORY REMARKS

Actualizing Therapy, whether employed in an individual or group setting, is a system for helping people to get in touch with themselves. A basic tenet of Actualizing Therapy is that most people are other-directed rather than inner-directed. They look to the outside—to authorities and people they respect—for "shoulds," "have tos," and "musts," not realizing that they could better learn to come from the inside: to trust their own thoughts, feelings, and bodies. A second important principle in Actualizing Therapy is that of polarities. A polarity is a continuum of feeling whose opposing ends are really complementary. Anger and love are examples of such "complementary opposites." People who get angry at each other can eventually find love, as demonstrated in the following group session.

The process of Actualizing Therapy operates at three levels. One is thinking, another is feeling, and the third is bodily response. Actualizing

Therapists want people to talk about their thoughts but to make this more meaningful by talking with their feelings and, eventually, letting their bodies express themselves. An Actualizing Therapist will encourage his group members to look at each other—to look at each other's eyes and mouths and bodies—and to try to feel together and experience together. Experiencing oneself within and expressing oneself without: this is the process of actualizing.

THREE APPROACHES TO GROUP PSYCHOTHERAPY: "ACTUALIZING THERAPY"

[After spending ten to fifteen minutes "warming up" the group with light conversation, Shostrom begins to "zero in" on Sumner.]

Shostrom: My hypothesis about you is that your voice has been tearful ever since you started today.

Sumner: Yeah.

Shostrom: You feel rejected and that you are not really aware of the fact that you are permitting this to happen. These important people who decide not to be with you, or decide they don't want you—you could say that they have poor judgment.

[Comment 1. This interpretation is given to assist Sumner in understanding an important principle of Actualizing Therapy: inner- versus other-direction. Shostrom is suggesting to Sumner that most people do not permit themselves to be inner-directed but, instead, allow others to make their decisions for them. One who is growing toward actualizing does not permit others to be his judge; the motivation for his behavior must come from within.]

Sumner: This is something I won't allow myself to do. I can look at the woman I am relating to and I can see things I didn't like—things about her I didn't like—but I have a difficult time allowing myself to realize that—to accept that.

Shostrom: Because you give her the power to judge your worth.

Sumner: Yes, that has bothered me. It has bothered me that I allow her to do that. It bothered me that I would allow myself to do that.

Shostrom: Can you tell us? Say it about three times: "I am worthwhile."

Sumner: I am worthwhile.

Shostrom: Again.

Sumner: I am worthwhile. I am very worthwhile?

Shostrom: But you smile, and the second time you had a question mark after your sentence. Were you aware of that?

[Comment 2. This is a Gestalt technique, wherein Shostrom is noting Sumner's *feelings* rather than his *words*. He is pointing out that Sumner's smile and tone of voice contrasted with his words.]

Sumner: Yes.

Shostrom: It's still hard for you to believe that. It is really not *their* problem that they are rejecting you. It is *your* problem of believing in your own lovability and your own worth.

Mary Anna: I can't sit still any longer, I am going to explode!

Shostrom: Explode!

Mary Anna: Heart's pounding! There is something you just said . . . it is so easy, in the head, to say "Oh, I know their judgment is lousy. I am great!" Goddamnit! What goes on in here and what comes out in the world . . . it falls apart. Ev, I can't take care of it upstairs.

Shostrom: It is because we have been reared to give people the right projection. We have been programmed that way. We have to revise the computer. We have to get in a new system.

[Comment 3. Shostrom points out that people have been programmed, developmentally, to give others in authority the right to decide what is best for them. Children tend to do this with parents and other authority figures. Here therapy helps the individual take back that projection so that he has the right to make decisions for himself.]

Mary Anna: We've got to take all the systems out of the head.

Sumner: I do it to myself. I don't need anyone else to do it to me. I do it myself.

Mary Anna: We rerun the old tapes and we keep them ready.

Sumner: Yeah, I go through a fit.

Mary Anna: It makes me angry.

Sumner: I can be very inner-directed with myself. When I am by myself, and not having to relate with other people intimately, I can be strong within myself, and it does not matter what anybody says or what anybody does. I am me. I can take care of myself. But getting very close and very emotional—emotionally packed in a very close relationship, that slips away more—other-directedness comes in. It was that way with Nadine. I allowed myself to be manipulated in many ways. I allowed *her* more power to do things. I didn't give myself a lot of credit. That bothered me.

Shostrom: Could you make the cup Nadine and say, "I am—right now—taking away your right to judge me. I am going to be trusting my own 'inner Supreme Court.' To hell with your judgment!"

[Comment 4. Here Shostrom uses the Gestalt technique of making Sumner's girlfriend the cup and asking him to tell her that he is no longer going to let her judge him. The phrase "trusting my own inner Supreme Court," was a term Maslow used in relation to someone who is actualizing and who trusts his inner feelings as a basis for living.]

Sumner: Nadine, I am at a point where I don't want to be judged by you. I am a worthwhile person and I am taking away your power to judge me. I will not allow you to be a judge—to be a person on a pedestal—anymore.

Shostrom: Now, just say, "Get off my back."

Sumner: Get off my back.

Shostrom: Louder.

Sumner: Get off my back.

Shostrom: Scream it.

Sumner: Get off my back!

Shostrom: Once more.

Sumner: Get off my back, damn it!

[Comment 5. Here Shostrom's attempt to reinforce Sumner's independence by asking him to repeat the demand more and more loudly is primarily a bodily therapy technique. The vocal repetition tends to release a felt bodily pressure.]

Shostrom: Good, now give an answer. What is she saying?

Sumner: "I can get off your back and I will get off your back. I am willing to allow you to find yourself, to be the kind of person you want to be."

Shostrom: Answer her.

Sumner: Yes, I understand that, but I think also that you have been very manipulating. You have assumed a role in our relationship where you wanted very much for me to take over lots of responsibility—make a lot of money—and I couldn't do it. I tried, but I couldn't do it all the time. I wanted to be myself. I wanted to feel my tears like I feel now, but you didn't want that, you wanted a father. You wanted an authority figure, and it tore me up. I couldn't do that all the time. And right now, I just want you to realize that I do see you. I do see you for what you are. I accept you for what you are, yet there are things that I don't like about you.

[Mary Anna sobs.]

Shostrom: O.K. Can I interrupt you now? I want to get to Mary Anna's response—to see what is happening. Tell us what has happened.

Mary Anna: [crying and sobbing] Oh, Jesus! I thought that was over with. I was identifying Ed with Sumner and I feel—I am beginning to realize in so many ways that this is what he was saying to me: "Go on and be, it is really okay with me," and I didn't see it that way totally. I know that he has his hang-ups, too. They are almost impossible to live with.

But a good deal of the time, the things that he said to me—he was telling me, "Go and be yourself. You are a separate individual. You don't have to be in this role that you are putting yourself in."

Shostrom: When Sumner went through it, it somehow really came into perspective.

Mary Anna: It triggered it. It has been coming through the last few days for some reason and it triggered it. I haven't said it out loud. I have been increasingly aware of it, and I guess the feeling is that I am angry at myself for not appreciating it.

Shostrom: Can you put Mary Anna there and tell her that?

[Comment 6. Shostrom is asking Mary Anna to be both her top dog and her underdog. That is, he asks her to be her strong self and her weak self.]

Mary Anna: You dumb, stupid little bitch! Jesus Christ! You are such a little girl. You want everybody to take care of you. You won't put out any effort at all. You are afraid to *be.*

Shostrom: Can you say, "Stand on your own two feet"?

Mary Anna: Get off your dead ass and stand on your own two feet! The world doesn't owe you anything!

Shostrom: Again, louder.

Mary Anna: The world doesn't owe you a goddamn thing, lady!

Shostrom: Once more. Come on, give it to her!

Mary Anna: Who the hell do you think you are anyway? Good God Almighty! You live on this earth and you think the earth owes you a living and pleasure and comfort! It is time you straightened up and started giving something back. Nobody needs you to just stand there and exist.

Shostrom: Now be her. What is she saying?

Mary Anna: I know it, I know it. Leave me alone. I am getting there.

Shostrom: Now could you stand up and feel that, standing there. Could you do that? Just stamp your feet into the floor and really feel like Mary Anna is doing that. Take your shoes off. That's good. Very close relationship—the way your body feels—the way you feel yourself inside. Bend your knees . . . and breathe.

[Comment 7. Shostrom is utilizing a Bioenergetic technique: asking Mary Anna to stand on her own two feet, to bend her knees, and to breathe. In effect, one cannot "stand on his own two feet" emotionally until he can do so physically.]

Shostrom: O.K. Now get it in there—pound it in! Say, "I am going to stand on my own two feet."

Mary Anna: I am going to stand on my own two feet.

Shostrom: Again.

Mary Anna: I am going to stand on my own two feet!

Shostrom: "I *am* standing on my own two feet."

Mary Anna: By God, I *am*!

Shostrom: Say that to me.

Mary Anna: I am standing on my own two feet and I don't need you or anybody else! I can make it!

Shostrom: Say it to the rest of the group.

Mary Anna: I am standing on my own two feet and I don't need you and your overprotection. I don't need any of you. But I feel I want people.

Shostrom: So you really want to be independent and stand on your own two feet, but also you don't want to deny the other part, which is that you care, too. You don't want to care to where you have to "kiss ass"—to where you have to give in to people's needs. But you can still be an independent entity and still live in the world where other people are important as well.

[Comment 8. At this point, Shostrom introduces the principle of *inter-dependence*. He is telling Mary Anna that it is not enough to simply be dependent or independent; she must express her interdependence by moving rhythmically through these three positions.]

Mary Anna: That's what personhood is all about. But—Oh God, it's a long road.

Shostrom: Yeah, I know it is hard. We have to do it again, again, and again. Stamp it in, huh?

Mary Anna: Yeah. And there is still a little fear.

Shostrom: Oh, yeah.

Mary Anna: Yeah.

Sumner: You look very beautiful. You really do. More beautiful than when you first came in.

Mary Anna: [laughing] This messy old maid is beautiful, huh?

Shostrom: Let's hear what you all feel. It's very important when someone reaches you, that you share.

Marv: Yeah, I felt for you and with you and was cheering for you, then you said you don't need us and I didn't believe you.

Mary Anna: [laughing] You're right!

Shostrom: This is a paradox. You can stand on your own two feet and yet still need.

[Comment 9. Shostrom continues to focus on interdependence, illustrating this concept by focusing on Mary Anna's ability to feel herself on her own two feet while still feeling her dependence.]

Marv: Still need people. Yes. I guess that is where I am at.

Shostrom: Yeah.

Marv: I desperately need other people.

[cut to later.]

Marty: I know you don't need me, but I need you very badly.

Pat: I was feeling really cool toward you because you reminded me of someone I was in a group with, and I kept picturing a role you were playing.
When you were standing there, I just really felt that was you, that I
would like to know you, but I really don't think that you really have to
play that role. And I agree with Sumner, I thought you looked really
very, very beautiful. All the kind of tension that was in your neck and
stuff just disappeared. It really did.

Shostrom: Dennis, how do you feel? I see lots of tension in your jaws.

Dennis: I could relate intellectually to what was going on, but I was having
difficulty relating emotionally.

Shostrom: You wouldn't let yourself go with her.

Dennis: I have a great deal of empathy for what you were saying. I can
identify with it, but I couldn't let my emotions completely identify with
what you were going through.

Shostrom: Couldn't stand up and cheer. You were afraid to stand up and
cheer.

Dennis: I was. But you don't need everybody. Sometimes you don't and
sometimes you do. You need everybody, but you got to be interdependent.

Shostrom: Yeah. This is really where I differ with Perls—with my teacher.
Perls said that therapy really leads to autonomy, to independence. I
think you have to be independent, but I think you also have to admit
that you still need people. You can be standing on your own two feet
and yet still hold hands.

[Comment 10. Perls believed that therapy should lead to complete self-
support. Shostrom illustrates his disagreement with Perls by stating that

you can stand on your own two feet yet still hold hands—that you can be independent and dependent at the same time.]

Susan: I feel so totally relaxed now. I just feel kind of like, "Ah, everything is coming at me." God I feel better.

Dennis: Do you feel better because you were identifying with it, or better because . . .

Susan: I don't know if I am feeling what you are feeling or whether it is a breakdown of everyone's tension—the fact that you exposed yourself so openly. I don't know, but right now I just feel loose. I just feel so loose and like things are good. Things *are* good.

Shostrom: I think that is one of the beauties of group therapy, you can get a piggyback ride on somebody else, occasionally, and that is O.K. And we can all be with her and kind of grow with her . . . together.

[Comment 11. Refering to the nature of group therapy in the actualizing sense, Shostrom stresses the decided advantage of being able to benefit by listening to others, rather than speaking alone.]

Sumner: I am glad that I was able to start something that helped you to identify. I was really glad to see you stand up.

Mary Anna: I am out of group now and sometimes you need a trigger. You need something. And I am not getting it in my everyday life so I realize it is building up a little bit, and I appreciate it.

Pat: I see a lot of sadness in Marty's eyes.

Marty: Yeah, maybe Susan feels better, but I don't. I feel worse.

Shostrom: O.K., stay with it.

Marty: Well, I don't know where I am, Mary Anna—whether I'm behind you or ahead of you. I feel like I try so damn hard to prove to the world that I can stand on my own two feet, and it is hard. It is just goddamn hard.

Shostrom: I know.

Marty: I don't want to be a burden on anybody and I hide it. And I can do it, but it is just hard to keep it up.

Shostrom: Can I illustrate this with you? I know it is simple. Let's see if we can do it together. Just stand up with me. See, ordinarily we think that as soon as we start to need people, we are going to have an A-frame relationship. You lean on me and I lean on you, O.K.? Just your head.

[Comment 12. Using the body, Shostrom demonstrates dependency by showing two people leaning against each other with only their foreheads touching, in an A-frame relationship. In the following comments he shows how it is possible to "fall flat," psychologically, when one does not learn to stand on his own two feet.]

Shostrom: Now we've got a nice dependency going. Getting a headache yet?

Marty: Can't move.

Shostrom: All right, so if I really pull away fast, you know, you fall flat on your face, but you see how each of us stand on our own two feet. O.K., now go ahead and bend your knees and breathe. Do you feet that? Come on. Push your head in hard. That's right. You can't be just a rigid rock, you know. That's it, stay with what you are feeling. Talk about how it feels to be shaky.

Marty: I am just going to fall apart.

Shostrom: Uh-huh, just go ahead and give in to it and see what happens if things fall apart. Stay with that vibration. People are alive—they are human—and we need to vibrate and we need to give into this aliveness. You are not alive if you are sitting still. You are dead. You are in a coffin standing up.

[Comment 13. Here Shostrom introduces the Bioenergetic principles of aliveness and vibration. He challenges the assumption that mental health is equated with an absence of bodily anxiety. Bioenergetics teaches that it is necessary to be alive emotionally and to experience different vibrations.]

Shostrom: [laughing] Even though you stand on your own two feet, it is going to be shaky, you know. You always shake, if you are really angry. If you are not shaking, you are not really angry. How are you feeling?

Marty: Better.

Shostrom: Keep the knees bent, don't ever lock those knees.

Marty: I shake even when they are locked. I feel as though I am going to fall on the floor. There would not be anybody there to help me stand while I helped myself stand.

Shostrom: And, again, you assume somebody has got to be there to pick the pieces up.

Marty: Right. It is kind of in my mind, because I know that I have to stand on my own two feet. Yet, what happens when I fall?

Sumner: I just hope to fall, because then you can stand up on your own two feet. It is just getting there. You are right there ready to fall.

Shostrom: Yeah!

Sumner: Will I allow myself to do it?

Shostrom: Don't just talk about it, do it! Can you take your shoes off Sumner, and then stand and see if you can fall backwards? And let Susan and Pat kind of respond to you as you go.

[Comment 14. Here Shostrom initiates a weakness, or vulnerability, exercise: exhausting one's strength by leaning forward and, when the pain becomes too great, allowing oneself to fall backward—being vulnerable to those behind one. This exercise enables Sumner to feel genuine weakness, an important polar dimension in actualizing one's being.]

Pat: He is bigger than me!

[Group laughter]

Shostrom: O.K. Now, let yourself fall. Keep your knees bent . . . breathe. That's it. When you feel like falling, see if you can let yourself fall back.

[Comment 15. Deep breathing is considered an extremely important method of feeling. The lack of breathing creates anxiety, while breathing creates aliveness, and here it enables Sumner to get in touch with the feeling of falling, which correlates with the fear of surrender to one's own vulnerability.]

Sumner: I feel good now. I feel like I can stand on my feet.

Shostrom: All right. You begin to get shaky after awhile. Give in to that vibration. That's it. See if you can bend over a little more and touch the floor with your hands. That's it. Keep your knees bent. Bend them way down. Now, straighten up your knees and you begin to feel that shakiness. Keep your hands down. Feel that shakiness now. That's it. Stay there till you have to fall backwards. Get into that vibration. Get into it. Good. Breathe deeply. Head down. That's it. Now put it into your voice. Feel the pain.

[Comment 16. Shostrom illustrates, through Sumner, the polarities of pleasure-pain and joy-sorrow. The body, trying to remain rigid, becomes constricted. In order to become alive it must experience pain, as a frostbitten hand must feel pain before it feels life. Experiencing pain is an important process of psychological growth.]

Sumner: No real pain now. I am not really allowing myself to really feel it.

Shostrom: Bend your knees back a little more. You will feel it. Don't let them lock, but bend them back so you begin to feel them. That's it. Give into that. Now, if you are human, you will feel pain.

Sumner: I feel numbness in my chin.

[Group laughter]

Shostrom: Don't try to be a man—try to be a human being and feel the pain. Keep your knees straighter. Bend all the way over. That's it. Now you are getting into it. Feel that?

[Comment 17. Here Shostrom points out another important polarity: humanness versus perfection. He suggests that the psychotherapist is not an expert in perfection, but, rather, he helps people understand their anger as well as their love—their humanness as well as their fallibility. The understanding of humanness is a very important Actualizing Therapy goal.]

Sumner: I feel weak.

Shostrom: Get into that. That's it . . . good. Feel as long as you can then just fall back.

Sumner: Oh God, I feel weak.

Shostrom: That's it. It is human to feel weak. Get into it.

Sumner: Oh, God.

Shostrom: Good. Stay with it. Fall backward. That's it. O.K. now, Patty. Standing on your own two feet doesn't mean being the rock of Gibraltar. It means just being human.

Sumner: That's right! It *is* good to be weak sometimes.

Shostrom: Yeah!

Sumner: Thank you.

Shostrom: This is what we fear. We are just going to fold up and be a pile of shit, huh? How do you feel about the pile of shit over there?

Dennis: I like him.

Shostrom: Say it to him.

Dennis: I like you.

Sumner: Thank you. I like you. I like you for expressing it. It makes me feel good.

Mary Anna: I feel a great deal of joy somewhere at meeting you, at seeing you and everything that you are . . . and that you've been here. I don't know how to express it.

Sumner: I wanted very much to experience it, but it was tough for me to get into it. But once I did, I wanted to go with it. That's because of the polarity I feel. I feel like I want very much to experience all this because it will help me just be me. Yet, I saw how reluctant I was to get into it.

Shostrom: Uh-huh.

Sumner: And that hurts me sometimes that I want to feel—to *really* feel. There is so much that's blank in me.

Mary Anna: You know what it is? I feel reassured that there is a man walking this earth that will allow himself to be the way you have been here.

Pat: I think you are a pretty worthwhile person.

Sumner: More and more I feel that, more than I ever have before.

Shostrom: Yeah.

Sumner: That I can feel worthwhile in all my moods.

Shostrom: Yeah.

Sumner: All my pains.

Mary Anna: I feel a lot of love for you, I really mean it.

Sumner: Thank you.

Mary Anna: I appreciate you.

Shostrom: Group gives us the experience of what we might not get on the outside, but I think we can, if we can just trust that . . .

Sumner: I get all these folks. Right now they are sincere, but you are not willing to get this from people you walk with on the streets.

Dennis: You get this from the people who are important to your problems.

Shostrom: Yeah.

Pat: But you will never know unless you really risk it to find out.

Dennis: Risk is the right word.

Pat: That's right.

Shostrom: It is the only word that really expresses what we are trying to say to you. You can't do it by playing safe.

Sumner: And also, the fear I have now is that I can do that, and I can *be* here. But I can play it safe when I am with the people I am relating to now.

Shostrom: Yeah.

Marv: I thought you were "em-bare-assed."

Shostrom: [laughing] You have to be able to get embarrassed to show your "bare ass"—in order to really *be* that.

[Comment 18. Reflecting the pun on the word "embarrassed," Shostrom suggests that, in order for growth to take place, people must show their weaknesses and their vulnerability. Such play on words is an important teaching method.]

Sumner: [laughing] I have one.

Shostrom: It was really showing when you were shaking there—way up— and you fell flat on it!

[Group laughter]

[cut to later.]

Mary Anna: Dennis, I feel compassion for your fear. I know what it means. I have experienced it and I do feel for you. I don't know the magic word, but we are here.

[pause]

Shostrom: Dennis, are you still in a quandary? It looks like you are still biting that mouth.

Sumner: I feel as though there is an exercise that will help you feel your feelings, too.

Mary Anna: I think it is coming.

Dennis: Thanks.

Shostrom: Let it all out.

[pause]

Dennis: I was having a great deal of difficulty trying to actually put myself in the position of risk.

Shostrom: Can I do something with you? That chin is bothering me. Stay where you are, and let's see if I can reach you. Keep your jaw up. Now I want to see if I can get in touch with that anger inside your jaw and your shoulders, O.K.? Keep it way out, and when I push here, I want you to say, "Ouch!" O.K., put your jaw out—way out. You can put it way out—you can get it out further than that. That's it. Say, "Ouch!" Come on! Are you trying to win a contest or something? Feel it! Does that hurt you?

[Comment 19. Shostrom introduces the Bioenergetic principle that the areas of the jaw and shoulders reflect bodily tension and hostility. He is helping Dennis to release these feelings and to bring out his "ouch" so that he can feel human and alive.]

Dennis: Uh-huh.

Shostrom: Say, "Ouch!"

Dennis: [meekly] Ouch.

Shostrom: [laughing] This time I want you to scream. You see, I think you have been a big guy all your life, and you have had the masculine "Bobby Riggs" assumption that all men are superior and strong and adequate. And Billie Jean has proved that is not true anymore. Get that damn chin out and feel the pain when I give it to you! There is pain there and I want you to loosen it up. Come on—get it out! Feel the ouch!

Dennis: Ouch!

Shostrom: But you say the ouch like you are still holding it in. You are a big man—you have a big voice. Scream that. Say, "Ouch!" and then say, "Stop it!" Can you do that with me?

Dennis: Ouch!

Shostrom: "Stop it!"

Dennis: Ouch! Stop it.

Shostrom: Louder.

Dennis: Stop it!

Shostrom: Louder! Again!

Dennis: Stop it! It hurts, goddamnit!

Shostrom: That's it! Now you see, the world did not fall apart with that "goddamnit," did it?

Dennis: No.

Shostrom: [works on shoulders] Now I am going to pound this stuff out!

Dennis: Stop it.

Shostrom: Hmm?

Dennis: Stop it.

Shostrom: What?

Dennis: Stop it! Stop it! I don't like to be hurt.

Shostrom: O.K., but sometimes you have to experience hurt to feel you can handle the hurt, you see. I think one of the assumptions we make about life is that we don't have to feel hurt. We go through life with painless dentistry—no hurt. The point is, when you discover you can handle the hurt, it is going to loosen up the tension and you are going to be more alive. Now let me give it to your neck a little bit. And feel that pain and say, "Ouch!"

[Comment 20. Shostrom continues to emphasize his pain versus pleasure principle. Life is not like painless dentistry; psychologically, people must experience pain so that they can learn to be alive.]

Dennis: Ouch! Ouch!

Shostrom: Very good.

Dennis: Ouch!

Shostrom: Louder! Scream it!

Dennis: Ouch!

Shostrom: That's it.

Dennis: Ouch!

Shostrom: That's it. Now you can handle that hurt—you didn't fall apart. All right, how do you feel toward me now?

Dennis: I built a wall.

Shostrom: You built a wall. But you see, I think it is very important for us to look at you now because it seems to me that you are new in therapy and you really haven't learned that you've got to let that wall down— that when you let that wall down and feel that hurt and experience it, it is going to be a relief for you. Right now it is still all right here. Would someone like to react to what you were experiencing?

Marv: I want to kick the wall down. I want to get to you.

Dennis: I won't let people get to me.

Shostrom: "I *haven't* let people." Don't make a prediction.

[Comment 21. This is the important Actualizing principle of expressing oneself in the appropriate tense. Dennis is really saying that in the past he did not let people get to him, and his comment suggests that this will continue to happen. By correcting him, Shostrom keeps him from making a predictive reinforcement.]

Dennis: To hell with you then!

Shostrom: Good.

Mary Anna: You know when you were shouting and it was still "Ouch?" Instead of opening up you were still holding it back so much.

Pat: It bothered me that . . . that it was hard for you to really let it all out. Just the fact that your mouth was so closed.

Sumner: Yeah, me too.

Pat: The thing I saw was that you let yourself be hurt, except you didn't really admit it. I can identify with that because I was the same way, and I went through this exercise and I lasted much longer than you. I just let myself go right on being hurt, and I kept thinking he doesn't really mean to hurt me, so why should I yell "Ouch"? "He doesn't really mean to hurt me," instead of, "He *did* mean to hurt me." And there is nothing wrong with yelling "Quit it! You're hurting me!" But if you never tell the other person, if you don't let them know that maybe something they have done has hurt you, they don't know.

Mary Anna: You said that you had let someone get close to you a couple of times. Is that on your mind? What happened? I am curious about it.

Dennis: Yeah. Ironically, I think, I went through a marriage of about twenty years of not really letting my wife get close to me. When I was in college I was extremely hurt by a girl. I allowed myself to be hurt, and it was the type of thing where I was a big football player and everything else—190 pounds—and it was such a hurt that I dropped to 140 pounds. Left school because of it.

Shostrom: You are still hurt?

Dennis: Yes, I am very hurt. In fact, there are times, twenty-two years later, when I—I dream about this girl still.

Shostrom: The hurt is still there.

Dennis: Uh-huh.

Shostrom: You're free to let it out. Could you make her the cup in front of you and tell her how much she hurt you? Give into that.

[Comment 22. Shostrom again shows that by talking to people through the medium of the cup one can have a revealing dialogue, and can learn to understand some of the emotional interactions that produced the pain.]

Dennis: I really don't want her to know.

Shostrom: You don't want her to know? After twenty-two years, you still don't want her to know.

Shostrom: [mocking Dennis] Goddamnit! I will die before I let her know.

Shostrom: Come on. Get it out.

[pause]

Dennis: Mary, you really stuck it to me. I suppose you don't owe a responsibility to me—but, nonetheless, you really hurt me. I would have done anything for you. I was madly in love with you and I wanted you very badly for my wife—for us to spend the rest of our lives together.

Shostrom: Can I share a hypothesis with you? Say those words again, but this time angrily: "Goddamnit, you really let me down!" Underneath a lot of that hurt is a lot of anger you never admitted to.

[Comment 23. Hurt and anger are often confused. Anger is a strong feeling that rigidifies the body, while hurt expresses a weakness that has the body surrendering. These feelings should be made specific and experienced separately.]

Dennis: You spoiled little bitch.

Shostrom: Say that again to her.

Dennis: You spoiled little bitch.

Shostrom: Louder!

Dennis: What you need is a good quick kick in the ass! Some day I will take a paddle to you and put blisters on your goddamn ass!

Shostrom: Scream it again.

Dennis: You son of a bitch!

Shostrom: Again. Louder!

Dennis: I hope you get hurt when you get married as much as you hurt me. I hope you really hurt. I hope you get hurt and you never forget it. You deserve everything that is coming to you.

Shostrom: Just say, "I resent you," louder and louder.

Dennis: I resent you.

Shostrom: Louder! Come on, give into it. Yell it at her. "I resent you!"

Dennis: I don't resent her.

Shostrom: You love her, but you can resent her. That is the polarity. Come on. It's O.K.

Dennis: I resent you. I resent you for what I allowed you to do to me. I would have been out of my fucking mind to have ever married you. The best thing that ever happened to me was for you to kick my ass out. Oh God, I am glad. I resent you! I hate you!

Shostrom: "Get lost!" Can you say that?

Dennis: Get lost!

Shostrom: Louder!

Dennis: Get lost!

Shostrom: Louder!

Dennis: Get out of my life once and for all!

Shostrom: Come on. Louder!

Dennis: Just get out and stay out! I don't ever want to see you again, or talk to you or think of you again! I hate you!

Shostrom: Say it louder. Just don't say it. Come on, everyone is pulling for you. Can you say, "I hate you," louder? You have to experience it, not just intellectualize it.

Pat: I think in saying, "I hate her," he also wants to say "I love her," too.

Shostrom: That's right, but you can't feel your love until you speak out your hate.

Pat: But he doesn't think he can say, "I hate you" and "I love you."

Shostrom: Is that true, Dennis?

Dennis: Yeah, that's right.

Shostrom: O.K., but try it. See if you can revise that hypothesis: "I can hate you, you goddamn bitch, and yet I love you."

Dennis: I hate you, you goddamn bitch!

Shostrom: Now just keep the hate separate, and we will get to the love afterwards. You won't be able to love her in a real way until you have gotten to that. Trust that. Hate again, louder. The loudest you have ever screamed. And I know that is hard for a guy that is as cool as you are. Come on!

[Comment 24. Working with the anger-love polarity, or any polarity, requires that the client separate the two feelings, even though they are theoretically correlated. Dennis has made the assumption that because he loved Mary, he cannot hate her at the same time. This is a common misconception.]

Dennis: I hate you!

Shostrom: Louder!

Dennis: MARY ELLEN, I HATE YOU! GOD, I HATE YOU!

Shostrom: That's it. Once more. You can't feel that hurt until you have fully given in to your anger. Can you try it once more for me?

Dennis: [crying] No.

Shostrom: That is about all you can do? O.K., let's sit back. There is an important point I want to finish our session on: Group therapy is being your feelings in the here and now, yet sometimes we have to go *back* to these primary experiences through our feelings—when we feel them— to know how we have been influenced and how they still continue to influence the way we behave now. I kind of hope that maybe, today at least, you have opened up the part that has been missing: you know, the anger—the part of Dennis that is real and just doesn't take crap and assume it is virtuous. I don't know whether we will make it or not. We will have to probably work some more. But I am really very impressed, not only with Dennis, but with all of you, because we have really experienced our anger. We have also experienced our love and our weakness and our strength. We are all trying to be more inner-directed and not influenced by all these people outside. But, really, the thing which motivates change, when you get right down to it, is love. I guess I would like to give you a definition of love I learned up at Esalen, up in the Nepenthe Lodge, where I once visited. I think it really summarizes what we have been doing today. "Love is a comfort —the inexpressible comfort of feeling safe with another person, having neither to weigh thoughts nor measure words, but pouring all feelings right out just as they are, chaff and grain together, certain that a faithful friendly hand will take them and sift them, keep what is worth keeping and, with a breath of comfort, blow the rest away." Thank you.

[Comment 25. Shostrom concludes his work with the group by defining "love" as being what happens in group therapy. A true therapeutic relationship involves a "safe emergency" relationship, where clients are able to freely express themselves without fear of judgment or exploitation.]

ANALYSIS

In one sense, a well-conducted Actualizing Therapy session can be viewed as a spontaneous rhythmic integration of each of the three aspects of being.

The primary responsibility for this integration, of course, lies with the therapist, who must evenly balance his responses in terms of thinking, feeling, and bodily expression. He must see to it that no one aspect is emphasized at the expense of the others and, conversely, that no particular aspect is minimized or ignored.

Our breakdown of the twenty-five primary therapist responses in the above session reveals that nine were intellectual responses, eight were concerned with feeling, and eight involved bodily techniques.

The intellectual responses were those followed by Comments 1, 3, 4, 8, 9, 10, 11, 20, and 21. These responses were primarily concerned with the various principles of Actualizing Therapy (such as "other- versus inner-direction" or the principle of trusting one's "inner Supreme Court") or with the significance of the intellectual assumptions made by the group members and/or the therapist (such as the fallacious assumption that one should avoid all pain). Comment 21 refers to Shostrom's vigilance in correcting his clients' language when their statements are existentially incorrect—an important intellectual task of the therapist.

Comments 2, 6, 16, 17, 22, 23, 24, and 25 follow the therapist's feeling responses. These responses are concerned with the expression of the clients' experiences on the feeling polarities, reliving past experiences emotionally, identifying and differentiating feelings, and so on.

The bodily techniques, discussed in Comments 5, 7, 12, 13, 14, 15, 18, and 19, include the use of physical demonstrations (creating a two-person A-frame, for instance, to illustrate the dangers of dependency), pointing out the bodily effects of emotions (on posture, breathing, muscular tensions, and so on), and the use of certain physical activities or exercises to reinforce intellectual responses and to aid in the expression of feeling.

CHAPTER 10. SEX, LOVE, AND MARRIAGE

There is nothing in life that is so important as love, yet psychology has paid little attention to this vital area of human concern. As Maslow (1970) has said, "Particularly strange is the silence of the psychologists. Sometimes this is merely sad or irritating, as in the case of the textbooks of psychology and sociology, practically none of which treat the subject. . . . More often the situation becomes completely ludicrous. [As a rule] the word love' is not even indexed [in psychological and sociological works]" (p. 181). We suggest that the field of psychology has been silent on love because of the inability to give any sense of scientific respectability and clarity to this subject. This chapter attempts to begin the task.

There has been a recent upsurge of interest not only in the meaning of love but also in the meaning of an actualizing marital relationship. Many psychologists and clergymen have been conducting "marriage enrichment workshops" (Bustanoby, 1974), in which they use the Actualizing Assessment Battery (AAB) as a basis for discussion of the health or 'wellness" of the marriages of members of the workshop. The AAB is particularly well suited to workshops of this kind because it provides a quick evaluation of the actualizing status of the individuals themselves, by means of the POI, and of the actualizing status of the relationship, as measured by the CRI and the PAI. Implicit in these instruments are assumptions about the nature of actualizing persons and actualizing relationships.

The philosophical assumptions held by the marriage therapist are a major influence on his approach to love and marital problems. To put it simply, there are two basic views of marriage today. The traditional view holds that one gets married once and lives with it, whereas the contemporary view is that divorce need not be considered a failure but can instead be seen as a growth experience to enrich the potential for another marriage. The Actualizing Therapist will do everything he can to help save a marriage if that is the wish of the client, but he does not simply do marriage-saving therapy. He believes in an actualizing therapy for two people who happen to be married. The Actualizing Therapist believes in trying to help individuals decide *who* they are, *what* they are, and what they *want* from any relationship, and then to let each decide whether all those things add up to being married or not. He insists on their freedom to choose. This, of course, is in direct conflict with the concept of a marriage counselor as one who tries to talk clients into a rigid posture and who keeps track of the number of marriages he has "saved" as an indication of his effectiveness.

Fully 80 percent of married clients come to therapy because of some marriage problem, and this is where the actualizing approach, with its stress on the value of the person, is far superior to the approach of much "marriage counseling," which seeks only to repair the marriage, often at the expense of the individual.

In this chapter we are going to identify some theories and critical issues that we think are of great importance in a philosophy of sex, love, and marriage therapy. We believe they will illustrate our contention, stated in Chapter 3, that the values of the Actualizing Therapist play an important role as he functions to help people.

EXPECTATIONS AND MARRIAGE

One of the central problems in marital or partner relationships has to do with expectations. The following propositions illustrate:

1. *High expectations.* High expectations lead to high disappointment. Thus, in a relationship, a central problem results from the expectations that inevitably lead to disappointment and "faulting" the other partner.

2. *Low expectations.* Expecting negativity, or having low expectations, leads to equal difficulty. The phrase "Give me the name and I'll play the game" is an example of someone who has been labeled as "dumb," "foolish," "stupid," "dishonest," and so forth.

3. *No expectations.* We propose that the alternative to each of the above is *not* expecting, either high or low. This means creatively living in the moment and observing self and other, but without pressure or demands. This leads to a relationship characterized by the term "adventure," in which one never knows what will happen. The relationship is filled with joy sometimes and sorrow sometimes, and is unpredictably exciting.

THREE APPROACHES TO RELATIONSHIPS

Figure 48 is our attempt to describe two fundamental relationship patterns that are prominent in our culture today, and a third alternative that we believe is needed to replace the other two.

	TRADITIONAL RELATIONSHIP	HEDONISTIC RELATIONSHIP	ACTUALIZING RELATIONSHIP
1. **Emphasis:**	Contractual	Genital	Core to core
2. **Basic Principle:**	Obligation	Manipulation	Commitment
3. **Orientation:**	Role oriented	Body oriented	Person oriented
4. **Nature of Relationship:**	I-it	It-it	Thou-Thou
5. **Motivation:**	Security based	Fun based	Growth based

Figure 48. Three Approaches to Relationships

In the first column is the *traditional relationship,* which is a *contractual* relationship based on a theory of *obligation* imposed from without by state legislation. It is a relationship that is traditionally *role oriented.* That is, one partner has certain dominant roles and the other certain subordinate roles. Traditionally, the dominant role has been given to the man by state laws and by our culture.

In terms of Martin Buber's concept, the nature of the relationship is an "I-it" orientation. The motivation for such a relationship is usually the promise of economic and emotional *security* for life as a reward for maintaining the contract.

In the second column is the *hedonistic relationship,* which is the relationship of many "moderns." Here the emphasis of the relationship is *genital.* That is, sexual conquest is most important, with no obligation contractually. The basic principle is a mutual *manipulation* to achieve a sexual end. The primary orientation has to do with a fascination with the *body* rather than the person. Thus the relationship becomes what we call an "it-it" relationship. The underlying motivation is pleasure or fun, and the emphasis has little to do with the total personhood of either party.

A third alternative is what we call the *actualizing relationship.* Here the emphasis does not rest primarily on a genital or contractual base, although both these dimensions could be included in an actualizing relationship.

Core to core refers to the achievement of a level of intimacy that makes possible the expression of all three aspects of being: intellectual, feeling, and bodily response. In order to achieve this goal, the basic principle is one of *commitment.* There are two dimensions to commitment: first, a fundamental dedication to expressing *oneself* on the intellectual, emotional and bodily levels and, second, a dedication to expression with a significan other at all three levels coactively, which is almost involuntary in its tota freedom. There is a joining together in a relationship that is more fully expressive of one's total being than with any other person. An actualizing relationship has exclusivity not because one promises it, but because one *chooses* it freely and because the relationship is more enhancing of self and other than is any other relationship. There is a feeling of confidence that the relationship will sustain itself, through conflict and differences that may arise, because of the strength of the ties fed by continual core expressions.

Commitment is necessary because without it the relationship is no more significant than any other. An actualizing relationship requires a commitment of one's core energy, found in the thinking, feeling, and body levels. One's energies need to be "priortized." Unless one decides with whom one is going to focus one's energy, the energy becomes dissipated. *Commitment is the best way to focus one's energies, particularly love. Commitment is more than a moral issue and it is more than a convenience—it is a decision to use one's energies wisely.*

The basic orientation in the actualizing relationship is not on the body, or the sexual roles in the relationship only, but rather on each person's expression of his or her own unique *personhood* in the relationship. Thus, the actualizing relationship is a "Thou-Thou" relationship—not an "I-it," as is the traditional relationship, where one partner assumes the role of the superior "I" or the inferior "it." Likewise, in the hedonistic relationship both persons become "its," since their primary identity is with their genital organs and with their bodies—not with their total *person*alities.

Finally, the actualizing relationship is *growth motivated* in that the relationship is a "workshop for growth." In contrast, the traditional relationship is motivated by the security of staying together for life, and the hedonistic relationship is based on the pleasure of the moment and no other considerations.

The actualizing relationship is one of sharing. This starts with one's core—the home of one's being. When one shares his home with someone, he is sharing his personal dwelling place, the vital center of his existence. He is sharing the deepest center of intimacy. He is sharing where he is at the moment. He is sharing what is most significant to him.

An actualizing relationship means sharing the chamber within, which is protected from most other relationships. It means sharing the innermost shrine, which is separated by a veil from the rest of the world. It's where one is most at ease. It means sharing the most inaccessible. It is sharing the truth of one's being—sharing one's "isness" rather than "shouldness." It is sharing the *depth* of one's being as opposed to one's facade. It is the holy place—the sacred, spiritual part of one's being. Sharing it is sharing one's God within.

Actualizing is a process of sharing all of the above in a core-to-core relationship with a significant other, gradually and continuously. This process can last a lifetime and the excitement comes in the gradual unfolding. Sharing one's inner core is a happening rather than an achievement. It is giving oneself as a gift to another. It is sharing one's unique biography and destiny with a significant other and not simply anonymously. It means asking for no guarantees and no certainties, but simply trusting in the ability and desire of each to respond to one another. Grace is risking the sharing of what is most deeply significant. One cannot talk about what is deeply significant with another until one first knows oneself, and one can only trust the other and feel safe when one has faith that what is said will be handled gently and with compassion.

THE PARTIAL FULFILLMENT THEORY

Many men and women enter marriage because they are not able to stand alone, because they are frightened and dependent, or because they are lonely and insecure. Most make the choice between the ages of eighteen and twenty-five, when they are totally unaware of their reasons. Such individuals are not really in love but are seeking a partial fulfillment through someone else. They ask another to do what they must do themselves. Thus, as Figure 49 shows, they find only a temporary wholeness when they come together in marriage. When trouble ensues, and as they recognize the rigidity of their roles, the process of mutual blaming begins. Each asks the other: "Why aren't you like me?" or "Why aren't you what I want you to be?" Each shifts the responsibility for his or her own happiness to the partner. Such a relationship can become fulfilling and rhythmic only when the individuals involved accept responsibility for their own behavior—developing that part of themselves that has been unconsciously denied, or modifying the polar dimension that has been exaggerated. Figure 49 is actually a paradigm for all immature relationships, even though its application is more obvious in the case of the complementary or dependent relationship. The diagram suggests that the problem of polarities within cannot be solved by marrying someone outside and feeling temporarily fulfilled. What therapy requires is not that one simply be masculine (strong and angry) or feminine (weak and loving), but that one be "full-filled"—both angry and loving, both strong and weak. This requires that one love oneself fully, and this requires therapeutic *work*, because no one is *wholly* actualizing or free from polar deficiencies.

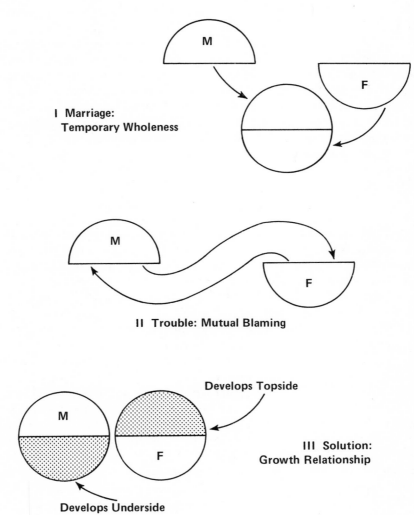

I Marriage:
Temporary Wholeness

II Trouble: Mutual Blaming

Develops Topside

III Solution:
Growth Relationship

Develops Underside

Figure 49. The Partial Fulfillment Theory

LOVE AS GROWTH IN ENCOUNTER

An area of prime concern in self-actualizing is the meaning of love. Unfortunately, too few people who are preparing for marriage have ever taken time to develop any understanding of love, much less to evaluate what love means to them as individuals. Most people are likely to say that they married for love; however, they cannot explain the nature of that original love, nor can they explain what they mean when they now say they love or do not love their mates.

Frequently, a person's concept of love does not distinguish between "romantic love" and "mature love" between man and woman. Romantic love has cultural roots in the past, but it survives in the present, nurtured by an endless barrage of fairy tales, told in slightly different forms in movies, magazines, novels, and television programs. The media cater to the susceptible daydreams of the immature and tend to make them "romantic emotionalism" freaks. This happens because most people, in their immaturity, appear unable to understand, let alone grow into, mature love relationships without assistance.

Love, in its experiential sense, may best be defined as *authentic human encounter*. Human encounter is defined as two persons *grasping* each other in emotional *contact*, having genuine mutual *concern* for the welfare and fulfillment of each other, and experiencing each other with attitudes of honesty, awareness, freedom, and trust.

Defined as encounter, love may be placed in a frame of reference comprising three elements: self, other, and context. Love, we posit, exists only when (1) *all three* of these elements are present, (2) none of these elements is *distorted*, and (3) there is awareness of all three elements in the *here and now*.

Three means by which love may be distorted are by transference, denial, and projection. *Transference* is defined as the *distortion* of encounter. This phenomenon is found in the therapeutic situation when, for example, a client sees his therapist as a father figure, a brainwasher, a devil, or a judge. Here it is likely that the client is distorting the here-and-now reality of a genuine encounter with projections from the past. Likewise, if the therapist sees the client only as a therapeutic label—as a schizophrenic, an obsessive, an anxiety neurotic—he is also distorting or oversimplifying and real encounter is lost.

Denial, the second means by which distortion of the human encounter takes place, is the refusal to admit the three essential elements of the encounter: the self, the other, and the context. If one denies that he himself is "being there" in the moment, if he denies the *other's* "being there," or if he denies the reality of the situation, encounter is not present.

Denial of self is refusing to believe the truth of one's own deepest feelings and expressing instead a socially acceptable comment. For example, one might say, "I like you" to a person whom one actually dislikes. Statements such as "You don't understand" and "You can't mean that" express denial of the other. References to the past ("You always make fun of me") or to the future ("You will think I'm silly") reflect denial of the context—of the "now" situation. In contrast, actualizing encounter is reflected in statements such as "I really am *afraid* now. I feel it deep inside me" (acceptance of self), "I really like you. I mean that!" (acceptance of the other), and "I really am aware of what's going on now. We are saying good-bye to each other!" (acceptance of the situation in context).

All emotions, whether positive or negative, contribute to encounter. The special form of denial most commonly seen is that of hostility—an attitude of negativity in which no contact is made with the other: for example, sarcasm or the silent treatment. Anger, on the other hand, is a *contact* emotion; because it is mixed with caring, it makes a direct encounter, lifting the barrier between the two persons.

The third means by which contact may be distorted is *projection*. Projection is commonly understood in its negative sense—a form of transferring negative dimensions of the self onto another. Less commonly understood is that projection can be positive—one can project or give to the other a power that really exists in oneself. For example, to give another the power of "teacher," "judge," "wise one," or "hero" is to give away one's worth or ability. Such an encounter is self-reducing and is therefore distorted.

THE CARING SEQUENCE

An Actualizing Therapist needs to be familiar with the common psychological interpretations of the forms of love and the processes of loving. The Caring Relationship Inventory helps to identify love's dimensions—the caring sequence—in objective fashion. The dimensions of caring that this inventory measures are very closely aligned to the characteristics of the human encounter that Rollo May called eros, empathy, friendship, and agape, or affection. These four characteristics correspond not only to the four life stages of man (see Chapter 5), but also to the parallel process of development during the marriage years: the relationship sequence.

THE RELATIONSHIP SEQUENCE

Just as the development of the human species may be said to be recapitulated in the development of the fetus, so the early developmental stages of the caring sequence are recapitulated in the four love dimensions of the relationship sequence.

The Eros Dimension

The first stage of romance and marriage may easily be identified as the *eros* stage. First attractions are often sexually based, and early courting is characterized by kissing, petting, depending, and fighting.

Eros is the romantic form of love, which includes such aspects as inquisitiveness, jealousy, and exclusiveness, as well as sexual or carnal desire. Jealousy is a very important element in romantic love. New spouses are very concerned about extra attentions given their partners by members of the other sex, and such attentions easily stimulate reversion to early oral dependent behavior and defensive mechanisms.

Eros usually involves a strong element of "positive projection." People project onto their partners idealized images of worth, beauty, and power that are not really there. Usually, during the first six years, all normal married persons face the developmental task of realizing that their spouses are not the idealized persons they married but, rather, are real human beings with normal weaknesses. Unless married couples accept the idea that marriage cannot be based on eros alone, the marriage is usually doomed to failure.

A manipulative eros relationship continues the same forms of oral manipulation, such as overdependency or overdefensiveness, that were used in relationship to one's parents. Not all eros is manipulative, however, and it would be inaccurate to say that eros is alien to a total love relationship. Eros is often misunderstood as being synonymous with *epithymia* (desire), and a similar lack of understanding attends Freud's treatment of the term *libido.* Freud proclaimed a half-truth when he said that libido is that which moves one toward release of tension, for libido is also a normal drive toward fulfillment of the self. Eros, in its positive sense, contains *epithymia* but goes beyond it. Eros is not simply desire for desire's sake—it can also be viewed as transpersonal, seeking to overcome the limitations of the individual life and to achieve union between lover and beloved.

An actualizing marriage means acknowledging one's needs, without foisting one's earlier projections, dependence, and defensiveness onto the partner. Such a marriage relationship stimulates self-support rather than excessive expectations.

The Empathy Dimension

As a marriage matures, it seems that empathy, or the ability to feel deeply the separateness and masculine or feminine nature of the opposite partner, becomes a paramount task. It involves compassion, appreciation, and tolerance for the unique personhood of the other.

The manipulative empathic relationship is one in which one partner assumes responsibility for the growth and change in the other person. This partner attempts to relate to the other in a way that will make that other person feel more masculine or more feminine. Such a partner forfeits loving his own center and becomes centered in the developmental tasks of his partner.

Empathy means appreciation of one's separateness and one's unique expression of masculinity or femininity. An actualizing relationship is one of mutually respecting individuals in contact. Kahlil Gibran likens marriage to the pillars of a temple—they are fused at the top, but they maintain their separateness. He says further that, like the oak tree and the cypress, marrieds do not grow in each other's shadows.

The Friendship Dimension

As a marriage deepens, the maturing years can be described as the "friendship years." Building on accumulated foundations of eros and empathy, friendship seeks to increase common interests—having more time to do things together, such as traveling or entertaining.

Our research with the CRI (Shostrom, 1966), contrasting successfully married couples with troubled couples and divorced individuals, shows that friendship is the feature that most troubled and divorced individuals want in a second marriage. They want a buddy, not just a sweetheart.

In the manipulative friendship pattern, one partner attempts to absorb the other in keeping with his or her own needs. Friends become objects that lend status or meaning to one's own strivings or goals. Fearing the loss of their own identity, manipulating persons withdraw from friendships that might make personal demands.

One of the most challenging tasks of actualizing a marriage in these maturing years is that of deepening the *identity* of each partner while still retaining the *intimacy*. Actualizing persons, having found identity within themselves, are now free to establish and maintain mutually nourishing relationships with their spouse and with others. This often means active searching out of new interests to which each can find allegiance. It may also mean making friends with another couple, enabling friendship to develop in a four-way relationship.

The Agape Dimension

Agape love is the love that God supposedly has for man. In human beings it is the helping, nurturing form of love that characterizes the mature assisting the less mature. It involves an identification with nature and an appreciation of man's humanness, as well as an appreciation of his potentialities.

In a manipulative marriage, agape love equals playing God with one's partner. Its basis is an overexaggeration of one's *need to be needed.* It expresses itself in reluctance to allow one's partner to seek meaningful nourishment outside the relationship. It is threatened by intimate supportive growth groups and situations in which one's partner's dependency needs may be met by somebody other than oneself.

In an actualizing marriage, agape is evident in the couple's love for each other and in their identification with the achievements and failures of their children, who are now recapitulating the processes with which they once struggled.

The actualizing relationship, in terms of agape, accepts and encourages each partner's own self-interests. The actualizing partner finds a sense of completion in the spontaneous joy and achievements of the other. Agape, as the term is used in the New Testament, is an unmotivated love; it has nothing to do with the quality of the beloved. It is not self-seeking, but altruistic in a healthy way. It seeks to replenish the emptiness of the other rather than the void within oneself. In an actualizing relationship, agape is an emotional investment in which the return is sheer pleasure in the acceptance of another's uniqueness. Agape love usually begins after age twenty-one and increases in maturity throughout the years of adulthood.

Actualizing marriages that reach the "silver anniversary" stages of twenty-five years are the ones that are sterling in character and are easily identified. Those that are leaden and that remain together through the years out of fear or obligation are transparent and phony.

It should be noted that the foregoing dimensions are not listed as absolute developmental stages or in absolute sequence. Their experience in marriage depends a great deal on how well they were first experienced during the original developmental years. In an actualizing marriage, however, it is assumed that certain years foster certain dimensions more than others. For example, eros is obviously dominant in the early years of marriage, while agape probably develops more deeply in the later years. Empathy usually follows eros, as the relationship deepens, and friendship is characteristic of a mature relationship. A relationship, therefore, needs some of each of these forms of love if it is to grow. The absence of any of these forms reduces the chances for the success of a relationship.

THE RELATIONSHIP OF THE DEVELOPMENTAL FORMS OF LOVE TO THE POLARITIES

In a real sense, the anger-love and strength-weakness polarities represent communication continua, because they are ways in which people affect each other interpersonally. "Affect" means *emotion*—the ways in which people "move" each other. An actualizing person's rhythmic movement between the polar dimensions is representative of the processes of nature: the beating of the human heart, the continuous succession of day and night, the procession of the seasons. Each polarity has an active, as well as a passive, dimension of expression. The relationship between the fundamental forms of love and these two polarities is shown in Figure 50. The anger-love polarity expresses the eros and friendship dimensions of love, and the strength-weakness polarity expresses the agape and empathy dimensions.

Thus, eros is expressed dynamically in its tendency to manifest itself actively and passively—angrily as well as caringly. When eros is angry, it takes the form of lust, passion, and seduction. But when eros expresses itself dynamically in terms of the opposite polar dimensions, love manifests itself more passively as tenderness, warmth, and creativity.

Likewise, friendship is often expressed by the criticalness of the anger pole—by assertively saying "no" to requests of friends. Yet, at the same time, friendship expresses itself in the "yes" of brotherly love, appreciation, and relatedness.

The strength-weakness polarity expresses the agape and empathy dimensions of love in the following ways. Agape is exemplified in the love of God for man, and manifests itself actively in the human realm through giving (or charity), responsibility, and commitment. It represents the concern for the other's welfare through the use of one's own resources or power. At the same time, however, it means the ability to receive more passively, because if one cannot receive, one dominates his or her partner. Thus agape, in the weakness sense, requires that one feel one's humanness in unconditional surrender, openness, and the experiencing of need.

Finally, empathy expresses itself in strength through feeling with others—through understanding and identifying with others—and at the same time expresses itself passively through experiencing one's own vulnerability—one's need to withdraw from contact—and one's awareness of his finiteness.

All the above leads to the important polarization of *manipulation versus love*. As Rollo May says, the manipulative man can take care of others without caring for them, can give money but not his heart, can hear but not listen. But love, in its fullest expression, requires the power and tenderness of eros, the assertion and relatedness of friendship, the responsibility and receptivity of agape, and the understanding and vulnerability of empathy. When any of these forms of love is missing, one's relationships become increasingly manipulative.

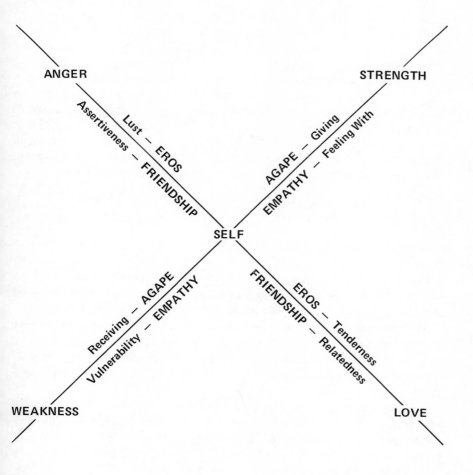

Figure 50. The Relationship of the Dimensions of Love to the Polarities

THE ACCUMULATION THEORY

Thus, we return to the original hypothesis of this chapter: that life may be described as an accumulation of levels of love. This is shown diagrammatically in Figure 51, where the sequence from eros, through empathy and friendship, to agape, represents the life stages of love and these same four forms of love are experienced in a similar sequence in marriage and caring relationships. Thus, people are given at least two chances for the development of each form of love: first, in their developmental history, and second, in their romantic relationships. Those stages that are learned weakly during the growth process may be learned more intensively in mature developing relationships. Thus, the actualizing person is given a second chance to develop actualizing love in significant interpersonal relationships.

In an actualizing relationship, each person focuses first on his own growth, but each can do this individually *within* the relationship. The relationship, therefore, provides the person with a living laboratory of growth. The relationship grows only if the individuals are growing. This is why, in marriage therapy, the focus is continually on the importance of each person's taking the responsibility for his or her own personal growth, which then facilitates the interdependent growth of the relationship.

THE RELATIONSHIP OF NEED SATISFACTION AND DEPRIVATION TO DEVELOPMENTAL GROWTH

All of the foregoing lends credence to the idea that, in *experiencing* love developmentally, people also *learn* to love. It is in being loved that one learns to love. But it also appears that deprivation sometimes causes one to love deeply: That which one is denied seems sometimes to be that which he or she appreciates and can give to others.

For example, the person who was denied the opportunity to express weakness as a child seems able to accept and love the weaknesses of others as an adult; the person who was denied opportunity to express strengths as a child seems able to foster and develop the strengths of himself and others as an adult.

It seems possible, then, that both satisfaction and deprivation of needs are teachers of love. It is not simply what happens developmentally that creates one's personhood, but it is in *knowing* oneself that one becomes a creative human being. It is self-knowledge that enables people to discover their needs and wants and to make them known in the loving relationships of later years, thus giving them the second chance to actualize themselves as fully dynamic human beings.

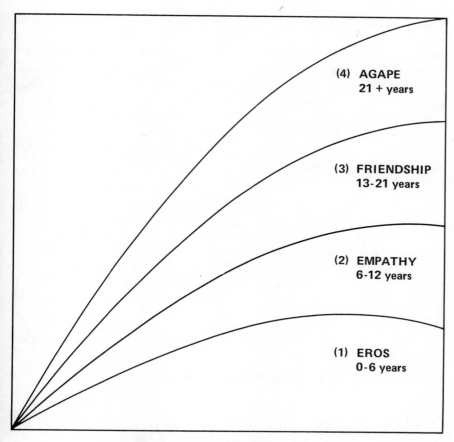

Figure 51. The Accumulation Theory of Love

MANIPULATION AND LOVE

When love becomes distorted, the result is some form of manipulation. The four dimensions of love may be viewed as bridges between two persons, as shown in Figure 52. If a person simply takes one of these forms of love and relates to another person only on that basis, then he is manipulating the relationship. For example, suppose somebody comes to you and says, "I'm only interested in agape; I'm only interested in your welfare. I have no personal interest in you, I have no eros interest in you, and I don't want friendship with you. I'm only interested in saving your soul." You would probably become very suspicious and angry with this person for playing

God with you. Agape, or affection, is the pure love that God has for man or the pure love of a parent for a child. If someone wants to relate to you, you would want them also to have empathy for you so that you would feel understood by them. In addition, you would want them to have some friendship and to be concerned about you in the future. If any of these elements of love is missing, the relationship weakens and manipulation exists. If someone just wanted you for eros, or sexual, reasons, you would simply feel used. Or if someone tried to "psych" you out by using empathy, you would be insulted. The absence of *all* of the dimensions of love is manipulation in its grossest form.

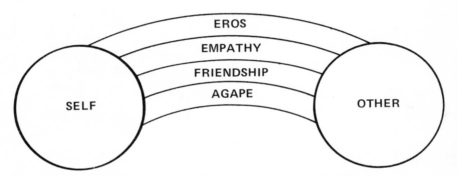

Figure 52. The Four Dimensions of Love in Encounter

The Obsessional Exploitation of Sex

One of the most detrimental aspects of our contemporary cultural view of marriage and love is the deterioration of eros. For example, as May says, *Playboy* magazine presents the most vivid example of people engaging in sexual titillation with no other human beings present. In our enlightened modern era no one wears a fig leaf over his or her genitals, but the women pictured in *Playboy* have "fig leaves" over their faces—faces without expression, faces without empathy, faces without any invitation to relate. Now this, of course, is what the men who look at *Playboy* often unconsciously want: the experience of sex as a kind of pseudorelationship, without really having to put one's heart into it—without having any encounter, any dedication. Such attitudes stem from modern American man's fear of impotence. American men and women have developed a great preoccupation with whether or not they can have orgasms, as though orgasms were all there is to sex. As a matter of fact, the encounter, the intimacy, and the meaningful relationship mean a great deal more than the technical performance of the sexual act. Many people can perform the sexual act very well but feel apathetic, without passion, and as though they are not human beings. When they have sexual relations with other persons, they feel that they are simply objects being manipulated.

Shostrom (1967), expanding on Buber, has described the contrast between a manipulative and an actualizing relationship as the difference between an "I-it" relationship (manipulative) and an "I-thou" relationship (actualizing). This is an important difference, because it suggests that the person who regards another as a "thou" becomes a "thou" as well, while the person who regards another as an "it" becomes an "it."

Appreciation of each other comes about through expression: Each person expresses preferences instead of ordering, each expresses acceptance of the other rather than tolerance, and each is even willing to genuinely surrender to the other's wishes instead of "playing submissive." The relationship is one of closeness, as opposed to one of distance.

Thus, the actualizing person, in efect, may be seen as appreciating himself and others as "thous" or valued human beings, rather than as "its" or "things" found in the attitudes of the manipulating person.

Masculinity versus Femininity

Until recently in our culture, the factors that constituted "maleness" and "femaleness" were thought to be obvious. Psychologists, for example, could speak simplistically of man as aggressive, penetrating, and active; woman as receptive, submissive, and passive. Man was the hunter and fighter, woman, the mother and nest builder; man, the theorist and warrior, woman, the healer and peacemaker. The Jungians saw man in terms of the *logos* principle (wisdom, logic) and woman in terms of the *eros* principle (relatedness, feeling). To some, woman was Mother Earth and man, Father Spirit; man was protector, woman was nourisher. But each authority fell into the trap of attempting to define as "natural" what the culture had created and shaped. Genesis called Eve the helpmate to Adam, St. Paul asked wives to "obey" their husbands, and the Christian marriage ritual incorporated such attitudes in nuptial celebrations. Labor laws, divorce laws, and social customs and institutions helped to make such biases sacred and permanent. A "feminine" man or "masculine" woman was considered to be a tragic distortion, or even perversion.

Now, such definitions seem closed and arrogant. Absolute certainty about sexual differences—beyond physical characteristics—is impossible to maintain. Masculinity is what the male discovers it to be in the process of living. Femininity is also the personal discovery of the female. Actualizing is being a full-filled *person*, expressing both polar dimensions.

PAIR ATTRACTION PATTERNS

Research utilizing the Pair Attraction Inventory (PAI) has confirmed six patterns, or pair relationships, that characterize the behavior of most couples in interaction. These relationships, shown earlier in Figure 45 (page 212), are: the nurturing relationship (mothers and sons), the supporting relationship (daddies and dolls), the challenging relationship (bitches and nice guys), the educating relationship (masters and servants), the confronting relationship (hawks), and the accommodating relationship (doves).

Each of these pair relationships can be exploitative or manipulative, or each can be creative or rhythmic. When a couple either consciously or unconsciously allows their relationship to freeze or rigidify in any one of these ways, it becomes manipulative. When a couple instead understands that their relationship can be a continuous workshop for growth, their relationship becomes actualizing or rhythmic.

The first four pair relationships are dependent, or complementary, because they consist of individuals who are trying to find, in their relationship, what is missing in themselves. These pairs support the theory that "opposites attract." Thus the master and the bitch have, to a greater or lesser degree, denied themselves the expression of love. Consequently, their anger or control is exaggerated. They relate in a complementary way to the servant and the nice guy, respectively, both of whom express a fawning and manipulative love because they have unconsciously denied their anger. The daddy and mother play the role of strength and unconsciously deny their weakness. They complement, and are complemented by, the doll and the son, who exaggerate their own weakness and deny their strength.

The remaining pair relationships, hawks and doves, are termed independent or symmetrical because each member independently fights for control. Hawk and dove relationships are both examples of "like attracting like." The hawks—any male-female combination of individuals shown at the top of Figure 45—unconsciously compete with one another because they deny their weakness or love and exaggerate their strength or anger. The doves—any male-female combination of individuals at the bottom of Figure 45—deny their anger or strength to control each other with weakness or manipulative love.

Although the pair typings of the Pair Attraction Inventory may appear to be stereotypical in nature, our research shows that they are the most common patterns found among pair relationships. A profile completed for each person tested reveals the ability of each to be rhythmic, or total, in his or her ability to express each of the patterns to some degree in the relationship.

A further way of using this test, as well as the CRI, is to use the "criss-cross technique." Here the wife, for example, responds as she sees the relationship and then takes the test again, responding this time as she believes her husband would. A comparison of these profiles reveals interesting patterns for discussion and suggests the degree to which each is aware of the other person's views of the relationship.

CREATIVE CONFLICT

In any marriage relationship, conflicts—negative feelings arising out of differing needs or goals—are not bad, but necessary, for out of conflict people can grow together. Conflict requires expression of *feelings*, not just logic. The feelings need to be expressed deeply, and one does not need to give reasons for their expression. Conflict involves an attitude of faith—faith that one's efforts will prove adequate to the resolution of the conflict. In *creative conflict*, the warring of marital partners can lead to creative solutions. Actualizing marriage partners respect differences in their spouses, just as the creative scientist welcomes disproving evidence. Indeed, the actualizing marriage partner is grateful for conflict.

The healthy marriage is one that recognizes the importance of creative fighting and conflict. It is a working relationship for conflict and resultant growth. Love doesn't mean not fighting—people who love each other and are close need to fight occasionally. Many people mistakenly fear expression of strong feelings in the marriage relationship, assuming that they should be rational and logical—trying to convince each other with facts rather than by expressing their feelings. The real fear of expressing anger or disagreement, however, is a fear of being hurt, or a fear of feeling guilt for inflicting hurt, or even a fear of abandonment. This fear causes people to deny their natural hostile feelings, with the result that they experience guilt, nag about unimportant things, or develop psychosomatic complaints. A marital fight involves the expression of strong feelings, and strong feelings need to be regarded as normal.

If people can believe that their feelings are natural and worthwhile expressions of the developing self, then they can learn to express *all* of them—the negative, hostile ones as well as the positive ones. When angry feelings are expressed, the opposite polar dimension, love feelings, can then be allowed into the consciousness. This leads to the view that expression of negative, hurtful feelings is necessary for an actualizing marital relationship. When one partner feels hostile toward the other, these feelings may represent an active desire for the other to realize more of his potential. This is an expression of true caring. The desire to communicate and be close can transcend the fear of being hurt in return.

THE RHYTHMIC RELATIONSHIP

The rhythmic relationship is shown in Figure 53. (We have simplified the personality by using the same polarities, or tensions, for the sake of clarity, as other chapters have dealt with each component more elaborately.) In the ideally rhythmic relationship there are no denials or exaggerations of the polarities. Each partner has his or her own identity or core and thus is able to express strength or weakness, anger or love. Each is free to relate as he or she really is. There are no frozen roles. The arrows in the diagram indicate that each partner is different at different times but that the entire personality is open and free enough to relate to the other in a real way. Thus, each can be a variety of things to the other, and nothing in either personality needs denial or distortion. It goes without saying that there are endless possible degrees of rhythm, and marriage becomes a kind of "workshop for growth." Actualizing couples are not really dependent or independent. We call them *interdependent.* They are continually in contact, and take the risk of expressing their innermost feelings without rehearsal or tailoring. Like two revolving pinwheels, they are constantly "in touch."

We have all known couples who enjoy such a relationship, in greater or lesser degree. They are not stereotypes, clinging in fear and dependency to their constricting roles; they are not slashing at each other, holding each other up, leading each other through life. But neither are they rigidly independent. They are men and women who can be a variety of things to each other. At different times they can be as a mother or father, son or daughter, consoler or confidant. They can be many things but, most of all, they are friends.

The rhythmic relationship is not simply a protection of personal uniqueness, nor is it the safeguarding of mutual independence. It is the creation of a new reality that neither individual could produce alone. It is the creation of two strong people growing stronger and together rather than two weak people clinging to each other for life or battling each other in aggressive competition or passive rejection. It gives meaning to the term "soul mates," who share with one another at ever greater depth and move beyond themselves into a new creation, to become more loving, aware, compassionate, creative, and joyous than they could ever be alone.

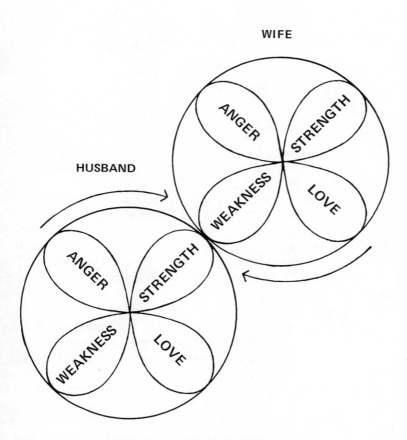

Figure 53. The Rhythmic Relationship

CHAPTER 11. ACTUALIZING AS A PERSONAL VALUING PROCESS

The emphasis of Actualizing Therapy is directed toward helping an individual develop a philosophy of functioning in life (a *scientific ethic* for living) rather than simply solving current problems. In a similar vein, more and more therapists are agreeing with Viktor Frankl's (1963) idea that therapy is a search for meaning and that "meaning" may be defined as personal values.

In Chapter 6, we said that when the person begins to actualize, he develops a personal priority system, or a hierarchy of personal needs or personal values. Personal values probably develop primarily from experience but also partly from an examination of the universal values found in religions and philosophical systems.

In this chapter, we share concepts of religion and philosophy that have relevance to the actualizing process. The proper relationship between psychology and religion is, of course, a question that transcends this book. It is an extremely difficult issue to deal with and a sensitive one to write about. Empirical psychology, perhaps necessarily from a historical perspective, has, by and large, chosen to ignore this issue, and it is only recently that the more "scientifically minded" psychotherapeutic theorists and researchers have seen the necessity of addressing themselves to the influence and the importance of the role of values in their field of practice.

ACTUALIZING THERAPY AS A VALUE DISCOVERING PROCESS

Many persons come to therapy with a disintegrated sense of values. The old, rigid systems of values by which they were raised no longer have meaning. And yet most clients have no sense of a way to rebuild their values. They often come with a sense of expediency or survival as their basis for choice in value-oriented situations. Or the more sophisticated client has a "situational ethic," as proposed by Joseph Fletcher (1966). Fletcher suggests an ethic wherein the *end* justifies the means, and one principle, such as "love," can cover all situations.

Actualizing Therapy suggests a theory we call *value discovering*: selecting a value, such as "love" or "honesty," by the process of polarity building—*discovering* opposite polar values that will also have *relevance* to living. The process leads to a system of values that is in constant evolution, but that builds on a central principle.

For example, a person can build on a dedication to Buber's "I-Thou" principle and then balance that with a concept of "I-it" as manipulation, defining certain situations in which manipulation may be *appropriate*.

The emphasis is on *process*—a willingness to experiment with the idea that for *every* truth there is an equal and opposite countertruth. The Actualizing Therapist must be sharp enough to encourage the client to consider his alternatives, or countervalues, to those proposed by the client. The emphasis is on *means* more than *ends*—teaching the client the ability to *fish* rather than providing him with a *meal*.

A second example that we have found common in young people today is the adherence to a one-value system—such as belief in *honesty only* as an ethic for living—then carrying this value to an extreme, justifying any form of behavior as long as one is open and honest about it. An alternative value that often comes up in Actualizing Therapy is *kindness*. When honesty is balanced by kindness, it becomes a more viable value. Such balancing always leads to an integration of polar values, but the process takes *time* and creativity.

A Valuing Exercise

An exercise in synergizing values is presented below from a publication called "For Humans Only." In each case, oppositional values are presented and then the game is to discover a "third way," or "tertium quid," that embraces and synergizes the original two terms. Because this exercise so embraces the theory of this book we feel it will be fruitful to those trying to understand the process of actualizing values.

> Dualities are opposites, standing against each other, equally repelled and attracted, with no resolution. A dualistic mentality tends to identify with one side against the other. A paradox, on the other hand, is a different way of looking at opposites, a way of encompassing both halves in a third process, which transcends the opposition.

A basic example of opposites is inhaling and exhaling. If either side is preferred at the expense of the other, the result is death. If both sides are encompassed without preference, then we have something called breathing—life.

The same process occurs with any pair of opposites. Duality-consciousness leads to death, and paradox-consciousness leads to life. To take this one step further, let's consider death and life as opposites: death without life is just death, and life without death is life motivated by fear of death, which is deadening. The third way, which has no name in our language, (and that's the case for most pairs of opposites—which says a lot about our culture) is life renewing itself by dying to itself.

A few more examples of opposites:

Creativity and **receptivity**: creativity without receptivity is actually aggression; receptivity without creativity is actually passiveness leading to apathy.

The *third way* is active receptivity, responsive action.

Maleness and **femaleness:** (within one person; regardless of physical gender): maleness without femaleness is hard, callous, and naive; femaleness without maleness is smothering.

We call the *third way* 'androgynous consciousness' (androgynous: Greek; 'andros' means 'man,' 'gynos' means 'woman').

Perception and **compassion:** perception without compassion leads to dry, pretentious intellectualism, and to isolation, if not schizophrenia and paranoia;

compassion without perception leads to mediocrity, conformism, if not hysteria and violence.

The *third way* is called 'wisdom.'

Humbleness and **exaltation:** to be humble while denying exaltation leads to oblivion, limbo;

to be exalted while denying humbleness leads to obnoxious self-centeredness.

The *third way* is the whole challenging and rewarding adventure of responsive living.

Gentleness and **firmness:** gentleness without firmness is wishy-washy; firmness without gentleness is rape.

It seems that the *third way* would be to be firmly gentle and gently firm in all situations.

Pain and **joy:** pain without joy is melodrama;

joy without pain is sentimentality.

The *third way* is feeling.

Seriousness and **humor:** seriousness without humor is heavy, pedantic; humor without seriousness is flippant, even insolent.

We cannot find words for the *third way* . . . we're open to suggestions, or rather the direct expression of it . . .

Good and **bad:** these are value-judgments depending on various mental criteria, but whatever the criteria: good without bad would be mellowly dull, and bad without good would be . . . well, mellowly dull, too; they obviously cannot exist without one another, like all other opposites . . .

So, good as opposed to bad is: afraid of being contaminated, is self-righteous, defensive-oppressive, naive or schizophrenic; and bad as opposed to good is afraid of being denied, and is equally self-righteous, defensive-oppressive, naive and schizophrenic.

The *third way* is: better—because bad, or evil, when integrated as such, sharpens consciousness and renders simplistic good into intelligent good.

Light and **dark:** where there is the sun, there is shadow: focusing on only one and denying the other is simply denying what is.

Being and **doing:** being without doing is a kind of aloofness which tends to deny the animal body as a part of the cosmos, refusing the adventure of incarnating, of taking risks, of making a fool of oneself (the lesson of humor);

doing without being is just plain absurd, like a dog chasing its tail; it's being busy for the sake of being busy, to avoid boredom, by fear of death; it's acting as a programmed robot, traditionally, mechanically, superficially; it's believing oneself to be only incarnation without spirit, without awareness of oneness, of the silent creative source, of the invisible; it's making a fool of oneself but being ignorant or proud of it (humorless); it's prepetuating a world "full of sound and fury, signifying nothing."

The *third way* is silence becoming music; it's what one really is, taking form.

VALUING AND CORE ACTUALIZING

The psychology of achieving a sense of core being is predicated on the theological theory of Kierkegaard that "purity of heart is to will one thing." In terms of polarity theory, this means actualizing the core is bringing together, in a synergistic fashion, the heart, the gut, and the brain, as well as creating a synergistic whole through the expression of the polarities of strength-weakness and anger-love, so as to empower or potentiate one's being.

To will one thing means to feel a sense of unity in the expression of one's polarities. The center for that energy comes from within, through the expression of what one truly *wants,* what one truly *prefers,* what one truly *wishes,* and what one truly *feels.* Each of these expressions of being represents a unity in that what one wants is an expression of one's strength, with the awareness of one's weakness in what one loves to do, and with the awareness of one's frustrations and anger in not always being fully able to do what one loves to do.

The polarities are not competitive, but cooperative, and they are experienced as unified. This is what we refer to as being inner-directed, or energized from the core and polarities within. This is opposed to being other-directed, or energized by the power of those to whom one gives authority to be stronger or weaker than oneself, more loving or more actualizing than oneself.

The polarities are synergized and potentiated into one thing, which can be referred to as the courage to be, or the freedom to be. But there is a feeling of being together with oneself as one experiences the various polar dimensions as a "family" rather than as "warring factions." Another way to say this is that the goal of therapy is to help one be the self that one truly is, rather than to be the self that others demand. "Isness" equals core actualizing.

CONCEPTS OF RELIGION COMPATIBLE WITH ACTUALIZING

In this chapter we will examine some concepts of religion and human growth that have been of most help to Actualizing Therapists in their professional attempt to help man understand the meaning of life—concepts that most technical manuals of our field fail to consider.

From the rich legacy of Jewish Hasidism come ideas much in the tradition of Actualizing Therapy. Consider the following from Kopp (1971):

> What is more, even the urge to evil is a kind of vitality, a life source to be reclaimed rather than rejected. We need to be in touch with and hopefully to *own every part of ourselves* so that we do not continue to be at war within ourselves. If a thief comes in the night, and we cry out and so scare him off, nothing is accomplished beyond the moment, and we must remain in fear. But if we do not alarm the thief, but let him draw near enough so that we may lay hold of him and bind him, then we have the chance of reforming him. So, too, our own willful impulses can become a rich source of renewal of imaginative powers. Our stubbornness can be transformed into determination, and our struggle with the other can surrender into intimacy. Each man must confront himself in order to accomplish these transformations, this *turning of the self.* (p. 41)

This passage could easily refer to the creative struggle with, and the transformation of, the polarities within.

Kopp further states:

> If others offend, a man must be prepared to deal with this too—
> not with widely destructive rage, but with a kind of tamed anger
> which he keeps in his pocket. When he needs it, he must be sure
> to take it out. (p. 44)

What better way of stating the importance of being able to express the
modulations of affect on the anger dimension?

In the Judaeo-Christian tradition, the statement that most fully expresses
Actualizing philosophy is, "The Kingdom of God is within." The theologian
Martin Buber best expresses this position with his "I-Thou" philosophy; if
one really sees the other person as a "Thou," then one sees the Kingdom
of God within that other person as well as within oneself. If one truly loves
his neighbor, one finds himself in contact with God in a very personal
sense.

Buber (1951) put it this way:

> Every person born into this world represents something new,
> something that never existed before, something original and
> unique. "It is the duty of every person . . . to know and consider
> that he is unique in the world in his particular character and that
> there has never been anyone like him in the world, for if there had
> been someone like him, there would have been no need for him to
> be in the world. Every single man is a new thing in the world, and
> is called upon to fulfill his particularity in this world." Every
> man's foremost task is the actualization of his unique,
> unprecedented and never recurring potentialities, and not the re-
> petition of something that another, and be it even the greatest,
> has already achieved. (p. 16)

The great Rabbi Zusya (in Kopp, 1971, p. 38) was once asked, "Rabbi,
tell us, why do you teach in this way when Moses taught in another way?"
"When I get to the coming world," answered Rabbi Zusya, "there they will
not ask me, 'Why were you not more like Moses?' but instead they will ask
me, 'Why were you not more like Zusya?' "

Both Buber and Zusya are saying that the personality of a person is more
significant than his doctrine; individuality is more important than imitation. This is another beautiful way of saying what self-actualizing is. It is
being oneself—something no other person can be!

From Oriental philosophies comes the psychology of Yin and Yang, the
two interacting forces of the universe. The original meanings of these words
were "shaded" (Yin) and "sunlit" (Yang). Symbolically, they stood for
dark, terrestrial, cool, and submissive (Yin) and all things bright, celestial,

warm, and aggressive (Yang). Everything in the universe shows the interplay of these forces: the seasons, the daily rhythm of light and dark—everything is in rhythm. Such rhythm is a key principle of Actualizing Therapy.

From Buddhism comes the Taoism, or the Way of Life of Lao Tzu. He emphasized the burdensomeness of the conventional concept of good versus bad. He said that it is the concern for right and wrong that is the sickness of the mind. Rather, man can seek what his Way is after his own nature. Thus the Master of the Tao teaches that life is a totally free and purposeless *journey.* Instead of *striving* and *reasoning*, we must stop trying. The first solution is to *give up* struggling against our own nature. Then we must *give in* to our own individual beings. "If you cannot get the better of your feelings," says Chauag Tzu, "then give play to them. Nothing is worse for the soul than struggling not to give play to feelings that it cannot control" (Waley, 1956, p. 48).

All manipulations are masked attempts to sustain the illusion that one can control oneself and others and to try to reason oneself into certainty. To learn to flow with life, like a cork on water, is the most difficult task of all. Appreciation of the wholeness of one's own homeostatic being helps avoid this false illusion.

Thinking in terms of complementary polar dimensions, rather than contrary opposites, is a mark of the actualizing person. As illustrated in Figure 54, right-wrong, good-bad, and ours-theirs are opposites that confuse because they are contrary, either-or, and unintegrative. Acceptance of such schemes leads to rejection of one's supposed "bad self" and creates an internal civil war, leaving one split—being only half his potential.

It was once said of King Charles V, "There is a soul of goodness in things evil." This intermingling of the good and the bad, the noble and the dishonest, the harsh and the gentle is a universal principle of actualizing. No person, no matter how much strength he has, is without his weaknesses and vulnerabilities. But it is the very awareness of one's weaknesses that gives a person the courage to be a fully human being.

Dualism has roots in both non-Christian and Christian religions, and the dichotomies it has fostered impede the process of self-actualizing in the individual. In Zoroastrianism, the Good God, Ahura Mazda, is opposed by the Evil Spirit, Angra Mainyu, who later was called Shaitin (a forerunner of the English word "Satan"). Mani, an Iranian, brought forth a system combining elements from Buddhism, Christianity, Zoroastrianism, and Gnosticism. His system taught a dualism of spirit and matter: The soul of man is good, but it is a prisoner of the vile matter of the body.

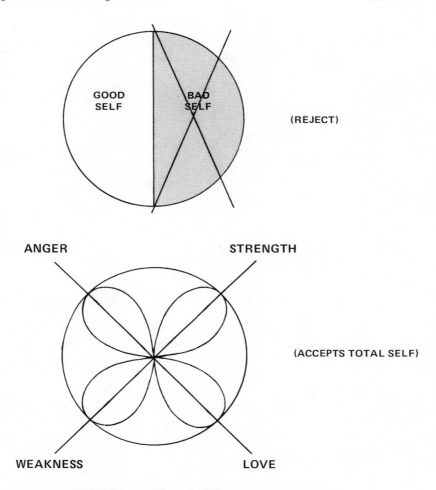

Figure 54. Splitting versus Accepting the Total Self

Dualism, in history and in the human personality, can be put into perspective by considering the two columns of the Pythagoreans: The "good" one had warmth, light, harmony; the "bad" one had coolness, darkness, and discord. A dualist living in upper Alaska might put warmth in the "good" column, but a dualist living in Needles, California in August, might put warmth in the "bad" column.

Appreciation of the polarities (or dualities) within ourselves leads to accepting the *whole-someness* of ourselves and avoids the trap of rigid thinking. Just as in Gestalt psychology the two sides of the coin, or figure and ground, must always go together, so in personality the individual derives his identity from the reconciliation and integration of the complementary poles within himself.

What this really means is that each person must trust his own organism or "inner Supreme Court." This does not mean that one should ignore society but rather that one must struggle to integrate the conflicting values he faces. The authors believe that most of these struggles are related to inner conflicts between the major polar dimensions. For example, most people are taught to "stand up and be counted," and yet they are also told, "Blessed are the meek." They are admonished to "love thy neighbor," and yet that they must not "let the sun set on our wrath."

The struggle to try to integrate the dimensions of one's polarities is the unique task of discovering the truth of one's own being. It requires a deeply spiritual attitude in which the *self* is regarded as a trustworthy, homeostatic control system. To affirm this truth about oneself is to have the most profound faith in one's total being.

AN ACTUALIZING ANALYSIS OF THE BEATITUDES

The truth of man's existence as expressed by Jesus in the Beatitudes of his Sermon on the Mount is most relevant to Actualizing Therapy. We have interpreted the Beatitudes in the light of the principle of synergy—not as "either-or," but as rhythmic, oscillating principles.

In the following analysis, each Beatitude is shown to have both an active and a passive dimension. This is the creative nature of Jesus' teaching; He did not recommend a lockstep control of life but a free, spontaneous range of rhythmic expression in which one may find one's freedom to be. The deep wisdom expressed in the Beatitudes is the recognition of this implicit rhythm of life. Just as the human heart must function by active and passive movement, just as day is active and night passive, just as spring is active and winter passive, so man, considered God's finest creation, must have his natural rhythm to be fully expressive of his potential.

The following discussion from Dunnam, Herbertson, and Shostrom (1968) is an attempt to describe the implicit rhythmic pattern of man's basic nature:

I.   Actualizing persons express themselves rhythmically on the continuum of *strength* and *weakness*.

    A. In the first Beatitude, Jesus says that the "blessed," or the joyous actualizing person is "poor in spirit." To be poor in spirit means the opposite of having pride. Man is human, not God, with all the strengths of man and all the weaknesses as well. He must be aware of his strength ("a little less than the angels"), and yet he must also be aware of his weaknesses. Jesus was tempted and felt His weakness in the wilderness, and yet in the temple, as He rebuked the moneychangers, He was aware of His strength.

B. In the second Beatitude, Jesus says, "Blessed are those who *mourn.*" Here it is clear that to mourn means to feel hurt, to experience suffering. To experience hurt means that we must be aware again of our human weakness—aware that we can be "gotten to." It also means to trust our capacity to experience hurt; it therefore leads to an increasing belief in our capacity to take misfortune or suffering, and therefore paradoxically helps us experience our strength. On the other hand, the courage to mourn with others empathetically provides them courage as they discover their strength. Through the pain He experienced as He wrestled with His destiny, even to the point of sweating blood, Jesus found the courage to face His own crucifixion.

II. Actualizing persons express themselves rhythmically on the continuum of *dependency* and [*self-support*].

A. In the third Beatitude, Jesus described the actualizing life as one characterized by *meekness*. To be meek is to be open to our limitations. It means expressing our dependency when it is felt and yet at the same time being aware of our self-sufficiency and independence. Jesus said, "He who has seen me has seen the Father." He spoke as one having authority. Yet at the same time He did not judge. He did not even need to "play God" and forgive. He merely said, "Go, and do not sin again."

B. In the fourth Beatitude, Jesus characterized the actualizing person as *hungering after righteousness*. To hunger after righteousness means ethical awareness. It means asking for what we need or want, but being aware of what we do not need for fulfillment. As with Maslow's actualizers, the religious actualizing person knows what is right and wrong and seeks what is right for him. Jesus expressed His hunger after righteousness, even at an early age, as He visited the temple and talked with the priests. He also knew what He did not need—the power and security which was promised Him by the Tempter in the wilderness.

III. Actualizing persons express themselves rhythmically on the continuum of [*evaluation*] and [*compassion*].

A. In the fifth Beatitude, Jesus talks of the importance of being *merciful*. To be merciful means to be understanding of others and to have compassion. It means being able to forgive injuries, but at the same time to express strong negative feelings regarding the behavior of those whom we love and disagreement with others without judging their rightness or wrongness. Expressing feelings still keeps the dialogue open, while making judgments closes it. Jesus was merciful when He said, "Let him who is without sin among you be the first to throw a stone." Yet He rebuked the Pharisees when He felt strongly negative toward their critical self-righteousness.

B. In the eighth Beatitude, Jesus said, "Blessed are those who are *persecuted.*" Here, He implies that from misunderstanding and disapproval we can grow. We can learn from our enemies. We can develop a creative indifference to persecution. We can guide others without making their decisions for them. Jesus loved Judas, even though Judas betrayed Him, and by His affirmation on the cross Jesus was *creatively* indifferent to persecution—"Father, forgive them; for they know not what they do."

IV. Actualizing persons express themselves rhythmically on the continuum of [*assertion*] and *caring.*

A. The seventh Beatitude describes the actualizing person as a *peacemaker.* To make peace means to make peace not only with others, but with ourselves, to assert our convictions, yet be compassionate and caring. Jesus was a peacemaker; He would not let Peter fight His enemies, and yet He Himself was willing to die for what He believed. He aggressively stated His convictions in the Sermon on the Mount, and yet He asked God to forgive those who crucified Him.

B. The sixth Beatitude described the religious actualizing person as *pure in heart.* In a real sense, this Beatitude integrates all the others. As Kierkegaard has so succinctly stated, to be pure in heart is to will one thing. This suggests the ability to integrate one's awareness of potential along with the acceptance of one's limitations. The actualizing person is synergistic; he has resolved his dichotomies. Jesus was a centered person. Though He humanly prayed, "Let this cup pass," He subordinated that desire to God's will for His life. "Nevertheless, not as I will, but as Thou wilt." He aggressively cared to fulfill His life's mission. (pp. 99-104)

The Beatitudes not only describe the polarities of human existence, but *invite* us to participate in the process of actualizing and blessedness through an increasing awareness of the natural polarities created within our beings.

PSYCHOLOGY AS SCIENCE VERSUS PHILOSOPHY

Therapists have always been reluctant to accept or acknowledge "religious" responsibilities and functions. There are many reasons for this, but the primary ones include the strong historical influence of the empirical tradition, the alleged hypocrisy and emotional extremism in much religious behavior, and frequent inner conflicts or ignorance concerning spiritual matters within the therapist himself.

The scientific models and procedures of the late nineteenth century were mechanistic and Darwinian theory, in particular, had considerable influence on psychologists, who saw man simply as a continuation of the animal world and as subject to the same natural laws. A strong effort was made (and still is being made) to divorce psychology from its earlier philosophical roots—to make the investigation of human behavior a strictly "scientific" enterprise. In light of this, it is interesting to note that William James—who was equally at home in both the philosophy and psychology departments at Harvard—is still considered by many to be the greatest psychologist America has produced. This is in spite of the fact that even though he had great regard for the experimental method, he was thoroughly committed to the study of philosophy.

Actualizing Therapists do not propose abandoning the careful observation and experimentation of the scientific approach, but they do suggest that psychologists examine their assumptions and techniques in terms of their usefulness for understanding basic human problems and for helping individuals to deal with these problems effectively. A major difficulty with psychology today is that hunger for increased knowledge about human behavior and for improved methods to assist people with their problems is making premature and unrealistic demands on this fledgling science. Actualizing Therapists are committed to looking beyond scientific methods and psychological techniques and to helping clients with those value problems that transcend the mere techniques.

Of course, one must not forget the fact that there is such a thing as a philosophy of science; in fact, there are several philosophies of science. Even though some may say that a philosophy of science falls into the same category as "Catholic University," which George Bernard Shaw once called a contradiction in terms, neither of these combinations is, in fact, contradictory. Although we do not have the space for a full discussion of the philosophy of science here, a paragraph from Michael Polanyi (1973) will serve to illustrate the relationship of science to philosophical assumptions:

> The propositions of science . . . appear to be in the nature of
> guesses. They are founded on the *assumptions* of science
> concerning the structure of the universe and on the evidence of
> observations collected by the methods of science; they are subject
> to a process of verification in the light of further observations
> according to the rules of science; but their *conjectural* character
> remains inherent in them. [Emphasis added.] (pp. 31-32)

Despite the predominance of the scientific approach, there is precedent
for the role of psychology in the areas of traditional religious concern (see,
for example, White, 1953, and Kunkel, 1955). More therapists seem to be
recognizing that religious sentiments and feelings are powerful positive or
negative motives in their clients' lives.

William James (1958) in his Gifford Lectures, titled *The Varieties of
Religious Experience,* provided an example of the use of personal docu-
ments in psychological science. In this treatise, James examined such subjects as religion and neurology, the reality of the unseen, healthy minded-
ness, the sick soul, and religious conversion. This work is both scientific
and philosophical, but it clearly indicates an appreciation for, and an
acceptance of, the connection between psychology and religion.

Therapists must recognize that religious concepts and actualizing concepts are not mutually exclusive. Of course, one must not assume that
either religious concern or actualizing interpretation is the sole solution to,
or explanation of, man's problems. Many people make this assumption and
feel inclined either to reject therapeutic interpretations and explanations of
behavior or to reject their religious belief system. There seems, however, to
be a third position: to accept the idea that *there is considerable overlap
between the actualizing and theological views of man.* One example of this
overlap in contemporary literature is found in a passage from Tournier
(1957), the eminent Swiss psychiatrist:

> The person is a potential, a current of life which surges up con-
> tinually, and which manifests itself in a fresh light at every new
> blossoming forth of life. At the creative moment of dialogue with
> God or with another person, I in fact experience a double cer-
> tainty: that of "discovering" myself, and also that of "changing." I
> find myself to be different from what I thought I was. From that
> moment I am different from what I was before. And yet at the
> same time I am certain that I am still the same person, that it is
> the very same life which is welling up anew, that it was contained
> in my being as it was yesterday, even though then there was
> nothing that could lead me to suspect what I am discovering
> today. (p. 232)

One should recognize these points of overlap and then look assiduously for areas where the meanings are congruent and where they seem to give greater combined insight into man's existence and the solution of his human problems. In any event, the view one holds about the nature, purpose, and origin of man influences his approach to any "I-Thou" concept. The Actualizing Therapist generally operates on the more humanistic assumption that ultimate values are rationally determined and are found within the person. It is possible, however, to resolve this issue at the technique level, since both religion and humanism are concerned with helping suffering humanity. Actualizing Therapists can evaluate their techniques on the basis of their effectiveness in reaching limited goals, quite apart from the basic philosophical assumptions and basic purposes involved.

RELEVANT RESEARCH

Traditionally, a church has been a community of people enhancing one another's growth. However, critics of current highly institutionalized churches feel that this *koinonia*, or fellowship of persons, has been lost. In a major study of the American Catholic Priesthood, Andrew Greeley (1970) has reported a number of significant relationships between priests' levels of self-actualizing and amounts of perceived institutional support. In responding to questions concerning conflict between real and ideal distribution of power in the Church, the more actualizing priests perceived a greater conflict and expressed a greater need to reform the Church. Higher levels of actualizing were associated with exercise of initiative and with unfavorable reaction to the birth control encyclical. As these associations would suggest, higher levels of actualizing are negatively related to adherence to traditional values within the Church, and, as would be expected, they are associated with general dissatisfaction with the Church. The correlation between self-actualizing, as measured by the POI Inner-Direction scale, and professed plans to stay in the priesthood was significant and negative. Supporting the latter relationship are data comparing POI scores of a sample of 917 active priests with those of 270 resigned priests. Scores were higher among the resigned priests on every POI measure of self-actualizing. Data from this important study clearly indicated that changes within the Church are necessary if an objective of the Church is to maximize the growth and actualizing of its clerical community.

Mowrer (1964, pp.17-19) has shown that the original Christian Church was a small-group movement. The faithful would meet secretly in caves to discuss their mutual concerns. However, in the fifth century A.D., the pope weakened the small-group aspect by requiring that Church members confess their faults to a professional priest rather than to one another. Martin Luther further complicated the issue when he maintained that Protestants need not confess to a priest but rather should speak directly to God in prayer. Thus, by fiat, the Christian Church ceased to be a small-group movement. As Dunnam, Herbertson, and Shostrom (1968) have maintained, the modern Church must revitalize the spirit of the small-group approach if it is to remain relevant for modern man.

It is our thesis that the actualizing process is a way to recapture this spirit. Actualizing Therapy groups conducted by understanding and trained clergymen can provide the vehicle for priests to experience the rewards of peace, joy, and a renewed sense of community and commitment. Introduction of the actualizing process through encounter group techniques has produced results in several church-affiliated studies. Reddy (1972) has reported the effects of a five-day, residential, human relations sensitivity training program for forty interdenominational missionaries preparing for foreign service. He found overall significant increases in self-actualizing. As a further refinement of this study, ministers were separated for analysis into four groups according to their premeasured compatibility for affection. As described in the section on group composition in encounter (Chapter 8), those in the two incompatible affection groups gained comparatively more on POI scales of Inner-Direction, Feeling Reactivity, Spontaneity, and Capacity for Intimate Contact.

Additional data with implications for the assessment of principles of Actualizing Therapy in the church setting have been provided by Byrd (1967). His studies were designed to evaluate the effects of several short-term laboratories upon assumed initiative and upon emotional expression. The sessions were attended by interdenominational groups of persons identified as key agents of change within their organizations. As in the Reddy studies, responses of participants in groups receiving one type of experience (the classical T-group) were compared with those in an experimental, creative risk-taking "Nongroup," a creative experience in which individuals tested their potential by expressing themselves through unfamiliar media and in unfamiliar styles. As in the Reddy studies, overall gains were reported in self-actualizing as measured by the POI. Significantly greater gains were obtained in the creative risk-taking group on those POI scales suggesting greater increases in personal autonomy (I), holding of values of self-actualizing persons (SAV), expressing feelings in spontaneous action (S), affirming a constructive view of the nature of man (Nc), and accepting aggression in oneself as natural (A).

Similar results have been obtained by the Navy Chaplain Corps in experimenting with an eclectic transgenerational workshop program with Navy personnel (Knapp & Fitzgerald, 1973). This program was established with the particular objective of building an increased sense of community among those persons whose feelings of alienation had led to such unsatisfactory behavioral expressions as drug abuse or alcohol addiction. Again, results from administration of the POI before and after the workshop demonstrate the positive effectiveness of programs of this type. Through such experiences, conducted by trained and sensitive clergymen, each participant had the opportunity to reexamine his personal values to rediscover and enhance his dignity and worth, and to regain his respect for the "thouness" of others.

All these studies demonstrate that the POI is a relevant instrument in the measuring of values in various kinds of church or community settings. If therapy is a process of personal valuing, the POI is an important adjunct to the process of therapy.

CONCLUSIONS

In this chapter we have explored some of the ways in which religious values have contributed to Actualizing Therapy. We have shown how views from Judaism, Christianity, and Buddhism contribute to the concepts of actualizing psychology. We believe this is religion in its finest meaning, which is to "bind again" man and all his beliefs and values. One possible tributary of the larger stream of self-actualizing might be an ecumenical approach akin to creative synthesis in psychotherapy. The establishment of such an approach would build on the work of Freud, James, Jung, Fromm, and others, and would provide another example of the inclusiveness of the self-actualizing model. Religion is a way of perceiving truth. One need not sacrifice the scientific side of psychology to include the resources of religion in the total process of self-actualizing as it relates to theory, research, and the practice of psychotherapy.

CHAPTER 12. ACTUALIZING THERAPY AS CREATIVE PROBLEM SOLVING

Creative synthesis is a form of creativity based on integration of the ideas of many, rather than of one. Too often, people think of creativity in an *intra*dimensional way, whereas in reality, it is stimulation by others that creates creativity. Creativity is *inter*personal first and *intra*personal second. Thus, therapy may be seen as a creative enterprise in the sense that each new contact with a client is a new adventure in creativity. The interaction of the state of particularity of the client, the state of particularity of the therapist, and the state of particularity of the moment all form a new gestalt. This gestalt can potentiate growth if the therapist is willing to be fully aware of the dimensions present, as well as the dimensions that are possible from the interaction in the moment. Thus, creativity is not a looking forward so much as it is an organizing of the dimensions of the moment as they interact before one's eyes.

Fritz Perls was a very creative therapist, and it was only a focus of the moment—of what was going on—that enabled him to be the genius of a therapist that he was. However, clients did not *always* find Perls to be a creative therapist, particularly when he was tired or ill, for example.

THERAPEUTIC CREATIVITY

In terms of Murphy's (1958) model, creativity springs from the alive elements of the moment, and not from a vacuum. The creative synthesizer *immerses* himself with all data available and then permits an *incubation period,* in which the creative forces of the organism *organize* and *reorganize* the data. This leads to "inspiration," or creative "leaps." The creative synthesizer then goes through a process of *evaluation* and working through, trying out various techniques that finally become original in the sense that they become a new gestalt, organized from old and new experiences.

In most intellectual areas creativity is not like the process of working with a block of clay, but rather it is more like the process of working with an erector set, erecting a new structure from elements that are already present in the moment. But the growing therapist never stops constructing and reconstructing. Sometimes it is a good idea to let the parts of an erector set that have been built into a system fall, and let the pieces loosen from one another. In this way a new gestalt can be formed that may be more effective and creative than the original.

Applying this idea to therapy techniques, it is possible to build on a body technique (such as stamping one's feet) as a foundation, then to build to a feeling technique (shouting "No!" as one stamps one's feet), and finally to move to a thinking technique (perhaps telling the parent, in fantasy, what has made one angry). Thus all three techniques are integrated into one.

Similarly, one may start with the construct that it is a good idea to feel one's vulnerability on the weakness dimension. One can begin to feel this vulnerability by sounding groans that express a childlike need for a parent. Finally, one can reach upward with the arms and give physical expression to this polar dimension.

Thus, therapy is a constant process of reformulating a therapeutic gestalt —moving from different viewpoints or perspectives. Learning takes place best through a variety of experiential and experimental approaches.

The recent emphasis on continuing education for therapists is a synthesizing principle. All creative synthesizers have been undergoing "continued education" for years. There is always an uncomfortable need to integrate the old with the new, no matter how diverse the new procedure may be. But this is an exciting discomfort, not an irritating one. Clinical and counseling psychologists will grow only if they admit to, and permit, the natural flow and change of the evolution of ideas.

Creativity occurs peripherally. The best ideas seem to come when one is driving a car, shaving, watching a ballgame, waiting in line for a movie, or relaxing after having sex. When the mind is free to wander into the nooks and crannies of one's existence, ideas are discovered that are not usually available through directly forcing oneself to think of something. This principle of indirection is important to recognize. Applying the principle to therapy, much growth occurs between sessions, when the ideas and experiences of individual or group therapy can be applied to the arena of living. Too often therapists do not give enough credit to the experiences outside of therapy, which are as important as the experiences inside of therapy in that they provide the workshop for the application of therapeutic learning.

THE KALEIDOSCOPE CONCEPT OF CREATIVITY

An analogy that illustrates the meaning of creativity is to liken its processes to the workings of a kaleidoscope. A kaleidoscope is an instrument containing loose fragments of colored glass so arranged that changes of position exhibit its contents in an endless variety of varicolored changing patterns. Similarly, creativity is basically the organizing of divergent elements into a relevant whole. Each interaction of a therapist in individual therapy is parallel to turning the kaleidoscope, as is each interaction in group therapy. Phrases such as "Here's a new twist!" and "Why don't you look at it this way?" or the changing of the outside frame of reference (shown in Figure 36, page 143) are illustrative of this idea.

It is important to see that (Figure 32, page 137) actualizing consists of a rhythmic movement from the core level to the actualizing level of interaction of interpersonal relating. The arrows symbolize the ability of the actualizing person to be deeply in touch with his core level, which means to be deeply in touch with the involuntary feelings that arise from within himself and his being. This also means being deeply aware of one's feelings that arise in interaction with others. The actualizing person rhythmically expresses both inner feelings and feelings that are responsive to others' reactions to him. He is a living kaleidoscope, turned by an inner gyroscope and responsive to colorings of external significant others.

THE PARADOX OF CREATIVITY

The paradox of creativity has its roots in the basic polar dimensions of strength and weakness. For example, the Human Potential Movement has stressed man's potential, whereas man has traditionally stressed his own weakness and impotence. The synergy of these points of view, however, leads to creativity. Creativity can come out of an awareness of one's potential *and* one's limitations. It has been said that people would never create unless they knew they have to die. Gestalt psychology has always stressed the potential creativity in the incompleted situation and the joy and ecstasy that come from knowing one has completed a worthwhile task.

It is the thesis of this chapter that creativity springs from an awareness of the dialectic between strength and weakness within oneself and that actualizing comes not simply from an awareness of the human potential but from an awareness of one's human limitations as well.

RESISTANCE AND THE IMPASSE

In therapy, the impasse provides the therapist with a daily reminder of his own limitations. When client and therapist get "stuck," both experience the limitations of their human abilities.

Actualizing Therapy is not a process of helping people to solve problems but rather one of helping people to become creative problem solvers. To illustrate this process, we would like to present an analysis of one of the central problems of therapy, which we define as "resistance." By resistance we mean the phenomenon of paying for therapy (or education), and then working diligently to get out of it.

In education, for example, one avoids writing term papers, complains about teachers, skips classes, does not check up on missed assignments, and complains when he fails. Similarly, in therapy one misses appointments and does not expect to pay for them, complains about the therapist and the group, and remains silent and expects the therapist to do the work. The problem of the therapist is to learn to handle resistance creatively.

This phenomenon is illustrated in Figure 55 with what we call the impasse, or "hour glass." Here, therapy is shown to be an inner journey from manipulating to actualizing. But this journey is characterized by many impasses, or places where one gets stuck along the way—as at the narrows of the hour glass.

Perls (1969) used the birth process as an example of the impasse:

> Look upon the unborn baby. It gets all its support from the mother—oxygen, food, warmth, everything. As soon as the baby is born, it has already to do its own breathing. . . .[At this point] we find the *impasse*. The *impasse* is the crucial point in therapy, the crucial point in growth. The impasse is the position where environmental support or obsolete inner support is not forthcoming any more, and authentic self-support has not yet been achieved. The baby cannot breathe by itself. It doesn't get the oxygen supply through the placenta any more.
>
> When we find the place where the person is stuck, we come to the surprising discovery that this impasse is mostly merely a matter of fantasy. It doesn't exist in reality. A person only *believes* he has not his resources at his disposal. (pp. 28-29)

Metaphoric Concepts for Actualizing the Impasse

Metaphors are figures of speech that shed new light on a problem and that encourage thinking about a problem in an intuitive way. Jesus, considered by many the greatest teacher of all, often used parables, a form of metaphor, as Zen Masters use koans, another form of metaphor: to stimulate thinking in pupils. In therapy, the use of metaphors is a valuable method of challenging the client to "see" his impasses in new and different ways.

We agree with Perls' idea that being "stuck" is an attempt to maintain the status quo and to avoid standing on one's own two feet. People become deadlocked because they do not have creative parallels to help them understand the dynamics of such an impasse.

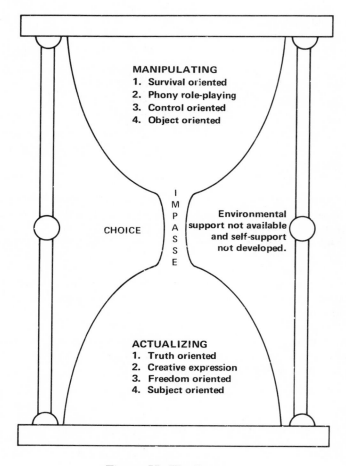

Figure 55. The Impasse

Like the word "crisis," "impasse" has two meanings: the danger of being "stuck," and the opportunity to grow. The trick is to view the impasse in such a way as to make it a growth experience and to afford oneself the opportunity to enter into the excitement of creative problem solving.

The following concepts and metaphors are helpful in actualizing or creatively coping with the many impasses that occur in therapy.

1. *Rebirth Concept.* To be reborn, one must be willing to die, in the sense of giving up old ways of living and discovering new ways to live more fully. To actualize is to experience a kind of rebirth: to allow the old patterns of manipulating and character styles to die so that the core self may be reborn like the phoenix, the beautiful bird that rises in youthful freshness from its own ashes.

2. *Decision Making.* Ultimately, all therapy requires that people grow by making decisions for themselves. Facing and making difficult decisions is itself an actualizing process. Greenwald (1973) says that this is true even if the person makes the "wrong" decisions. All forms of manipulating and character styles can be thought of as partial or inappropriate decisions on ways to live made early in life. To actualize one's being is to make new decisions for living based on a richer understanding of the nature of life.

3. *Law of Reversed Effort.* Watts (1951) has said that the harder you try, the more you fail. Thus "trying is often very trying." The solution is to stop trying. For example, if one tries to float, one will sink because of the constriction of his muscles. Conversely, if one tries to sink, one will float. Therapy often requires giving up trying in order for insight to occur. For example, many people have had the experience of going to bed after having given up on a troublesome problem, only to awaken in the morning with an obvious solution in mind.

4. *Judo Concept.* A person taking judo lessons learns the trick of going with and then reversing his opponent's momentum, using it to his own advantage, to direct the opponent as he chooses. Similarly, the Actualizing Therapist may say, "You say you don't want to hurt anybody. Let me experiment with you. There is something I'd like to tell you, but I'm afraid it would hurt your feelings." The client usually responds, "Go ahead. I can take it." The client has been "tricked" into seeing that, if he can take it, so can other people. Actualizing Therapy may be thought of in this context as a form of psychic judo.

5. *The Rut Concept.* When a car is stuck in the snow or sand, one can rock it back and forth and, by using reverse gear and moving *backward,* can ultimately move forward from the momentum that develops. The analogous process in therapy, termed "paradoxical intention" by Frankl (1963), is to attain results the opposite of the stated intention. For example, in Masters and Johnson's (1966) sexual training method, the therapist implores the couple experiencing sexual impotence to play "teenager"—that is, to explore all forms of sexual foreplay but to refrain from actual intercourse. By going backward to an earlier form of expression, the couple usually develops the momentum of desire for actual sexual relations and consequently overcomes impotence.

6. *Natural Growth Theory.* A gardener knows that trying to pull the petals outward on a rosebud to make it grow is the worst thing he can do. The rose needs natural growth, which takes time, and so does the developing individual. For example, the Actualizing Therapist may say, "You have taken thirty-five years to get here. Don't expect to change everything in one day."

7. *Experiencing Pain as Creative Growth.* This concept relates to the Bioenergetic concept of pain. When there is a physical block in the muscles, they are in a locked state of contraction. Massaging the muscles loosens them from this chronic constriction, but the massaging process causes pain. Pain, in this sense, is part of a creative process. The concept of the value of pain is in opposition to the usual principle of medicine, which advocates the diminishing of pain.

8. *The Slough of Despond.* This idea is one suggested by the novel *Pilgrim's Progress.* In order to cross the pit, one has to go to the bottom and back up again. Similarly, in therapy one has to go down first, through the nadir, in order to rise to a new peak.

9. *Obstetrics Theory.* To aid a child in the birth process, a doctor may feel it necessary to use forceps, despite his awareness that their use may be dangerous to the child. An alternative is natural childbirth, as taught in Lamaze classes. Here women learn to exercise their muscles to facilitate movement downward, so that the baby can be born naturally. In therapy, Greenwald (1973) suggests "joining the resistance" rather than trying to force thought. When the client is encouraged to carry his thinking to its ultimately ridiculous conclusion (through proddings such as "What's wrong with that?"), he makes a decision for change, but if the therapist tries to force change prematurely, the client strongly resists.

10. *Frustration.* Perls (1969) used the technique of frustrating people to get them to mobilize their anger long enough to get through the impasse. In attempting to counter-manipulate, the therapist often must be more skillful at manipulating than the client. For example, the therapist can say, "You expect me to be your poppa. You be me, the therapist, and scold yourself for what you are doing." By requiring the client to take the role of the authority, the therapist is actually telling the client to tell himself what to do.

11. *Unconditional Positive Regard.* This technique is the opposite of the frustration technique just described. The theory, as Rogers (1961) developed it, is that the client will eventually grow if the therapist gives him unconditional love and understanding. The therapist may say, "I often tell my children I would love them even if they committed murder. That's the way I feel about you. Whatever you choose is O.K."

12. *Rational Assumptions Theory.* Ellis (1962) developed the idea that if one can expose the unreasonableness of beliefs or assumptions that cause people to get stuck, the person can then get unstuck by revising his assumptions. Actualizing Therapy can be seen in one sense as a process of revising one's assumptions about life. For example, in Chapter 9 the therapist says to Dennis, "It's O.K. to be angry at someone you love." Dennis had made the assumption that he could not be angry at a person he loved. In reality, being angry at someone is one way of showing love.

13. *Sense of Humor.* Being able to laugh at oneself, and on a broader scale, at the human situation, is a valuable asset. Maslow calls this "Lincolnesque" humor, and it puts life into perspective. The therapist may say, "Can you see the humor in what you are doing?" Learning to laugh at oneself is an important actualizing attribute.

14. *Cooperating with Nature.* The key to this idea is not to fight nature but rather to join the resistance in a creative way, with an understanding of nature's principles. For example, any experienced fisherman demonstrates his finesse with this concept when he lets the fish that has taken the bait swim with the slack line until it is tired and can be reeled in easily. Similarly, the skilled sailor, or even the novice who has to learn the hard way, sails into the wind by tacking, zigzagging across the wind. In the same way, a swimmer caught in a riptide is wise to swim diagonally across the riptide. Indirection is often the best direction. Likewise, the significant questions of therapy are often best dealt with by indirection rather than by trying to solve them immediately. Therapy leads one to discover the answers by living the questions.

15. *Creative Synthesis.* One can be creative by simply joining old things into a new pattern or gestalt, as shown in Figure 56. The therapist is a creative synthesizer when he is able to bring together thinking, feeling, and bodily responses into a new gestalt, as illustrated by Gendlin's system of "focusing," discussed in Chapter 7. In the interview itself, the therapist can creatively synthesize by pointing out to the client the pattern emerging from the great variety of material the client presents. For example, he might say to the client, "Do you see the pattern emerging in the way you treat her?" In group therapy the therapist may say, "Are you aware that there is a consistency in the way you are responding to everyone here?"

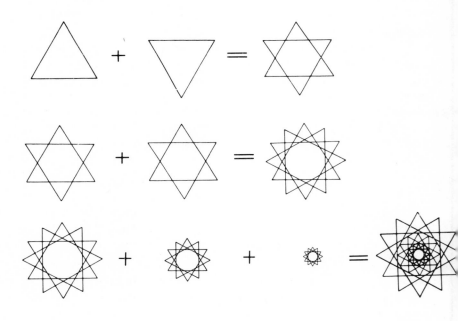

Figure 56. Creative Synthesis

16. *The Incompleted Situation.* Gestalt psychologists have postulated the theory of the incompleted situation, or "closure." In Figure 57, one tends to perceptually close the gaps and see a diagram of several

circles. This is analogous to the tendency of an electric current to jump a small gap in a circuit. The gap represents a state of unbalanced tension and closure brings equilibrium. Applying this principle to psychotherapy, a troubled person may also be illustrated as a series of incomplete circles, as in Figure 57.

In therapy, a husband is often best advised to let his wife finish an affair in her own way and her own time rather than demand that she immediately stop seeing the other person. If the husband requires that she complete the situation on his demand, she may always resent him. She must be the one to finish the situation by her own choice, or the decision is premature and the situation is not really finished.

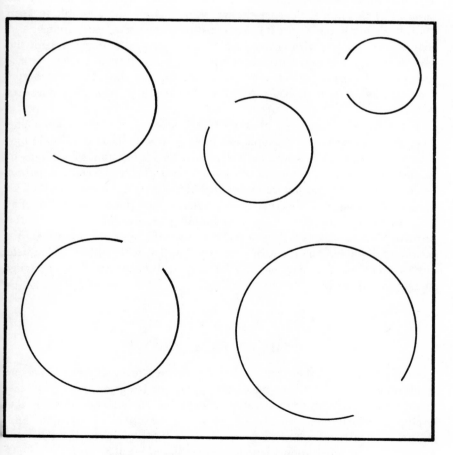

Figure 57. The Incompleted Situation

ACTUALIZING AS A PROCESS

No one ever achieves actualization. It is not an *end,* it is a *process.* The goal of Actualizing Therapy is to produce the actuali*zing* person, a person in constant change and growth. Such persons are forever trying to "get it all together," to integrate their being, while at the same time being *aware* that "there's a lot there that doesn't fit" and that life is a process of always trying to get it all together.

There is an old home in San Jose that illustrates the point. This home is called the "Winchester House" because it was owned by Mrs. Winchester, heiress to the rifle company. Mrs. Winchester became obsessed with the idea that there was a relationship between the longevity of her life and the building of this home. Because she was very wealthy, she was able to keep "building" her home—with stairways leading to nowhere, extra rooms, and fixtures and gadgets with no purpose. She felt that as long as she kept the workmen busy, her longevity was assured. One day, it seems, all the workmen stopped working at the same time, and on that day Mrs. Winchester died. The house still stands in San Jose and is visited by curiosity-seekers daily.

The symbolic meaning of the Winchester House for Actualizing Therapists is that creative people are those who are constantly "building" their lives. Although it would be foolish to keep adding unneeded rooms to a finished building, actualizing a *person* is never finished. People must not become stagnant, rigid, and uneducable. Actualizing demands that they be curious—seeking new dimensions for talents, new ideas for contemplation. Actualizing persons never stop building or growing. It is as if the creative tendency keeps trying to put the parts of the gestalt figures into a meaningful whole. The creative tendency "needs" to complete incomplete circles. In contrast, nonactualizing persons can be characterized as having many incomplete situations in their lives.

THE TERTIUM QUID

Figure 58 depicts the application of polarities to creativity. A person stuck on strength must first make the often agonizing journey (1) all the way across the polarity to the weakness condition. He moves (2) through the weakness polarity and finally (3) to the integration of strength and weakness, which we define as *courage.* This "third something" that has grown from an integration of polarities we define as the "tertium quid." Life for the creative person, it seems, is a continuous developing of tertium quids. A child is the product of a love relationship between a man and a woman, and so is the creation of a relationship that lifts the being of each to a level unattainable by one's self alone. Paradoxically, the best relationships develop without effort. The very determination to try inhibits success—the more effort, the more likely a failure. It is the excitement of two beings in harmony that creates a new symphony of becoming. This is a relationship that is a "workshop for growth" and that does not discriminate between work and play.

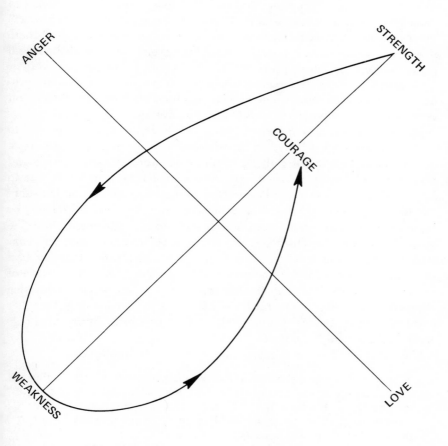

Figure 58. The Tertium Quid

CREATIVITY AS A PROCESS OF LOVING

Another way of defining creativity is to describe it as the process of "falling in love" with some kind of work. Many people, for example, find ceramics a pleasing avocation. The following passages examine how such a person develops a passing interest in looking at and perhaps owning ceramics into an urge to become more actively involved in fashioning images out of clay.

Creativity begins with eros, the first stage of love as defined in Chapter 10. Taking a course in ceramics may bring an initial flush of enthusiasm. The student begins to "love" the touch of molding an object with his hands.

When one moves further into the creativity process, he feels an "empathy" for, and identifies with, his product. It is possible to "feel with" the texture of a pottery form. When one goes further into learning all there is to learn about various pottery forms, one develops a "friendship" with pottery objects of various kinds.

Finally, in creating one reaches the agape stage, in which one has produced a product that can now be shared with the world. In a very real sense, the finished pottery is a child of a creative love.

Being creative is having a love affair with life. In some stages, people do better in their work when their mate is not around or not attended to, because he is so involved with the affair of his work. Ideally, a man and woman synergistically enhance each other's life energy and work, but in some circumstances loving someone is standing back and letting the other "do his thing." Bertha Maslow is an outstanding example of a woman who came to an accommodation with herself and her marital relationship. She sought to protect her husband, Abraham Maslow, from what she considered harmful demands on his time, but she soon learned that her best intentions for him had to be sacrificed in the pursuit of his career. One of the authors vividly remembers a visit with him in Maine when a scheduled afternoon chat was interrupted by Mrs. Maslow suggesting that her husband take his nap. Stimulating talk won out over rest, and the kind lady graciously accepted her defeat.

Maslow (1970) has some interesting comments on creativity:

> This creativeness of the self-actualized man seems to be kin to the naive and universal creativeness of unspoiled children. It seems to be more a fundamental characteristic of common human nature—a potentiality given to all human beings at birth. Most human beings lose this as they become enculturated, but some few individuals seem either to retain this fresh and naive, direct way of looking at life, or if they have lost it, as most people do, they later in life recover it. Santayana called this the "second naiveté," a very good name for it.

This creativeness appears in some of our subjects not in the usual forms of writing books, composing music, or producing artistic objects, but rather may be much more humble. It is as if this special type of creativeness, being an expression of healthy personality, is projected out upon the world or touches whatever activity the person is engaged in. In this sense there can be creative shoemakers or carpenters or clerks. Whatever one does can be done with a certain attitude, a certain spirit that arises out of the nature of the character of the person performing the act. One can even *see* creatively as the child does. (pp. 170-171)

An example of creativity involved in the actualizing process is the current trend among automobile manufacturers to try to instill a creative spirit in workers who have traditionally been saddled with boring, repetitive one-step jobs. Workers are now being trained as teams, constantly shifting from one part of the assembly line to another and working together to assemble one whole unit of the finished product. A dozen people will be involved in, say, all phases of motor assembly, giving each individual a feeling of having played a creative role in the manufacture of a car. As a result, employee turnover and absenteeism are both down, as the worker begins to "love" the automobile because of his creative role in bringing it into being.

In any endeavor, as one moves from the eros stage to the agape stage, he can be said to move from the "d" (deficiency) involvement to the "b" (being) involvement. One moves from a deficiency relationship, in which one knows little about the object of interest, to a relationship in which one loves the object in and of itself—it becomes fun to be a part of it. As such diversely employed persons as William James and Willie Mays have put it, people paid them to do what they would have gladly paid to be allowed to do.

It is in adolescence that the relationship between actualizing and creativity first makes itself felt. The actualizing teenager is a creative rebel. He has the courage to rebel in a healthy manner—not by outward symbols, such as long hair and exotic clothing, but by the purpose, direction, and meaning of individual behavior. Rebellion can thus be creative rather than destructive or negative.

Damm (1970) compared the relationship of self-actualizing to creativity and intelligence in high-school students. The subjects were 95 boys and 113 girls drawn from a high-school student body. Using the POI and other measuring devices, Damm found that the group of students who had obtained high scores on both intelligence and creativity were superior in self-actualizing to those who had obtained a high score on only intelligence or creativity or low scores on both intelligence and creativity. He concluded that if education has as its goal the productive self-fulfillment of every student, the curriculum should focus on development of both intellectual *and* creative abilities, rather than on one to the exclusion of the other. In other words, the students should be encouraged to work through the eros to the agape stages of whatever endeavor they undertake.

MURPHY'S STAGES OF CREATIVITY

Gardner Murphy (1958) has described four stages of creativity: *immersion* (the long and fulfilling involvement in a particular person, place, idea, symbol, or sensation); *organization* ("sorting out" basic patterns and experiences and organizing them into more structured units); *inspiration* (the sudden creative leap based on the storehouse of experience); and *evaluation* (a period of refining, evaluating, and perfecting the results of the creative leap).

Murphy's *immersion* corresponds to *friendship*; with long involvement in a project one becomes totally immersed, observing its incubation and anticipating its fruition. In writing this book, for example, the authors occasionally experienced the frustration of not being able to select the proper material for a particular chapter. However, after becoming more immersed in a specific topic, a period of incubation took place and the creative process dramatically asserted itself; an abrupt flow of ideas made the finished product seem satisfyingly well-rounded.

MASLOW'S CONCEPTS OF CREATIVITY

Using writing or any of the arts as an example of the creative process can be misleading. A woman who rears a successful family may be considered more creative than a competent musician who merely plays what someone else has written. Maslow was fond of recalling that he expanded his own thinking on the subject of creativity while watching his mother-in-law make soup. He reasoned that what she was doing was an eminently creative act, much more so than, say, the work of a second-rate painter. His mother-in-law made the best soup he had ever tasted, whereas the painter was merely going through the motions of his craft. In *Toward a Psychology of Being,* Maslow (1962) expanded on this theory:

> I first had to change my ideas about creativity as soon as I began studying people who were positively healthy, highly evolved and matured, self-actualizing. I had first to give up my stereotyped notion that health, genius, talent and productivity were synonymous. A fair proportion of my subjects, though healthy and

creative in a special sense, were *not* productive in the ordinary sense, nor did they have great talent or genius, nor were they poets, composers, inventors, artists or creative intellectuals.

Furthermore, I soon discovered that I had, like most other people, been thinking of creativeness in terms of products, and secondly, I had unconsciously confined creativeness to certain conventional areas only of human endeavor, unconsciously assuming that *any* painter, *any* poet, *any* composer was leading a creative life. Theorists, artists, scientists, inventors, writers could be creative. Nobody else could be. Unconsciously I had assumed that creativeness was the prerogative solely of certain professionals.

The consequence was that I found it necessary to distinguish "special talent creativeness" from "self-actualizing creativeness" which sprang much more directly from the personality, and which showed itself widely in the ordinary affairs of life, in a tendency to do *anything* creatively. (pp. 135-137)

Maslow's self-actualizing creativity could really be considered as the development of excellence in work or in love. Maslow's work reinforces the idea that creativity, self-actualizing, and love are interdependent. Furthermore, it is frequently forgotten that the end products of creativity are often the result of nothing more esoteric than hard work. The old bromide that genius is 90 percent perspiration and 10 percent inspiration applies very directly to this concept of creativity.

It is important to realize that there is a general tendency to idolize the creative process, the supposed sudden flash of enlightenment that leads to the announcement of some great discovery or the solving of a long-standing problem. What is often lost sight of are the weeks, months, and often years that stand between the great dawning and the implementation of the idea. "The fact," Maslow said, "that the people who create are good workers tends to be lost."

This concept, that "getting the idea is not enough," has been elaborated upon by Gowan (1972). Acknowledging the essential creativity of self-actualizing, he defines it as "a state of continual becoming in which one is thrown forward or caught up in the process of manifesting one's potentiality."

"A creative opening," Gowan continues, "is best conceptualized as a merging of the conscious and preconscious minds in which a flood of material previously catalogued by the conscious mind is reorganized by the preconscious and then expelled into the conscious domain." But not without effort. Here are some suggestions for creative expression:

1. Creativity is not so much the having of good ideas as the process of nurturing them. Like women who find it easy to conceive but hard to carry

to term, people continually get ideas, but they continually abort them. Like most things just born, good ideas need to be nurtured, loved, and cleaned up.

2. People need to develop a quiet time, when ordinary routine may be stripped away. In short, they need to nurse their creativity. There are two rhythms here—a daily rhythm and a much longer one. There is some time every day, usually around the time of sleep—just before or just after—when the gates to the preconscious seem to fall open. The other rhythm is a much longer one of alternation of work and travel. Traveling, especially outside one's culture, evokes a creative response. A rhythmic alternation between work and vacation is an extremely useful actualizing principle.

3. Inevitably, in any creative functioning there will be a down cycle. The worst possible thing is to resist this tendency. Forcing creativity results in the production of noncreative products.

4. Be sensitive to dissonance and discontinuities in material that otherwise seem to fit well. The discontinuity shows where the fit is less than perfect. It is the imperfections or flaws in a present theory that point to the genesis of a new or better theory.

Actualizing is not a static state, a once-and-for-all goal to be achieved at age fifty-five, but rather a continuous process of being child, parent, and adult. Barron (1972) applies this rhythmic relationship to the creativity process. "All of us," he writes, "are both creatures and creators, but we vary both in our quality as a creation and our power to create" (p. 42). Barron addresses himself to the "perspiration factor":

First of all, we must note the fact that a considerable amount of training and discipline is necessary for most sorts, if not indeed all sorts, of work that can reach a high level of creativeness. This certainly is true of the outstanding products of our culture, whether we think of musical compositions, painting and sculpture, problem solving and theory construction in mathematics and the sciences, architecture, or such performances as ballet dancing and operatic singing. Long years of discipline, training and devotion are necessary. Moreover, such work is generally directed towards an audience capable of understanding and receiving or appreciating the work, while children's inventiveness and spontaneous creativity do not have these characteristics, either in demand or in intention. In brief, a certain amount of maturation of the talent, and discipline in its exercise, must precede its full expression. Since this also *takes time,* the complex creative act can be expected to occur only rarely in childhood, or before maturation has taken place. (p. 42)

It follows that the therapeutic view of actualizing, involving the rhythmic swing between the adult and child in everyone, leads naturally to a condition combining the best of both worlds and that its continued swinging encourages an ongoing creativity. This, in turn, implies a constant adaptability to change, a capacity for innovation that Maslow (1971) fully perceived. He said of creative people that

> they must be people who will not fight change but who will antici- pate it, and who can be challenged enough by it to enjoy it. We must develop a race of improvisers, of "here-now" creators. We must define the skillful person or the trained person, or the educated person in a very different way than we used to (i.e., *not* as one who has a rich knowledge of the past so that he can profit from past experiences in a future emergency). Much that we have called learning has become useless. Any kind of learning which is the simple application of the past to the present, or the use of past techniques in the present situation has become obsolete in many areas of life. Education can no longer be considered essentially or only a learning process; it is now also a character training, a person-training process. We need a new kind of human being who can divorce himself from his past, who feels strong and courageous and trusting enough to trust himself in the present situation, to handle the problem well in an improvising way, with- out previous preparation, if need be.

The creative person, then, must not only be innovative and effective but must also project his own *beingness*, rather than merely taking a rigid stance and doing what someone else tells him to do. Manipulative people are continually striving to do the "right" thing or the "good" thing; actualizing persons feel free to express themselves in a "being" way, being themselves.

When one is being his mission, for example, he is being his uniqueness in the world in the Buber sense. When one is being existentially honest, he is saying that no one principle is appropriate but rather that a bipolarity exists in most situations. This is the essence of the creative love process.

The general key to creativity in life would seem to be the same as that for the patient in psychotherapy: Through being oneself as one is in the moment, one gradually becomes all that he or she is capable of becoming.

Rainer Maria Rilke (1934) has said it another way:

> Do not now seek the answers, that cannot be given you because you would not be able to live them. And the point is, to live every- thing. *Live* the questions now. Perhaps you will then gradually, without noticing it, live along some distant day into the answer. (p. 24)

CHAPTER 13. THE INNER JOURNEY

Kopp (1971), in his book *Guru*, says, "The searching of the heart must involve a genuine willingness to *face up to our losses*, to bury our dead, and to mourn their passing as we helplessly give them up. Otherwise, there is only a sterile self-torture, a stubborn holding on which leads to the despair of not living with things as they are" (p. 42). This expresses a very important message about self-actualizing. Too often, students identify with the self-actualizing theory because it seems to hold a promise of greatness without pain, of a here-and-now heaven without a struggle. In our work in Actualizing Therapy, we have found the reverse to be true. Self-actualizing is the product of struggle and pain.

ACTUALIZING AS ACCEPTANCE OF LOSSES

Transactional Analysts have spoken simplistically of being "a winner instead of a loser." As James and Jongeward (1971) say in their book *Born to Win*, "People are born to win, they are also born helpless and totally dependent on their environment. Winners successfully make the transition from total helplessness to independence, and then to interdependence. Losers do not. Somewhere along the line they begin to avoid becoming self-responsible" (p. 3).

Actualizing people "win" *and* "lose" many times in life. It is handling, or coping with, losses, not simply always winning, that is important. Simply being "winners" or "losers," however, seems to imply artificial dichotomies that are imposed on the structure of life. In reality, the structure of life is more like protoplasm, with an indefinite form that does not readily adapt to the either-or rigidity that the terms "winners" and "losers" imply.

Abraham Lincoln, in so many ways a winner, left us a cogent lesson when he spoke at New Salem, Illinois, after being defeated in his early try for Congress. "If the good people, in their wisdom, shall see fit to keep me in the background," he said, "I have been too familiar with disappointments to be very much chagrined." He accepted that losing is something that everyone must face again and again, as he, himself, had experienced many times in his life.

Most people who become self-actualizing do so as a result of a struggle to overcome problems in their lives. For example, although it is common to refer to a divorcee as a loser or to a divorce as a tragedy, divorce might easily be considered a growth or learning experience. People tend to simplistically think that divorce always results in a broken family, when, in reality, many families are shattered emotionally and physically at the expense of keeping a marriage intact. In contrast, a recent graduate of therapy characterized herself as "happily divorced."

As long as people keep using terminology that implies loss or brokenness, that suggests a negative permanency rather than a continuous learning process, they will remain bogged down in outdated concepts. Every loss represents an opportunity for growing and moving forward rather than a cue for assuming a stuck or defeated posture.

The "three-time loser" syndrome can easily get people into a rut from which they have great difficulty emerging; it represents a built-in predisposition to identify everyone as either winners or losers and implies that one cannot be both. Actually, all of life is winning and losing. The idea that life is an either-or process is essentially limiting.

ACTUALIZING AS AN INNER JOURNEY

The roads we travel in life follow an irregular terrain. The mountains, rivers, and coastlines of the world are not neat and square and regular; they all vary erratically. Man lives in an erratic universe, and life is a process of moving up, down, and sideways in strange ways. Alan Watts (1966) has suggested that life can be ordered—that order can be imposed on chaos just as a system of *latitude* and *longitude* can be imposed on the earth to give us a useful map. We have prescribed such order through the *polarities* described in this book. It is good to remember though, that the world is not *really* that way; a natural rhythm of life requires experiencing its "wiggliness."

In *Man's Search for Meaning* Viktor Frankl (1963) says that the role of the therapist is like that of an eye specialist as opposed to that of a painter. Whereas a painter tries to present a picture of the world as he sees it, an ophthalmologist tries to help his patient see the world *as it really is for him*. The therapist broadens his client's visual field and so helps him see a full spectrum of actions, feelings, meaning, and values. According to Frankl, one's journey in life can be enhanced by doing a deed, by experiencing values or feelings, and by finding meaning in suffering. He talks a great deal about love as providing meaning in life, and he also talks about finding meaning in suffering. One of the basic tenets of Frankl's therapy, called Logotherapy, is man's need to find meaning in life.

As Frankl's ophthalmologist analogy suggests, self-actualizing is not an end in itself but a means—a process. One must be careful not to see self-actualizing in too much of a goal-oriented way. Goals can be a *curse* in that one can feel ever dissatisfied with oneself for always being short of achieving them. One of the most important principles of the actualizing life is to live fully in the present. Many people make plans for the future that they never enjoy when they mature, because by then they are living for still another future.

As Alan Watts (1966) has pointed out, first people attend kindergarten to prepare for elementary school; then in elementary school they prepare for secondary school, where they subsequently prepare for college; even graduation is no fulfillment because new quotas have been established, and now they must progress from sales manager to vice president. Eventually the insurance and investment people help them plan for retirement. When they reach it, they find that their anxieties, exertions, and urgings toward the future have left them with a "weak heart, false teeth, prostate trouble, sexual impotence, fuzzy eyesight and vile digestion." None of them has ever learned to live in the moment, to win *and* lose in their journey to becoming an actualizing person.

Self-actualizing requires understanding the paradox that both psychotherapy and growth require a capacity to accept one's own disabilities. People must accept the fact that they all are, to some extent, disabled because of early parental training and environmental exposure. This, however, makes them anything but losers; on the contrary, knowledge of these deficiencies makes their development possible. Thus, by their very existence, these deficiencies enable growth.

Actualizing Therapy believes in the ever-changing nature of humankind. This is best stated in the following passage, the author of which is unknown:

> There is an old superstition that men have certain definite qualities; that a man is wise, stupid, kind, cruel, and so forth. Man is not like that. He is more like a river: here fast, here slow, here narrow, here rough, here smooth. Each man is all of these, in

an everchanging rhythm. And a man becomes unlike himself while still remaining the same.

A similar attitude is implied in the book title *Don't Push the River*. Each person is like a river in that he must flow at his own speed and in his own direction. Psychotherapy is a process of facilitating the flow, but not directing the flow. Each individual varies in speed and direction in an ever-changing rhythm.

ACTUALIZING AS LIVING ONE'S TOTAL BEING

The following personal account by the senior author may serve to illustrate much of what Actualizing Therapy is all about:

Not long ago I worked as a group therapist attempting to help a young lady face the possibility of having cervical cancer. None of the usual therapeutic "answers" seemed to help. Instead, I asked her to see me in individual therapy. I believe it was a creative session for both of us. How I approahced this problem will, perhaps, summarize much of what we have had to say in this book.

My client was a beautiful young lady of twenty-two and was asking, with strong intellectual curiosity, "Why?" As I probed into my own core, I believed there to be a universal principle involved, if I could but discover it. My answer was that this girl's problem was not simply that of facing possible cancer, but rather one of *fragmentation*. She was blessed with an unusually bright mind, and when we spoke of the need for her to face this concern not only with her mind, but also with her heart and body, deeper insights occurred. Her father had died of cancer at an early age, and she was obsessed that somehow he "caused" this premature death by his own approach to being. And now she faced the possibility that perhaps she, too, was following in his footsteps.

I believe that the core of our being, which is the only thing we can ultimately trust, requires that we understand the principle of *synchronicity*, which has been expressed by Jung as the principle that all things can work together for good if we but let them. I posited that my client had possibly become *fragmented*, and that her mind (her thinking), her heart (her feelings), and her body (her physical sensations) were not synchronized. I asked her if this had any meaning to her. She then began to recall that a few months ago, she had broken off a relationship with a man because it just "seemed so carnal." I reflected her feeling: "You felt that you weren't committed to him with your total being? You loved him with your vagina, but not your head and heart?" "Yes," she replied, "that's it!"

Cryosurgery cleared up the rebellious cells. But I believe her malignant attitude, which changed to an actualizing attitude (with a *love* for her mind, feelings, and body) at this point, was equally responsible for her new *life* orientation.

A key tenet of Actualizing Therapy is that we have a criterion within for judging our own behavior: whether our head *and* our heart *and* our body all seem to agree; whether they are all *synchronized*. In contrast, my client was relating to her boyfriend with only one element of her being, as Figure 59 illustrates.

Synchronized Relating

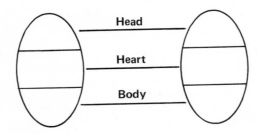

Partial Relating

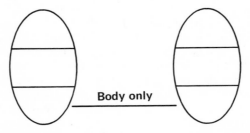

Figure 59. Synchronized Relating versus Partial Relating

In terms of our definition of love, only eros was present, not empathy, agape, or friendship. Thus, my client was not "together" with herself or with her friend. There was not a total commitment in this relationship, only a partial eroticism. It seems that in our liberally oriented world of free sex, this is a problem with young people more often than they wish to admit.

As we have stated earlier, the Chinese have two definitions for the word "crisis": "danger" and "opportunity." The word for us has only one meaning: "decisive moment." "Thus," I explained to my client, "you can either accept this as a dangerous point, or as an opportunity. Which of these you choose is up to you."

At this moment, the young lady brightened up and said, "I *know* the meaning of this illness: it is a turning point where I can choose to live partially with my being or fully with my being. I choose to live fully!"

Some therapists, medical men, and philosophers who read this volume may question the tenets herein. We are troubled by the strife that exists in the various helping professions today. No one seems to agree with other points of view. Medical men see man chemically, psychiatrists see him symptomatically and diagnostically, behavior therapists see him mechanically, marriage counselors see him as part of a relationship, religious men see him as a soul to save, and even humanistic psychologists see him as only a self-help system. The patient flounders as professionals attempt to destroy each other. The *creative synthesis* of Actualizing Therapy is an attempt to heal the wounds of our differences.

If there is one tenet of Actualizing Therapy that stands above all others, it is that we must accept that there is no one best way to help people. The Buddha is said to have stated, "There are many roads up the mountain." Until all the helping professions can appreciate their own differences and permit the use of various modalities, they will continue to selfishly proclaim their own false infallibilities. It is the hope of Actualizing Therapy that all therapists can come to appreciate, rather than try to destroy, different approaches. For example, in the above case of the young lady with possible cancer, even her physician respected her wish to postpone surgery and to attend consciousness classes in an attempt to "cure" her malignancy. He apparently did not believe that this was "The Way" but he at least respected her decision to try this route. When all of the helping professions can take such an attitude, perhaps professionals will have reached a new stage of maturity.

When therapists can say to their clients, "Trust your total being and do as you will," they will be coming close to a deeply spiritual view of man's being. They will begin to understand, in its deepest meaning, that "the Kingdom of God is Within."

Creativity, in the fullest meaning of the word, therefore, is an attitude that one takes in approaching all of life's problems. As Rilke (in Lindbergh, 1974), has said, "Be patient toward all that is unsolved in your heart and try to *love the questions themselves* like locked doors and like books that are written in a foreign language." (pp. xxiii-xxiv)

EPILOGUE: ACTUALIZING AND THE WIZARD OF OZ

(This section is a revision of Everett Shostrom's Presidential Address to the Division of Humanistic Psychology, Division 32, of the American Psychological Association. It was originally presented at the August 1974 meeting of the APA, in New Orleans.)

A primary difficulty in teaching actualizing as a process is to find a model that is easily understandable. Kopp (1971), in his attempt to describe the complex processes of therapy, has used many metaphors from various religions and cultures and from science, poetry, fiction, and children's stories. One of the stories he refers to is *The Wizard of Oz,* by L. Frank Baum. Kopp uses the story as a general description of the therapeutic process. In this analysis, we will particularly center on the dimensions of Actualizing Therapy implicit in this American fairy tale.

The reader will remember that Dorothy, the tale's heroine, is separated from her foster family in Kansas and is whirled by a cyclone into the Land of Oz. Her only concern is to go back home, but she finds herself necessarily involved in a long journey before this is possible. As in group therapy, her journey is shared by three others whom she meets on the Yellow Brick Road. (Yellow, incidentally, is described by Lüscher, 1969, as a color of adventure, which they all experience while traveling on the road.)

The Characters

Dorothy's first encounter is with the Scarecrow, whose stated problem is that he has no brain. In manipulative terminology, he is a *withdrawer and avoider,* or at the character level he is a *schizoid personality.* He is fragmented and disjointed and, since he is made of straw, he cannot feel. His phony painted-on face denotes he is "out to lunch"—he is not *there.* His wish is that he might have "brains," but being afraid to feel, he can only conceive of relating in a thinking way, and therefore needs more than only brains. He is fearful and needs to *trust.*

The second person Dorothy meets is the Tin Woodman. She finds him to be a *rigid character,* pieced together from tin because, in his enthusiasm for his work, he would cut himself up again and again. His assumed problem is that he needs a heart because he had lost his love for the girl he had hoped to marry. In manipulative terminology, he is a *striver and producer.* He is a workaholic, trying to prove himself through work, and his entire body is rigid and tight. Having lost the girl he hoped to marry, he is afraid to love—to give his heart.

The third character Dorothy meets is the Cowardly Lion. He pretends anger, but admits to being a big coward. As with manipulative persons of this type, he is a *pleaser and placater,* or at a character level an *oral dependent personality.* Unable to stand on his own two feet, he has become excessively dependent on others. He uses his sadness and longing, rather than his aggressiveness, to relate to others.

The fourth character Dorothy encounters is the Wizard himself. When they finally meet, he appears as a giant Head, without a body, but with eyes, ears, and a nose—huge and awful. He blurts out, "I am Oz, the Great and Terrible." When he meets the others, he changes his manipulative masks to become a lovely Lady for the Scarecrow, a most terrible Beast for the Woodman, and a Ball of Fire for the Lion. Thus, Oz, at first, is the master manipulator, playing different forms of strength and weakness, anger and love.

At a deeper level, the Wizard may be seen as a *masochistic character.* Life for him is a burden. He had taken on the burden of becoming the Wizard of all of Oz, and all the duties and responsibilities thereof. He is in a double-bind: He wants to express his aggression and anger, as he did in his original encounter with Dorothy, but then his tender feelings emerge and block his anger. When these tender feelings emerge, they, in turn, get blocked by the anger.

Although Kopp sees Dorothy as Small and Meek, preferring the security of misery to the misery of insecurity; we see her as "playing" Small and Meek to the Wizard. In reality, she is a quietly determined little girl. She is undoubtedly the leader of the group of adventurers, and the others would be lost without her. She is a therapist in her own right.

Dorothy used the age-old underdog manipulation of "playing weak and helpless" with the Wizard as a ploy to overcome him. It was the crisis of being whirled off to Oz that led her to the Wizard. In her back-home world, she is an orphan living with foster parents in a dull, gray existence. Her primary problem is her unwillingness to tolerate the insecurity of her Oz existence. Dorothy, like most people, has not yet learned the "wisdom of insecurity" and still believes that "security" is being back home, even though her unsmiling Aunt Em and her solemn Uncle Henry hardly provided a fulfilling atmosphere. Her problem is that she had not yet learned that "You can't go home again."

It is only when the Wizard is exposed by Toto, Dorothy's dog, that he is really found out to be a little old man with a wrinkled face. He then admits he is a common man making believe; a humbug, who had fooled everyone by his multiple faces. It is only when he admits to his manipulative masks that he can help each of the others with the problems they say they have. As the therapist himself needs therapy to understand his own foibles, so the Wizard of Oz needed to admit to his own humanness before he could help others.

The Miracle of Experiencing

At this point, the Wizard reveals the miracle of the experiencing of thinking, feeling, and bodily expression: In their adventures, Dorothy had repeatedly turned to the Woodman for comfort, to the Scarecrow for advice, to the Lion for protection. It was in the living of their experiences that they had already arrived at their goals! The Tin Woodman did not need a heart, but a willingness to suffer through crises. The Scarecrow did not need brains, but the willingness to risk experiences to get wisdom. The Cowardly Lion did not need courage, but the confidence to risk facing danger.

The mistake that most people make is that their "goals" are really attempts to short-cut the process of experiencing. Each of Baum's heroes wants a simple solution to his problems: a heart, a brain, courage, and an external home. But each has a hard time understanding that life never offers such simple solutions. Only by experiencing can one gain maturity, and such experiencing comes from *living* in the here and now, fully and completely. Goals can be a curse when they substitute for living.

Most people play the manipulative games of Baum's heroes. Like the Scarecrow, they refuse to take responsibility for themselves, withdrawing and avoiding so people won't expect too much of them. Like the Tin Woodman, they need someone to care about them, rather than caring for themselves. Like the Cowardly Lion, they say, "How can I help it?" and expect others not to frighten or challenge them. Each person expects others to satisfy their needs for them. They refuse to "come home" into themselves and to trust their own "inner Supreme Courts" and their "courage to be." They become other-directed rather than inner-directed.

To be able to go into a strange land and to accept each moment as it comes and for what it brings, is to live totally now, unconcerned about the future or the past. The willingness to risk being *vulnerable* and *weak*, being *loving* and *tender* even if it hurts, being one's *anger* in the face of danger, and being one's *strength* to face the dangers of living fully: These are the polarities that need to be experienced if one is to live his journey of life fully and completely.

The Group Process

To achieve this process, people need to face themselves individually, as in individual therapy, to understand that their problems may not be as they have personally diagnosed them to be. People also need group therapy to see others as persons with problems of their own and whose search for meaning is only different in certain ways from their own.

In *The Wizard of Oz,* some problems had to be solved individually by each of the characters; others were worked on jointly. Similarly, therapy needs both of these emphases. But the "Aha" experience is the necessary mode for personal growth. No amount of resolutions, contracts, or good intentions will substitute. Clients must be willing to enter into spontaneous dialogue with a therapist; dialogue that is unplanned and goes where it will. Group therapy must similarly be an exercise in *being* strong and weak, angry and loving—not simply talking about it. *People must talk the talk, but they must also walk the walk.*

The realization that the answers to life's problems are in experiencing life, rather than seeking goals, is the most difficult one to accept. Each person needs to know that, like Dorothy, he already has the Silver Shoes on, but he must also be willing to risk using them to walk the walk. Each person has within himself the power to actualize his own being, but too frequently, people prefer to give others the responsibility for helping them rather than accepting the power within.

But even when they walk the walk, many people fear making mistakes, being foolish, experiencing unhappiness. They want an easy trip, rather than an exciting and challenging one. They want a rose garden without thorns. It is only when they accept the lonely road, the rocks upon which they will stumble, that they can learn to enjoy the trip, rather than vainly seeking illusions.

L. Frank Baum wrote *The Wizard of Oz* in 1900, when it was generally considered inappropriate to express one's anger. In fact, Baum makes it a point in his stories never to express violence. When Dorothy deals strongly with the Lion, for example, she succeeds by simply patting him on his face. Modern psychological theory is not quite so kind. Actualizing requires the expression of anger on the outside congruent with the degree of intensity felt on the inside. Anger is an expression of love between friends. Anger is frustrated love.

This is not to deny, however, the validity of love's therapeutic value. Actualizing Therapy sees love on a polarity with anger and both as representing dimensions of honest expression. The opposite of each is fear or indifference, which is found at the center of all polarities. Indifference, or fear, is the unwillingness to risk the expression of either anger or love, strength or weakness. It represents the passivity of the Munchkins, who are depicted as cardboard characters. Actualizing involves the risking of our honest feelings, whatever they may be, in interaction.

Perhaps the most significant dimension of the story of the Wizard of Oz has to do with the "therapeutic task" given to the principals before the story can end—the task of killing the Wicked Witch of the West. Instead of simply being given the brain, heart, courage, and a home, they were given a job to do that required active participation with others. As in group therapy, they had to *help each other* instead of simply receiving help. They got *involved* in a *process* rather than getting a *solution*. Therapy, both individual and group, does not give solutions; it enables a person to discover his own humanness by experiencing others as human beings also seeking meaning. In so doing, one discovers that he has been *demanding* from others what he already possesses. As the song "Tinman" points out, Oz never gave anything to the Tin Man that he didn't already have. But the discovery that, like the Tin Man, one has potentials within comes only when one can experience *using these powers*. Humanistic Psychology is an attempt to help man find himself and his potentials through his *involvement* with others, for it is just such *involvement* that nourishes individual and collective potential.

CONCLUSIONS

In a manner of speaking, each character in *The Wizard of Oz* was right, but only in a partial way. Actualizing requires more than simply a physical home or a heart or a brain or courage. Like the Prodigal Son, people must "come to themselves." "Coming to oneself" means trusting one's whole being—bodily, intellectually, and emotionally. Only then will one find that his journey has lead him in a circle back to himself.

Dorothy thought she needed a physical home, a place where she could find personal security. But a person's home is his body, and he must go wherever it goes. Thomas Wolfe says, "You can't go home again," and while this may be true of a physical home, one can discover one's own home in an existential way. One can discover the comfort of believing in one's own being as a reliable vehicle for meeting the daily stresses and challenges of life. Each person can learn to *be at home* with his own core being, and people can share their cores.

Lowen has said that, for him, self-fulfillment is having enough self-esteem to risk disappointment and enough courage to stand alone. For me, risking disappointment means reaching to others for *love,* realizing it may not come, and yet being in touch with one's *anger* enough to say "no" to those from whom one cannot receive affection honestly. Standing alone means accepting our *strength* to be alone in the world and at the same time being able to face our *weakness* and accept that we cannot manipulate others to love us. Love must be freely given and truly received. The *actualizing core* is a home in which we are *comfortable,* with doors that can open and close rhythmically to the world.

When Robert Graves (1971) asks the ultimate question, "What is Love?" he may well be asking, "What is actualizing":

> Is it a re-attainment of our centre, a core of trustful innocence come home to?

This is the meaning of actualizing!

BIBLIOGRAPHY

Albee, G. The short unhappy life of clinical psychology. *Psychology Today,* September 1970, pp. 42-43; 71. (a)

Albee, G. The uncertain future of clinical psychology. *American Psychologist,* 1970, *25*(2), 1071-1080. (b)

Allport, G. W. *Personality: A psychological interpretation.* New York: Holt, Rinehart and Winston, 1937.

Allport, G. W. *Becoming.* New Haven, Conn.: Yale University Press, 1955.

Allport, G. W. *Personality and social encounter.* Boston: Beacon Press, 1960.

Allport, G. W. *Pattern and growth in personality.* New York: Holt, Rinehart and Winston, 1961.

Alperson, B. L., Alperson, E. D., & Levine, R. Growth effects of high school marathons. *Experimental Publications System,* February 1971. (Ms. No. 369-56)

Ansbacher, H. L., & Ansbacher, R. R. (Eds.). *The individual psychology of Alfred Adler.* New York: Basic Books, 1956.

Bach, G. *Intensive group psychotherapy.* New York: Ronald, 1954.

Banmen, J., & Capelle, R. Human relations training in three rural Manitoba high schools. Paper presented at the Convention of the National Council on Human Relations. Winnipeg, Canada, April 1971.

Banmen, J., & Capelle, R. Human relations training in three rural Manitoba high schools: A three-month follow-up. *Canadian Counsellor,* 1972, *6*, 260-270.

Barron, F. Is creativity akin to madness? *Psychology Today,* July 1972, p. 42.

Baum, L. F. *The wizard of Oz.* New York: Grosset & Dunlap, 1900, 1956.

Bebout, J., & Gordon, B. The value of encounter. In L. N. Solomon & B. Berzon (Eds.), *New perspectives on encounter groups.* San Francisco: Jossey-Bass, 1972.

Bleuler, E. Cited in J. F. Brown, *Psychodynamics of abnormal behavior.* New York: McGraw-Hill, 1940.

Brammer, L. M. *The helping relationship: Process and skills.* Englewood Cliffs, N.J.: Prentice-Hall, 1973.

Brammer, L. M., & Shostrom, E.L. *Therapeutic psychology: Fundamentals of actualizing counseling and therapy* (2nd ed.). Englewood Cliffs, N.J.: Prentice-Hall, 1968.

Braun, J. R. Effects of "typical neurotic" and "after therapy" sets on the Personal Orientation Inventory scores. *Psychological Reports,* 1966, *19*, 1282.

Braun, J. R. Search for correlates of self-actualization. *Perceptual and Motor Skills,* 1969, *28,* 557-558.

Braun, J. R., & LaFaro, D. A. Further study on the fakability of the Personal Orientation Inventory. *Journal of Clinical Psychology,* 1969, *25,* 296-299.

Brown, J. F. *Psychodynamics of abnormal behavior.* New York: McGraw-Hill, 1940.

Buber, M. *I and thou.* New York: Scribner's, 1937.

Buber, M. *The way of man.* Chicago: Wilcox and Follett, 1951.

Buhler, C. Maturation and motivation. *Journal of Personality,* 1951, *1,* 184-211.

Buhler, C. *Values in psychotherapy.* New York: Free Press, 1962.

Buhler, C., & Massarik, F. (Eds.). *The course of human life.* New York: Springer, 1968.

Bunyan, J. *Pilgrim's progress.* New York: E. P. Dutton, 1972.

Bustanoby, A. The pastor and the other woman. *Christianity Today,* August 30, 1974, pp. 7-10.

Byrd, R. E. Training in a non-group. *Journal of Humanistic Psychology,* 1967, *25,* 296-299.

Cattell, R. B., & Eber, H. W. *The sixteen personality factor questionnaire.* Champaign, Ill.: Institute for Personality and Ability Testing, 1957.

Comrey, A. L. *Comrey personality scales.* San Diego: EdITS/Educational and Industrial Testing Service, 1970.

Counseling Center Staff, University of Massachusetts. Effects of three types of sensitivity groups on changes in measures of self-actualization. *Journal of Counseling Psychology,* 1972, *19,* 253-254.

Crampton, W. How U.S. men can live longer. *This Week,* February 20, 1955, pp. 7-26.

Crosson, S., & Schwendiman, G. *Self-actualization as a predictor of conformity behavior.* Unpublished manuscript, Marshall University, 1972.

Culbert, S. A., Clark, J. V., & Bobele, H. K. Measures of change toward self-actualization in two sensitivity training groups. *Journal of Counseling Psychology,* 1968, *15,* 53-57.

Damm, V. J. Creativity and intelligence: Research implications for equal emphasis in high school. *Exceptional Children,* 1970, *36,* 565-570.

Dollard, J., & Miller, N. E. *Personality and psychotherapy.* New York: McGraw-Hill, 1950.

Dunnam, M. D., Herbertson, G. J., & Shostrom, E. L. *The manipulator and the church.* Nashville: Abingdon Press, 1968.

Ellis, A. Rational psychotherapy. *Journal of General Psychology,* 1958, *59,* 35-49.

Ellis, A. *A guide to rational living.* Englewood Cliffs, N.J.: Prentice-Hall, 1961.

Ellis, A. *Reason and emotion in psychotherapy.* Seacaucus, N.J.: Lyle Stuart, 1962.

Epstein, S. The self-concept revisited: Or a theory of a theory. *American Psychologist,* 1973, *28,* 404-416.

Erikson, E. H. *Childhood and society.* New York: Norton, 1950.

Erikson, E. H. *Childhood and society* (Rev. ed.). New York: Norton, 1964.

Eysenck, H. J., & Eysenck, S. *The Eysenck personality inventory.* San Diego: EdITS/Educational and Industrial Testing Service, 1963.

Eysenck, H. J., & Rachman, S. *Causes and cures of neurosis.* San Diego: EdITS/Robert R. Knapp Publisher, 1965.

Fenichel, O. *The psychoanalytic theory of neuroses.* New York: Norton, 1945.

Fink, P. F. (Ed.). *The challenge of philosophy.* Scranton, Penn.: Chandler, 1965.

Fisher, G. Felons' conception of societal self-actualization values. *Corrective Psychiatry,* 1973, *19,* 3-5.

Fisher, J. *A few buttons missing.* Philadelphia: Lippincott, 1951.

Flanders, J. N. A humanistic approach to inservice education. Project Upper Cumberland, Title III ESEA. Livingston, Tenn.: Overton County Board of Education, 1969.

Fletcher, J. *Situation ethics: The new morality.* Philadelphia: Westminster Press, 1966.

For humans only. Ashland, Oreg.: Human Dancing Company, 1974.

Foulds, M. L. Self-actualization and the communication of facilitative conditions during counseling. *Journal of Counseling Psychology,* 1969, *16,* 132-136.

Foulds, M. L., Guinan, J. F., & Hanningan, P. S. The marathon group: Changes in a measure of self-actualization. In press.

Foulds, M. L., & Hannigan, P. S. Effects of gestalt marathon groups on measured self-actualization: A replication and follow-up study. *Journal of Counseling Psychology,* in press.

Foulds, M. L., & Hannigan, P. S. Gestalt marathon group: Does it increase reported self-actualization? *Psychotherapy: Theory, Research and Practice,* in press.

Foulkes, S. H. *Introduction to group-analytic psychotherapy.* New York: Grune & Stratton, 1949.

Fox, J., Knapp, R. R., & Michael, W. B. Assessment of self-actualization of psychiatric patients: Validity of the Personal Orientation Inventory. *Educational and Psychological Measurement,* 1968, *28,* 565-569.

Frankl, V. E. *Man's search for meaning.* New York: Beacon Press, 1963.

French, T. *The integration of behavior.* Chicago: University of Chicago Press, 1952.

Freud, S. *The future of an illusion.* New York: Liveright, 1928.

Freud, S. *An outline of psychoanalysis.* New York: Norton, 1949.

Fromm, E. *Man for himself.* New York: Holt, Rinehart and Winston, 1947.

Fromm, E. *Psychoanalysis and religion.* New Haven, Conn.: Yale University Press, 1950.

Fromm, E. *The art of loving.* New York: Harper & Row, 1956.

Fromm, E. *The art of loving* (2nd ed.). New York: Harper & Row, 1962.

Gallwey, W. T. *The inner game of tennis.* New York: Random House, 1974.

Garfield, S. L., & Kurtz, R. Clinical psychologists: A survey of selected attitudes and views. *The Clinical Psychologist,* 1975, *28*(3), 4-7.

Gendlin, E. T. Focusing. *Psychotherapy: Theory, Research and Practice,* 1969, *6*(1).

Gesell, A. *Child development.* New York: Harper & Row, 1949.

Gibb, J. R. The effects of human relations training. In A. E. Bergin & S. L. Garfield (Eds.), *Handbook of psychotherapy and behavior change.* New York: Wiley, 1970.

Gibb, J. R. Sensitivity training as a medium for personal growth and improved personal relationship. In G. Egan (Ed.), *Encounter groups: Basic readings.* Belmont, Calif.: Wadsworth, 1971.

Gibran, K. *The prophet.* New York: Knopf, 1923.

Gilbert, J. G. *Understanding old age.* New York: Ronald, 1952.

Gilligan, J. F. Personality characteristics of selectors and nonselectors of sensitivity training. *Journal of Counseling Psychology,* 1973, *20,* 265-268.

Gowan, J. C. *Development of the creative individual.* San Diego: EdITS/ Robert R. Knapp Publisher, 1972.

Grater, M. R. *Effects of knowledge of characteristics of self-actualization and faking of a self-actualized response on Shostrom's Personal Orientation Inventory.* Unpublished master's thesis, University of Toledo, 1968.

Graves, R. *Poems, 1968-70.* Garden City, N.Y.: Doubleday, 1971.

Graves, R. Editorial. *Life,* April 21, 1972, p. 3.

Greeley, A. Personal communication, December 31, 1970.

Greenwald, H. *Direct decision therapy.* San Diego: EdITS Publishers, 1973.

Guidelines for psychologists conducting growth groups. *American Psychologist,* 1973, *28,* 933.

Guilford, J. P., & Zimmerman, W. S. *Guilford-Zimmerman temperament survey.* Los Angeles: Sheridan Psychological Services, 1949.

Guinan, J. F., & Foulds, M. L. Marathon group: Facilitator of personal growth? *Journal of Counseling Psychology,* 1970, *18,* 101-105.

Harlow, H. F. Nature of love. *American Psychologist,* 1958, *13,* 673-685.

Harvey, V., DiLuzio, G., & Hunter, W. J. Effects of verbal and non-verbal T-groups on personality and attitudinal variables. *Journal of Applied Behavioral Science,* 1975.

Hathaway S. R., & McKinley, J. C. *The Minnesota multiphasic personality inventory.* New York: Psychological Corporation, 1942.

Havighurst, R. J. *Human development and education.* New York: Longmans, 1953.

Hekmat, H., & Theiss, M. Self-actualization and modification of affective self-disclosures during a social conditioning interview. *Journal of Counseling Psychology,* 1971, *18,* 101-105.

Hilgard, E. R., & Atkinson, R. E. *Introduction to psychology* (4th ed.). New York: Harcourt Brace Jovanovich, 1967.

Hobbs, N. Group centered psychotherapy. In Rogers, C. R. (Ed.), *Client centered therapy.* Boston: Houghton Mifflin, 1951.

Hora, T. The process of existential therapy. *Psychiatric Quarterly,* 1960, *34,* 495-504.

Horney, K. *New ways in psychoanalysis.* New York: Norton, 1939.

Huxley, J. The coming new religion of humanism. *The Humanist,* February 1962.

James, M., & Jongeward, D. *Born to win.* Reading, Mass.: Addison-Wesley, 1971.

James, W. *The varieties of religious experience.* New York: Macmillan, 1958.

Jourard, S. M. *The transparent self.* Princeton, N.J.: D. Van Nostrand, 1964.

Jung, C. G. *Modern man in search of a soul.* New York: Harcourt, 1933.

Kaats, B. A. *Personality change as a function of group experience in drug education and counseling programs.* Unpublished master's thesis, Trinity University, 1972.

Kagan, N. Issues in encounter. *The Counseling Psychologist,* 1970, *2,* 43-50.

Kaufman, W. (Ed.). *The portable Nietzsche.* New York: Viking, 1954.

Keen, S. *To a dancing god.* New York: Harper & Row, 1970.

Keen, S. The golden mean of Roberto Assagioli. *Psychology Today,* December 1974, pp. 97-107.

Kelley, R. K. *Courtship, marriage, and the family.* New York: Harcourt Brace Jovanovich, 1974.

Kimball, R. & Gelso, C. J. Self-actualization in a marathon group: Do the strongest get stronger? *Journal of Counseling Psychology,* 1974, *31,* 38-42.

Kinnell, G. *The book of nightmares.* Boston: Houghton Mifflin, 1971.

Kinsey, A. C., Pomeroy, W. B., & Martin, C. E. *Sexual behavior in the human male.* Philadelphia: W. B. Saunders, 1948.

Kinsey, A. C., Pomeroy, W. B., Martin, C. E., & Gebhard, P. H. *Sexual behavior in the human female.* Philadelphia: W. B. Saunders, 1953.

Kirsh, C. *The role of affect expression and defense in the character.* Unpublished manuscript, 1973.

Klopfer, B. Personal communication, 1961.

Knapp, R. R. Relationship of a measure of self-actualization to neuroticism and extraversion. *Journal of Consulting Psychology,* 1965, *29,* 168-172.

Knapp, R. R. Effect of instructions to "fake good" on the POI. Unpublished manuscript, 1966.

Knapp, R. R. *POI scales in major encounter group studies.* Unpublished manuscript, 1973.

Knapp, R. R., & Comrey, A. L. Further construct validation of a measure of self-actualization. *Educational and Psychological Measurement,* 1973, *33,* 419-425.

Knapp, R. R., & Fitzgerald, O. R. Comparative validity of the logically developed versus "purified" research scales for the Personal Orientation Inventory. *Educational and Psychological Measurement,* 1973, *33,* 971-976.

Koffka, K. *Principles of gestalt psychology.* New York: Harcourt, 1935.

Kopp, S. B. *Guru.* Palo Alto, Calif.: Science and Behavior Books, 1971.

Krantzler, M. *Creative divorce.* New York: Evans, 1973.

Krumboltz, J., & Thoreson, C. *Behavioral counseling.* New York: Holt, Rinehart and Winston, 1969.

Kunkel, F. Growth through crises. In Doniger, S. (Ed.), *Religion and human behavior.* New York: Association Press, 1954.

Laing, R. D. *The politics of experience.* New York: Pantheon, 1967.

Laing, R. D. *The divided self.* New York: Pantheon, 1969.

Leary, T. *Interpersonal diagnosis of personality.* New York: Ronald, 1957.

Lederer, W. J., & Jackson, D. D. *The mirages of marriage.* New York: Norton, 1968.

Levy, A. *Authentics.* Unpublished manuscript, 1974.

Lewis, R. H. *Information processing, humanism, and the helping relationship.* Unpublished doctoral dissertation, University of Wisconsin, 1973.

Lidz, T. *The person.* New York: Basic Books, 1968.

Lieberman, M. A., Yalom, I. D., & Miles, M. B. *Encounter groups: first facts.* New York: Basic Books, 1973.

Lindbergh, A. M. *Hours of gold, hours of lead.* New York: Harcourt Brace Jovanovich, 1973.

Lindbergh, A. M. *Locked rooms and open doors.* New York: Harcourt Brace Jovanovich, 1974.

Litt, S. Shaping up or self-shaping: A look at modern educational theory. *Journal of Humanistic Psychology,* 1973, *13,* 72.

Lowen, A. *Betrayal of the body.* New York: Macmillan, 1967.

Lowen, A. *Training manual in bioenergetics.* Unpublished manuscript, 1972.

Lüscher, M. *The Lüscher color test.* New York: Random House, 1969.

McClain, E. W. Further validation of the Personal Orientation Inventory. *Journal of Consulting and Clinical Psychology,* 1970, *35,* 21-22.

Mace, D. Your marriage today. *Women's Home Companion,* April 1956, pp. 29-33.

Magden, R. Eight dimensions of group psychotherapy as they relate to three approaches to group therapy. Unpublished doctoral dissertation, United States International University, 1975.

Magden, R., & Shostrom, E. L. An adaptation of Yalom's curative factors in group therapy. Manuscript in preparation, 1975.

Mailer, N. A fire on the moon. *Life,* August 29, 1969, pp. 24-40.

Maliver, B. *The encounter game.* New York: Stein & Day, 1972.

Marks, S. E., Conry, R. F. & Foster, S. F. Comment: The marathon group hypothesis: An unanswered question. *Journal of Counseling Psychology,* 1973, *20,* 185-187.

Maslow, A. H. *Motivation and personality.* New York: Harper & Row, 1954.

Maslow, A. H. *Toward a psychology of being.* New York: D. Van Nostrand, 1962.

Maslow, A. H. *Toward a psychology of being* (2nd ed.). New York: Harper & Row, 1968.

Maslow, A. H. *Motivation and personality* (2nd ed.). New York: Harper & Row, 1970.

Maslow, A. H. *The farther reaches of human nature.* New York: Viking, 1971.

Masters, W. H., & Johnson, V. E. *Human sexual response.* Boston: Little, Brown, 1966.

May, R. *Love and will.* New York: Norton, 1969.

May, R., Angel, E., & Ellenberger, H. *Existence.* New York: Basic Books, 1958.

Meredith, G. M. Temperament and self-actualization. *Eits Research and Developments,* 1967, *1*(3), 1.

Mowrer, O. H. Some philosophical problems in psychological counseling. *Journal of Counseling Psychology,* 1957, *4,* 103-111.

Mowrer, O. H. *The crisis in psychiatry and religion.* New York: D. Van Nostrand, 1961.

Mowrer, O. H. *The new group therapy.* New York: D. Van Nostrand, 1964.

Murphy. G. *Human potentialities.* New York: Basic Books, 1958.

Nidich, S., Seeman, W., & Dreskin, T. Influence of transcendental meditation: a replication. *Journal of Counseling Psychology,* 1973, *20,* 565-566.

Noll, G. A., & Watkins, J. T. Differences between persons seeking encounter group experiences and others on the Personal Orientation Inventory. *Journal of Counseling Psychology,* 1974, *21,* 206-209.

O'Kelly, L. I., & Muckler, F. A. *Introduction to psychopathology* (2nd ed.). Englewood Cliffs, N.J.: Prentice-Hall, 1955.

Otto, H. A. *Human potentialities.* St. Louis: W. H. Green, 1968.

Pascal, B. *Penseés* and *The provincial letters.* New York: Modern Library, 1941.

Perls, F. S. *Gestalt therapy verbatim.* Lafayette, Calif.: Real People Press, 1969.

Perls, F. S., Goodman, P., & Hefferline, H. *Gestalt therapy.* New York: Julian Press, 1951.

Pfeiffer, J. W., & Heslin, R. *Instrumentation in human relations training.* San Diego: University Associates, 1973.

Polanyi, M. *Science, faith, and society.* Chicago: University of Chicago Press, 1964.

Polanyi, M. *Knowing and being.* Chicago: University of Chicago Press, 1973.

Reddy, W. B. On affection, group composition, and self-actualization in sensitivity training. *Journal of Consulting and Clinical Psychology,* 1972, *38,* 211-214.

Reddy, W. B. The impact of sensitivity training on self-actualization: A one-year follow-up. *Comparative Group Studies,* in press.

Riesman, D. *The lonely crowd.* Garden City, N.Y.: Doubleday, 1950.

Rilke, R. M. *Letters to a young poet.* New York: Norton, 1934.

Rioch, M. Personal communication, 1969.

Rogers, C. R. *Counseling and psychotherapy.* Boston: Houghton Mifflin, 1942.

Rogers, C. R. *Client-centered therapy.* Boston: Houghton Mifflin, 1951.

Rogers, C. R. *On becoming a person.* Boston: Houghton Mifflin, 1961.

Rogers, C. R. The increasing involvement of the psychologist in social problems. *California State Psychologist,* 1968, *9*(7), 29. (a)

Rogers, C. R. Interpersonal relationships: U.S.A. 2000. *Journal of Applied Behavioral Science,* 1968, *4,* 265-280. (b)

Rogers, C. R. *Carl Rogers on encounter groups.* New York: Harper & Row, 1970.

Rosensweig, S. An outline of frustration theory. In Hunt, J. M. (Ed.), *Personality and the behavior disorders.* New York: Ronald, 1944.

Rueveni, U., Swift, M., & Bell, A. A. Sensitivity training: Its impact on mental health workers. *Applied Behavioral Science,* 1969, *5,* 600-601.

Russell, B. *Portraits from memory.* New York: Simon and Schuster, 1951.

Satir, V. *Conjoint family therapy.* Palo Alto, Calif.: Science and Behavior Books, 1966.

Satir, V. *People makers.* Palo Alto, Calif.: Science and Behavior Books, 1973.

Schutz, W. C. *Joy.* New York: Grove Press, 1967.

Schutz, W. C. *Here comes everybody.* New York: Harper & Row, 1971.

Seeman, W., Nidich, S., & Banta, T. Influence of transcendental meditation on a measure of self-actualization. *Journal of Counseling Psychology,* 1972, *19,* 184-187.

Shepard, M. *Fritz.* New York: Saturday Review Press-Dutton, 1975.

Shostrom, E. L. *Personal orientation inventory.* San Diego: EdITS/Educational and Industrial Testing Service, 1963.

Shostrom, E. L. A test for the measurement of self-actualization. *Educational and Psychological Measurement,* 1964, *24,* 207-218.

Shostrom, E. L. *Caring relationship inventory.* San Diego: EdITS/Educational and Industrial Testing Service, 1966.

Shostrom, E. L. *Man, the manipulator.* Nashville: Abingdon Press, 1967. Bantam Edition, New York, 1968.

Shostrom, E. L. Group therapy: Let the buyer beware. *Psychology Today,* May 1969, pp. 36-40.

Shostrom, E. L. *Pair attraction inventory.* San Diego: EdITS/Educational and Industrial Testing Service, 1970.

Shostrom, E. L. *Freedom to be.* Englewood Cliffs, N.J.: Prentice-Hall, 1972. Bantam Edition, New York, 1973.

Shostrom, E. L. Comments on a test review: The Personal Orientation Inventory. *Journal of Counseling Psychology,* 1973, *20,* 479-481.

Shostrom, E. L. *Personal orientation dimensions.* San Diego: EdITS/Educational and Industrial Testing Service, 1974.

Shostrom, E. L., & Kavanaugh, J. *Between man and woman.* Los Angeles: Nash, 1971. Bantam Edition, New York, 1975.

Shostrom, E. L., & Knapp, R. R. The relationship of a measure of self-actualization (POI) to a measure of pathology (MMPI) and to therapeutic growth. *American Journal of Psychotherapy,* 1966, *20,* 193-202.

Shostrom, E. L., & Riley, C. Parametric analysis of psychotherapy. *Journal of Consulting and Clinical Psychology,* 1968, *32,* 628-632.

Shostrom, F. L. *A validity study of Shostrom's Pair Attraction Inventory.* Unpublished master's thesis, United States International University, 1973.

Shuttleworth, F. K. *The physical and mental growth of girls and boys age six to nineteen in relation to age at maximum growth.* Washington, D.C.: National Research Council, 1939.

Sjostrom, D. Clinical applications of the Actualizing Assessment Battery. Unpublished master's thesis, United States International University, 1975.

Skinner, B. F. *Beyond freedom and dignity.* New York: Knopf, 1971.

Stevens, B. *Don't push the river.* Lafayette, Calif.: Real People Press, 1970.

Strupp, H. H. The therapist's personal therapy: The influx of irrationalism. *The Clinical Psychologist,* 1975, *28*(3), 1.

Stuart, G. *Narcissus.* London: G. Allen, 1956.

Sullivan, H. S. *The interpersonal theory of psychiatry.* New York: Norton, 1953.

Suzuki, D. T. Introduction to *Zen in the art of archery,* by E. Herrigel. New York: Pantheon, 1953.

Thurstone, L. L. *Multiple factor analysis.* Chicago: University of Chicago Press, 1947.

Tournier, P. *The meaning of persons.* New York: Harper & Row, 1957.

Travis, R. P., & Travis, P. Y. Personal communication, June 13, 1975.

Treppa, J. A., & Fricke, L. Effects of a marathon group experience. *Journal of Counseling Psychology,* 1972, *19,* 466-467.

Trueblood, R. W., & McHolland, J. D. *Measures of change toward self-actualization through the human potential group process.* Unpublished manuscript, 1971.

Waley, A. *Three ways of thought in Ancient China.* Garden City, N.Y.: Doubleday, 1956.

Walton, D. R. Effects of personal growth groups on self-actualization and creative personality. *Journal of College Student Personnel,* 1973, 490-494.

Wareheim, R. G., & Foulds, M. L. Social desirability response sets and a measure of self-actualization. *Journal of Humanistic Psychology,* 1973, *13,* 89-95.

Wareheim, R. G., Routh, D. K., & Foulds, M. L. Knowledge about self-actualization and the presentation of self as self-actualized. *Journal of Personality and Social Psychology,* 1974, *30,* 155-162.

Watts, A. W. *The wisdom of insecurity.* New York: Pantheon, 1951.

Watts, A. W. *The book: On the taboo against knowing who you are.* New York: Collier, 1966.

Watzlawick, P., Helmick, J., & Jackson, D. D. *Pragmatics of human communication.* New York: Norton, 1967.

White, R. The concept of the healthy personality: What do we really mean? *The Counseling Psychologist,* 1973, *4*(2), 3-12.

White, V. *God and the unconscious.* Chicago: Regnery, 1953.

Winch. R. F. *Mate selection.* New York: Harper & Row, 1958.

Wolpe, J. *Psychotherapy by reciprocal inhibition.* Stanford, Calif.: Stanford University Press, 1958.

Wolpe, J., & Lang, P. J. *Fear survey schedule.* San Diego: EdITS/Educational and Industrial Testing Service, 1969.

Yalom, I. D. *The theory and practice of group psychotherapy.* New York: Basic Books, 1970.

Yalom, I. D., & Lieberman, M. A. A study of encounter group casualties. *Archives of General Psychiatry,* 1971, *25,* 16-30.

Young, E. R., & Jacobson, L. I. Effects of time-extended marathon group experiences on personality characteristics. *Journal of Counseling Psychology,* 1970, *17,* 247-251.

Zuckerman, M., & Lubin, B. *Multiple affect adjective check list.* San Diego: EdITS/Educational and Industrial Testing Service, 1965.

ACTUALIZING FILMS: A COORDINATED LIST

The following films, produced or distributed by the senior author, are available from Psychological Films, Inc., 1215 E. Chapman Avenue, Orange, California 92666. (Catalogues with prices are available upon request.) To assist instructors, each film is keyed to the chapter to which it is most relevant.

CHAPTER 1: ACTUALIZING THERAPY: AN EMERGING METHODOLOGY

The Humanistic Revolution: Pioneers in Perspective. 16mm. Black & white. 32 minutes.
Interviews with the leaders of the "unnoticed revolution" in psychology, including Abraham Maslow, Gardner Murphy, Carl Rogers, Rollo May, Paul Tillich, Frederick Perls, Viktor Frankl, and Alan Watts.

Search and Research: Psychology in Perspective. 16mm. Black & white. 30 minutes.
Through the medium of a story of a young lady seeking psychotherapy, this film attempts to describe the three forces in psychology: experimental, psychoanalytic, and existential (or humanistic). Intimate visits are provided with three prominent psychologists: Harry Harlow, Rollo May, and Carl Rogers.

Actualizing Therapy: An Integration of Rogers, Perls, and Ellis. 16mm. Color. 30 minutes.
Sequences from the film series *Three Approaches to Psychotherapy* illustrate the work of Carl Rogers, Frederick Perls, and Albert Ellis. Following the sequences, Everett L. Shostrom analyzes the three styles and describes his integration of these approaches into a working unity.

CHAPTER 2: RESEARCH FOUNDATIONS: THE ACTUALIZING ASSESSMENT BATTERY

Maslow and Self-Actualization, Film no. 1. 16mm. Color. 30 minutes.
Abraham Maslow discusses honesty and awareness as dimensions of self-actualization and elaborates on recent research and theory related to each.

Maslow and Self-Actualization, Film no. 2. 16mm. Color. 30 minutes.
A continuation of the previous film. Maslow discusses self-actualization in terms of the dimensions of freedom and trust and examines recent research and theory related to them.

CHAPTER 3: PERSONALITY CHANGE IN ACTUALIZING THERAPY

Frederick Perls and Gestalt Therapy. Two-film series. 16mm. Black & white. Film no. 1: 39 minutes; film no. 2: 36 minutes.
The most comprehensive overview films yet produced on Gestalt Therapy, representing the latest and best summary of Frederick Perls' theories.

In the Now. 16mm. Black & white. 45 minutes.
Three segments, from a ten-hour workshop conducted by James S. Simkin, demonstrating the individual application of Gestalt Therapy techniques with three different persons. Subject matter includes work with a dream, an incident of the recent past, and a current interaction—all in the "here and now."

CHAPTER 4: THE EXISTENTIAL CHOICE: FACADE LIVING OR CORE BEING

Experimental Neurosis by Control of Emotions. 16mm. Black & white. 30 minutes.

Produced by the faculty and graduate students in the Clinical Department of the Psychological Laboratory at the University of Amsterdam, this film demonstrates that feelings are learned in living, and that under post-hypnotic suggestion feelings may be shown to be experimentally produced.

CHAPTER 5: ACTUALIZING AS DEVELOPMENTAL AWARENESS

Childhood: The Enchanted Years. 16mm. Color. 52 minutes.
The studies of Jerome Bruner, Burton White, Jerome Kagan, Wanda Bronson, Jean Block, and others are highlighted as the growing process is shown from a child's eye view. In candid detail, the film shows how children—from infancy to age four—learn to reach, perceive, walk, and talk.

Rollo May and Human Encounter: Self-Self Encounter and Self-Other Encounter. 16mm. Color. 30 minutes.
May describes man's dilemma as having to see himself as both subject and object in life, and discusses the four elements of human encounter: empathy, eros, friendship, and agape.

Rollo May and Human Encounter: Manipulation and Human Encounter—Exploitation of Sex. 16mm. Color. 30 minutes.

May discusses how man is manipulated when any of the four elements of human encounter is missing, the problem of transference in psychotherapy as a distortion of human encounter, and modern man's fixation on sexuality as related to his fear of death.

Touching: Importance for Human Growth. 16mm. Color. 29 minutes.
A conversation with Ashley Montagu on the key concepts of his recent work, *Touching.* Utilizing psychological research and medical opinion, Montagu develops the case that touching is necessary for human life.

CHAPTER 6: THE PROCESS OF ACTUALIZING THERAPY

Target Five, Film no. 1. 16mm. Color. 26 minutes.
Virginia Satir and Everett L. Shostrom discuss the four manipulative response forms, which are then demonstrated by simulated family situations.

Target Five, Film no. 2. 16mm. Color. 22 minutes.
Satir and Shostrom describe the three essential qualities of an actualizing relationship, which are then demonstrated.

CHAPTER 7: THE TECHNIQUES OF INDIVIDUAL ACTUALIZING THERAPY

Three Approaches to Psychotherapy: Part One—Dr. Carl Rogers. 16mm. Color and black & white. 48 minutes.
Following a general introduction to this film series and a description of Client-Centered Therapy, Rogers conducts a therapy session with the patient, "Gloria."

Three Approaches to Psychotherapy: Part Two—Dr. Frederick Perls. 16mm. Color and black & white. 32 minutes.
After a description of Gestalt Therapy, Perls interviews "Gloria" and presents a summation of the interview.

Three Approaches to Psychotherapy: Part Three—Dr. Albert Ellis. 16mm. Color and black & white. 38 minutes.
This film presents a description of Rational-Emotive Psychotherapy as well as Ellis' interview with "Gloria" and his summation. "Gloria" is also seen giving an evaluation of her experiences with the three therapists.

Lowen and Bioenergetic Therapy. 16mm. Color. 48 minutes.
Alexander Lowen describes the key ideas of bioenergetic therapy and
demonstrates them in his work with a young female patient.

CHAPTER 8: GROUP THERAPY AND ENCOUNTER GROUPS

Encounter: To Make a Start. 16mm or videocassette. Black & white. 31
minutes.
Documentation of a day-long workshop-encounter session, conducted by
Joel Fort and Sara Miller, between seven policemen and seven young
people, most of whom described themselves as revolutionaries.

A Conversation with Carl Rogers. 16mm. Black & white. 30 minutes.
In conversation with Keith Berwick, Rogers comments on his own Client-
Centered Therapy, humanistic psychology, his own affinity for a phenomenological approach to human beings, the worth of encounter or
sensitivity groups, and many other topics.

The Actualization Group. Seven-film series. 16mm. Black & white.
Approximately 45 minutes each.
This series follows one group through seven sequential sessions of therapy
with Everett L. Shostrom and Nancy W. Ferry. Each session focuses on a
different general theme: "Risking Being Ourselves," "Freedom and
Actualization," "Aggression and Actualization," "Manipulation and
Actualization," "The Divorce from Parents," "Self-Disclosure of the
Therapist," and "From Deadness to Aliveness."

A Session with College Students: Gestalt Dream Interpretation. 16mm.
Black & white. 60 minutes.
Frederick Perls demonstrates his method for discovering and expressing
the meaning of dreams.

CHAPTER 9: AN EXAMPLE OF ACTUALIZING GROUP THERAPY

Three Approaches to Group Therapy. Three-film series. 16mm. Color.
Film no. 1: 38 minutes; film no. 2: 40 minutes; film no. 3: 38 minutes.
In these films, Everett Shostrom (film no. 1), Albert Ellis (film no. 2),
and Harold Greenwald (film no. 3) use a group setting to demonstrate
Actualizing Therapy approaches, Rational-Emotive Therapy approaches,
and Decision Therapy approaches, respectively.

CHAPTER 10: SEX, LOVE, AND MARRIAGE

Between Man and Woman. 16mm. Color. 33 minutes.
In conversation with Howard Miller, Everett L. Shostrom discusses various marital roles people play and professional actors demonstrate these modes of reacting.

CHAPTER 11: ACTUALIZING AS A PERSONAL VALUING PROCESS

Frankl and the Search for Meaning. 16mm. Color. 30 minutes.
Viktor Frankl describes man's search for meaning as a form of "height" psychology, as opposed to Freudian theory, which he describes as "depth" psychology. Frankl says that, in his continuous growth toward self-actualization, man discovers new meanings for himself. He describes meaning as a form of personalized valuing that each man must have in order to make his life meaningful.

INDEX

ABOUT THE AUTHORS

Everett L. Shostrom is Director of the Institute of Actualizing Therapy of Santa Ana, California, is a Diplomate in Clinical Psychology, American Board of Professional Psychology and is Past President of the Division of Humanistic Psychology (Division 32) of the American Psychological Association. He is Distinguished Professor of Psychology, United States International University. He is author or coauthor of six other books and numerous articles in the field of psychology and psychotherapy. He is President of Psychological Films and has produced or directed many films which are listed in the film list at the back of this volume. He is author of the four inventories collectively known as the Actualizing Assessment Battery. Actualizing Therapy represents the "creative synthesis" of his many years of work in the field of psychotherapy.

Robert and Lila Knapp, research psychologists, have worked extensively on the research dimensions of the Actualizing Assessment Battery with Dr. Shostrom; they have compiled and coordinated the extensive research base for Actualizing Therapy.